Essentials of Nutrition for Chefs THIRD EDITION

Catharine Powers, MS, RDN, LD
Mary Abbott Hess, LHD, MS, RDN, LDN, FAND

Culinary Nutrition Publishing, LLC
Chicago, Illinois

Library of Congress Cataloging-in-Publication Data

Powers, Catharine. Hess, Mary Abbott
    Essentials of Nutrition for Chefs / Catharine Powers, Mary Abbott Hess
      p.cm
    ISBN 978-0-9911788-1-0
    1. Nutrition

                                            201 129 2515

Cover photos: Front Cover: Back cover purchased through istockphoto.com, contributed by PeaFactory.

For more information or permission to reprint contact
Culinary Nutrition Publishing, LLC

www.nutritionforchefs.com

www.culinarynutritionpublishing.com

$65.00
ISBN 978-0-9911788-1-0
56500>

9 780991 178810

Table of Contents

From the Kitchen

Case by Case (Operational Vignettes)

Recipes

Foreword

Everyone, from energetic young children to adults in their sunset years, should have healthful food options wherever they eat. Schools, colleges and universities, employee dining rooms, entertainment venues, restaurants of all sorts, healthcare facilities, and congregate or group feeding sites share a responsibility to provide appetizing, healthful foods. As a culinary professional, you have an opportunity to show that planning, preparing and serving nourishing and appealing foods to guests is not only the right thing to do but also makes good business sense.

Adventuresome diners, innovative technology and an abundance of healthful ingredients – fruits, vegetables, whole grains, beans, lean meats, low-fat dairy products, nuts, seeds, herbs and spices – make this an exciting time to be a culinary professional. Basic nutrition knowledge mixed with creativity will position you to meet the needs of a challenging marketplace. We designed *Essentials of Nutrition for Chefs* as a roadmap for your journey with fundamental nutrition information plus charts, diagrams, sidebars and practical applications.

Today, I work with foodservice operators across the country, from school foodservice operators to restaurants, training others how to put healthful cooking into practice. The 14 years I spent at The Culinary Institute of America, Hyde Park developing and teaching the CIA's cutting-edge nutrition program gave me insight into what today's culinary students and professionals need to know about nutrition. We put this knowledge into practice at the institute's St. Andrew's Cafe, a living laboratory that tested and validated healthy cooking concepts.

So many individuals have inspired and motivated me and shaped my food and nutrition knowledge as well as my culinary skills. Special thanks and admiration go to my coauthor, Mary Abbott Hess, whose life motto, "Just do it!" inspires me to take risks and do more. Many culinary and nutrition colleagues, especially those at The Culinary Institute of America, have generously shared their expertise and passion for food with me throughout the years. All of you truly have enriched my life.

A very personal thanks goes to my mom, Charlene Powers Huber, a retired registered dietitian, for her constant support while I have pursued non-traditional dietetic roles and for her encouragement and role modeling each step of the way. A special personal thank you goes to my partner, Rebecca Coste, whose love and patience provides me a wonderful life-balance. Finally, I would like to acknowledge my sons, Andrew and William, who have taught me the practical side of preparing healthful foods for kids and who have always been eager taste-testers.

Catharine Powers
Akron, Ohio

As a former president of The American Dietetic Association (now The Academy of Nutrition and Dietetics) and former chairman of The American Institute of Wine & Food, one of my professional and personal goals to support the union of nutrition science and the culinary arts. Chefs can give us wonderful food that nourishes both body and soul, but to do so, they often need more science-based nutrition education. Thus, my focus became supporting the culinary expertise of fellow dietitians while also increasing nutrition knowledge among chefs.

Within the Academy of Nutrition and Dietetics, the Food & Culinary Professionals Dietary Practice Group has had a transformative influence on many registered dietitians. More and more dietitians are now working in the food industry, and a number of them have told me that we need better ways to share nutrition knowledge with chefs. As an author, educator and nutrition communications consultant, I saw this need as an opportunity to create a resource to help chefs, food writers, cooking teachers and other culinary professionals combine today's nutrition knowledge with their culinary skills to create healthful foods that meet high standards for taste and quality.

A few years ago, I became a restaurant owner and opened New Buffalo Bill's, a barbeque restaurant in New Buffalo, Michigan. Quite an undertaking as a Texas-style smokehouse is not a usual venue for a healthful meal. Offering a variety of healthful options integrated into the broader menu, controlling portion sizes, and meeting the needs of customers with particular dietary needs on a day-to-day basis has attuned me to the challenges that chefs face on a day-today basis. My solutions are within this third edition.

My coauthor, Cathy Powers, is the most accomplished culinary nutritionist I know. Her many years developing and implementing curriculum for the Culinary Institute of America, and more recently teaching school foodservice leaders nationally and internationally, has made her a master at creating useful and engaging materials supporting nutri-

tion education. In *Essentials of Nutrition for Chefs* we address contemporary nutrition issues and offer solutions to some of the daily "cooking healthy" challenges facing chefs. Within these pages are answers to hundreds of questions chefs have asked us over the years, the most current nutrition thinking and facts, and virtually everything chefs should know to create healthful foods. To go beyond the science and look at nutrition through the lens of food and food choices, we invited experts – chefs, fellow dietitians and food professionals – to share their advice, recipes and best practices. These experts add a unique dimension to the book.

We have been delighted by response to the earlier editions of *Essentials of Nutrition for Chefs*. The book has been adopted by many culinary programs and received top honors in the Health and Special Diets at the 2011 International Association of Culinary Professionals (IACP) book awards and was a finalist in the Professional Kitchens category. That year I was part of a team that used the first edition of *Essentials of Nutrition for Chefs* to teach a course on nutrition for chefs at the Washburne Culinary Institute in Chicago. With that experience, plus input from chef instructors and responses from students who have used our book, we have made the third edition of the book even better.

My thanks go to the amazing team listed in the acknowledgments. Special personal thanks go to Chef William Reynolds, my partner in New Buffalo Bill's, for enriching both my culinary education and my life as well as critically reviewing this book from the perspective of a chef; to The American Institute of Wine & Food and the memory of Julia Child who remains an inspiration and my guardian angel; and to the Food & Culinary Professionals Dietetic Practice Group, the International Association of Culinary Professionals and Les Dames D'Escoffier International – three strong networks of generous colleagues who have supported my culinary education and this venture.

Mary Abbott Hess, LHD, MS, LDN, RDN, FAND
Chicago, Illinois

Preface

Essentials of Nutrition for Chefs is unique because it offers a look at nutrition through the lens of food. This textbook provides essential nutrition information for culinary professionals as well as guidance on practical application. A longstanding criticism of healthful cooking is that removing fat, salt and sugar results in foods that are bland, boring and lacking in flavor and texture. Omitting these classic flavor-enhancing ingredients makes creating wonderful tastes and textures more challenging. *Essentials of Nutrition for Chefs* is designed to help chefs meet this challenge by preparing food that nourishes both body and soul.

Building on the positive response and acknowledged excellence of the first edition, which received the 2011 International Association of Culinary Professionals Cookbook Award in the Health and Special Diets category and the second edition, which is used by culinary schools across the country, the third edition is even better.

Chef William Reynolds, an experienced chef educator and winner of the Foodservice Educator Network International's 2011 Award for Excellence in Culinary Education, reviewed the entire text with a critical eye to what chefs need to know and understand about nutrition. He used the first and second edition in classes and provided valuable suggestions from the perspective of a chef and educator.

New information on *Dietary Guidelines for Americans, MyPlate*, the National Restaurant Association Chef Survey: What's Hot in 2018, and the International Food Information Council (IFIC) Food & Health Survey: Consumer Attitudes Toward Food Safety, Nutrition & Health and other sources are included. New charts, website resources, chef interviews and case studies are also provided.

What Lies in Store

Chapter 1, The Power of Food, focuses on marrying the science of nutrition with the art of preparing food and discusses the foodservice industry's responsibility to offer plenty of healthful food choices for today's consumers. The heart of the second chapter, Nutrition Guidelines and Tools, is the *Dietary Guidelines for Americans*, 2015-2020 Report and the applications of that document are reflected throughout the book. Additional tools include the Nutrition Facts panel on food labels and the *MyPlate* guide

to a healthful diet. Chapters 3 through 7 review the six classes of nutrients – carbohydrates, fats, protein, water, vitamins and minerals. Chapters 8 through 10 are all about putting nutrition into practice by planning healthful menus, recognizing the importance of flavor and using healthful cooking techniques. Chapter 11 focuses on communicating nutrition to guests and looks at the impact of healthcare reform on nutrition in restaurants. Finally, Chapters 12 and 13 deal with nutrition for various age groups and for those with special dietary and health needs.

Each chapter begins with learning objectives – the knowledge readers can expect to glean from the pages that follow. Throughout each chapter, charts, tables and sidebars present information in a concise, learner-friendly format. Chefs working in a variety of operations around the country talk about how nutrition fits into their life and work in features titled A Word from the Chef, which are sprinkled throughout the book. Another recurring feature, Case by Case, highlights practical applications from a variety of operational viewpoints, including schools, healthcare, restaurants, and business and industry. Each chapter concludes with Opportunities for Chefs, hands-on Learning Activities and a list of additional resources for more in-depth information. Key words are in bold italics for easy identification and definitions are found in the glossary.

Principles in Practice

Essentials of Nutrition for Chefs also contains recipes illustrating concepts discussed in each chapter. All the recipes, which the various chefs and dietitians featured in the book have been kind enough to share, have been standardized and tested. From starters to desserts, from summer to winter, from simple to complex, from fruits to nuts, the recipes reflect a range of cooking techniques and showcase nutrient-rich ingredients.

Select nutrient data (calories, fat, saturated fat, trans fat, cholesterol, sodium, carbohydrates, dietary fiber and protein) are listed with each recipe. These data are rounded using Food and Drug Administration rounding rules for labeling. Most nutrient data presented in charts are also rounded. Recipes for this book were analyzed using ESHA Genesis R & D software. Optional recipe ingredients are not included in the analyses. The analyses do not include suggested accompaniments. Recipes were taste-tested and many include salt; if lower sodium levels are desired, salt can be omitted.

Acknowledgments

It is hard to believe how many hearts, hands and minds have touched this text from inception to printing. Thank you to everyone who encouraged and supported us in writing and revising *Essentials of Nutrition for Chefs*, especially:

Jill Melton, MS, RDN, editor and publisher of *Edible Nashville*, provided new nutrition insights and a connection to an up-and-coming group of chefs who are embracing healthful cooking techniques.

Jane Grant Tougas, who assisted at every step of the process from brainstorming and shaping the book's vision to editing, writing and endless re-writing. Her skill and attention to detail gave this book one voice.

Tami Petitto, a superbly creative designer who gave color to ordinary words and brought energy to every page. Her aesthetic and functional sensibilities are outshone only by her patience. The cover photo is an example of her ability to see beauty in simple things and her eye for just the right angle.

William N. Reynolds, who shared his passion, his expertise and his critical eye. He offered a thorough and careful review of each page of the text from the viewpoint of the chef. One of three chefs who is an honorary member of the Academy of Nutrition and Dietetics, he has always given freely of his time in training dietitians and others on the importance of healthful cooking that is also delicious.

Deborah McBride whose copyediting skills made sure we crossed every "t" and dotted every "i" and offered guidance in publishing.

All the outstanding contributors who offered their expertise and experience to make this book more practical for chefs, foodservice operators, recipe developers, cooking teachers and other culinary professionals.

Chefs and Culinary Professionals

Jason Bruner, Executive Chef, 1801 Grille, Columbia, South Carolina

Samantha Cowens-Gasbarro, Chef/Nutrition Coordinator, Windham Raymond Schools, Windham, Maine

Justin Dean, Co-owner, Madhouse Vinegar, Co., North Bend, Ohio

Patty Erd, Owner, The Spice House, Chicago, Illinois

Jonathan B. Howard, Head Bartender, Henley Modern America Brasserie, Nashville, Tennessee

Max Knoepfel, Chef, Music City Center, Nashville, Tennessee

Deborah Madison, Chef/Author, Sante Fe, New Mexico

Susan E. Notter, formerly Program Co-Coordinator Pastry Arts, Pennsylvania School of Culinary Arts, Lancaster, PA

Rebecca J. Polson, CC SNS, Executive Chef, Spartanburg County School District Six, Roebuck, South Carolina

Nora Pouillon, Restaurant Nora, Washington, DC

Rakka, Chef/Owner, Café Rakka, Hendersonville, Tennessee

William N. Reynolds, Chef/Co-owner, New Buffalo Bill's, New Buffalo, Michigan

Barton Seaver, Chef/Author, Maine

Sarah Stegner, Chef/Owner, Prairie Grass Café, Northbrook, Illinois

Melanie Stewart, General Manager, Gourmetfile, Boca Raton, Florida

Scott Uehlein, Corporate Chef, Sonic, Oklahoma City, Oklahoma

Shawn Weed, Chef/Owner, The Acre, Albuquerque, New Mexico

Registered Dietitians and Food and Nutrition Experts

Jacqueline R. Berning, PhD, RD, CSSD, Associate Professor and Chair, Biology Department, University of Colorado, Colorado Springs, Colorado

Leslie Bonci, MPH, RD, LDN, CSSD, Director of Sports Nutrition, University of Pittsburgh Medical Center, Pittsburgh, Pennsylvania

Maria Caranfa, RDN, LDN, ACSM, EP, Chicago, Illinois

Nancy Clark, MS, RD, CSSD, Sports Nutritionist, Brookline, Massachusetts

Margaret Condrasky, EdD, RD, CCE, Associate Professor of Food Science and Human Nutrition, Clemson University, Clemson, South Carolina

Becky Dorner, RD, LD, Becky Dorner & Associates, Akron, Ohio

Patty Penzy Erd, former owner, The Spice House, Chicago, Illinois

Cheryl Forberg, RD, Chef and former nutritionist for NBC's "The Biggest Loser," Napa, California

Janet Helm, Chief Food and Nutrition Strategist, North America, Weber Shandwick Public Relations, Chicago, Illinois

Penny M. Kris-Etherton, PhD, RD, FADA, Distinguished Professor of Nutrition, Pennsylvania State University, State College, Pennsylvania

Georgia Kostas, MPH, RD, LD, President, Georgia Kostas & Associates, Inc., Dallas, Texas

Carolyn Leontos, MS, RD, CDE, Professor Emeritus Retired, University of Nevada Cooperative Extension, Las Vegas, Nevada

Marilyn Majchrzak, MS, RD, former Corporate Menu Development Manager, Canyon Ranch, Tucson, Arizona.

Mariam Majeed, formerly with Islamic Food and Nutrition Council of America, Park Ridge, Illinois

Jill Nussinow, MS, RD, The Veggie Queen™, Santa Rosa, California

Maggie Powers, PhD, RD, CDE, Research Scientist, International Diabetes Center at Park Nicollet, St. Louis Park, Minnesota

Tina Wasserman, BS, MA, Cooking and More, Dallas, Texas

Donna L. Weihofen, MS, RD, Retired Senior Clinical Nutritionist, University of Wisconsin Comprehensive Cancer Center, Madison, Wisconsin

Renee Zonka, CEC, RD, CHE, MBA, Chef and former Dean, Kendall College, Chicago, Illinois

Foodservice Operations/Experts

Boston Medical Center, Boston, Massachusetts

Burke County Schools, Waynesboro, Georgia

Canyon Ranch, Tucson, Arizon

InHarvest, Bemidji, Minnesota

New Buffalo Bill's, New Buffalo, Michigan

Sonic, Oklahoma City, Oklahoma

SPE Certification, Kristy Del Coro, MS, RDN, CDN, New York, New York

The Spice House, Chicago, Illinois

This Old Farm, Colfax, Indiana

University of New Hampshire, Durham, New Hampshire

Reviewers

Garrett Berdan, RD, LD, Consultant, Spokane, Washington

Susan Braverman, MS, RD, CDN, FADA, retired Director of Dietetic Internship, Department of Family, Nutrition, & Exercise Sciences, Queens College, Flushing, New York

Mary Kimbrough, RD, LD, Senior Director, Wild Hive, Dallas, Texas

Kathy King, RD, LD, Helm Publishing, Lake Dallas, Texas

Carolyn Leontos, MS, RD, CDE, Consultant, Las Vegas, Nevada

William N. Reynolds, Chef Educator and Owner of New Buffalo Bills, New Buffalo, Michigan, Chicago, Illinois

Janet Sass, MS, RD, Assistant Dean and Associate Professor, Hospitality & Nutrition, Northern Virginia Community College, Annandale, Virginia

Debbie F. Swanson, RD, CHE, Culinary Instructor, The Art Institute of Colorado, Denver, Colorado

Chapter One

The Power of Food

Learning Objectives | *After completing this chapter, you should be able to:*

- Summarize the factors that influence food selection
- Discuss the importance of providing healthier food options to your guests
- List general food recommendations for providing nutritious meals
- Discuss how American's eating habits have changed in the last 20 years
- List the operational implications of cooking healthfully
- Define essential nutrients
- List the six classes of nutrients
- Identify the nutrients that provide energy (calories)
- Describe the factors that influence daily calorie needs
- Explain nutrient density and list examples of foods that are nutrient dense and foods that have a low nutrient density
- Give five examples of how to implement "moderation" in restaurant food

Food, glorious food: Cooking it and eating it are as much a part of our culture as art, music, dance, theater, poetry, prose and other creative pursuits. We cook and eat not only to survive but also to celebrate, to mourn, to court, to impress, to console and to calm. Look closely and you will see that just about every human emotion has an associated food ritual or behavior. Granted, some may be more constructive than others; regardless, the depth of emotion tied to food speaks to feeding the soul as well as the body.

Long before the emergence of nutrition science as we know it today, people learned through experience that food and wellness share a close bond. Based on the four classical elements – fire, air, water and earth – early Greek physicians prescribed "hot, cold, wet and dry foods" to treat illness. Different foods or food combinations were thought to create disease-fighting substances in the body. It was the Greek physician Hippocrates who famously said: "Let food be your medicine and medicine be your food."

With the 20th century emergence of nutrition as a science, food garnered new respect as an evidence-based health promoter and disease preventer. But as history has shown many times, people don't always do what they know to be best for their health and well-being. So it has been with food. Although science has repeatedly demonstrated the health benefits of nutritious food eaten in moderation, our high-tech lifestyles and calorie-laden food options don't often support healthful choices and the physical activity needed to balance it.

Fortunately, however, we are living in a time of profound transition in the public's attitude toward food and health. Today, unlike in years past, it is recognized that tasty food and healthy food are not mutually exclusive. In fact, due to the farm-to-table movement of the past ten years, fresh, seasonal, local food, standing on its own and minimally embellished, is preferred by many diners. We will always want indulgent foods but also healthy foods. Few people eat the same foods every day or the same types of foods each day. As a chef who understands the role of nutrition and possesses the expertise to deliver food that is both healthful and delicious, you can offer a range of good choices.

But it's not quite that simple. According to Chef Tom Colicchio, restaurateur and food advocate, "if we want people to eat less meat and more vegetables—a generally recognized healthy habit—we need to allocate more funds to that. For example,

about 85 percent of agricultural subsidies now go to commodity crops and processed foods, and about 15 percent go to beef and dairy. One percent or less goes to "specialty crops"—better known as fruits and vegetables. A shift in priorities is needed.

Essentials of Nutrition for Chefs can help you understand issues and advocate for improvement. With knowledge and skills in place, you will be ready to meet the growing need for healthier food options while becoming a stronger, more versatile and better prepared foodservice professional. While this book is not a comprehensive nutrition text, it presents nutrition basics for culinarians and foodservice operators: what you need to know to cook and serve healthful, delicious food that guests want to purchase again and again. That is the bottom line – for you, for your patrons and for the success of your operation.

It's All About the Food

As a foodservice professional you cook food, not nutrients. Understanding which foods deliver valuable nutrients will put you well on your way to delivering healthful meals.

Although nutrition is a complex (and evolving) science, choosing and preparing healthier foods is, by contrast, really not that difficult. "Eat foods, not too much, mostly plants" is the mantra of Michael Pollan, author and food activist. Sounds simple, right? Then why do so many of us get bogged down with fad diets and misinformed eating plans. You will no doubt be asked to prepare gluten-free, dairy-free and carbohydrate-free dishes in your workplace, some of which may be medically necessary, some based on whims and misconceptions. But if you focus on foods that are inherently healthier with cooking techniques that are simple and fresh, you will be well equipped to deal with the needs of all of your guests.

Core food recommendations throughout this text include:

- Increase fruit
- Increase vegetables, including legumes
- Increase whole grains and substitute whole grains for refined grains when possible
- Substitute healthier fats for less-healthful fats and reduce total fats
- Increase fish and seafood
- Decrease foods with added sugars

- Limit sources of sodium, especially salt
- Decrease processed and packaged foods

The message is clear: Reducing fats and sugars helps diners lower the many health risks caused by over-weight and obesity, while increasing vegetables, legumes, fruits, fish and whole grains leads to better health. Your charge is to select, prepare and serve these important foods in ways that will satisfy our love of flavor, comfort and health.

From the Kitchen

Barton Seaver
Chef/Author
Maine

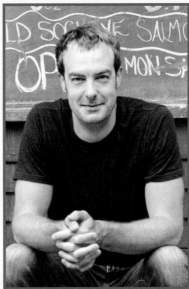

As a young chef I was driven to constantly push myself to be better, to bring more creativity and new techniques, explore bold flavors and constantly perfect my execution. I measured success by always pushing to improve myself and my team. But as I matured as a chef, I began to consider the context of the work that I was so passionate about and the meals I served.

As chefs we are fortunate to be given the opportunity to feed people and entertain them with our talents. But with this blessing comes an equal responsibility to sustain them. I came to believe that in order to achieve great food it must be made with ingredients that support the wellness of our guests. Nutrition doesn't equal sacrifice or diminished creativity. By expanding my knowledge of nutrition science and exploring healthier cooking techniques I didn't limit my repertoire or my approach to cuisine. Rather, I discovered new avenues of creativity, experimenting with and developing menus that were meaningful, healthful and exciting to my guests.

Our role as chefs has evolved. We are expected to do more than simply manage kitchens. We are increasingly responsible for stewarding our relationship with the environment and to consider how the food we serve contributes to the well-being of our guests. As professionals, we thrive when our guests thrive, and integrating principles of nutrition is a fundamental skill vital to your success and to the future of our industry.

Barton Seaver is on a mission to restore our relationship with the ocean, the land, and with each other—through dinner. He has translated his illustrious career as a chef into his leadership of the Sustainable Seafood and Health Initiative at the Center for Health and the Global Environment at the Harvard T.H. Chan School of Public Health. In this role, Barton spearheads initiatives to inform consumers and institutions about how our choices for diet and menus can promote healthier people, more secure food supplies, and thriving communities.

Barton is a firm believer that human health depends on the health of the ocean and that the best way to connect the two is at the dinner table. As an award-winning cookbook author, Barton pairs simple cooking techniques with a vast knowledge of seafood for a fresh take on sustainable eating.

As an executive chef, Barton opened seven restaurants awarded both for their cuisine and as environmentally-conscious businesses.

Barton is the author of five highly regarded books, including *Superfood Seagreens: A Guide to Cooking with Power-packed Seaweed*, which explores the health benefits of this emerging player in the superfood realm. His second sustainable seafood-centric cookbook is entitled *Two if by Sea*. His most recent book, *American Seafood: Heritage, Culture & Cookery From Sea to Shining Sea*, is an essential guide to more than 500 species, as well as a riveting history of one of our country's most iconic industries.

Barton currently resides in coastal Maine, a stone's throw away from a working waterfront, with his wife, son, and their 10 heritage chickens.

Arctic Char with Blistered Cherry Tomatoes in Garlic Olive Oil

Serves: 10

Barton Seaver
Harvard T.H. Chan School of Public Health

Arctic char is an easy fish for anyone to fall in love with. It's widely available, affordable and packed with Omega-3s. The simplicity of this preparation highlights the beauty of great ingredients. It's a healthful meal that is so convenient you'll keep coming back to it.

Extra-virgin olive oil	1 cup
Garlic	15 cloves, halved
Cherry tomatoes	10 pints
Salt	½ teaspoon
Arctic char fillet	10 (5-ounce) portions skin-on

1. A large cast-steel or cast-iron skillet is best for this dish, as it will do most of the work for you. Preheat the broiler.

2. Set the pan on the stove over high heat until it is smoking hot. Add the olive oil and garlic. Cook the garlic until it is blistered and golden brown. Add the tomatoes, but do this very carefully, otherwise searing hot oil will splash up onto you. Cook until the skins of the tomatoes begin to blister in the hot oil, about 1 minute, then season with salt.

3. Carefully place the char fillets, skin side up, on top of the tomatoes and transfer the pan to under the broiler. Cook for 6 minutes, then check on the fillets. The skin should be blistered and bubbling. Remove the char fillets to serving plates. Spoon the tomatoes onto the char fillets and serve immediately.

Per Serving

Calories	320		Cholesterol	117	mg
Fat	19	g	Sodium	210	mg
Saturated Fat	0.5	g	Carbohydrates	12	mg
Trans Fat	0	g	Dietary Fiber	3	mg
Sugar	7	g	Protein	26	g

From Barton Seaver's *For Cod and Country: Simple, Delicious, Sustainable Cooking,* Sterling Epicure, 2011.

Arugula, Mint, Apple and Seagreens Salad

Serves: 10

Barton Seaver
Harvard T.H. Chan School of Public Health

The peppery bite and texture of arugula, the crunch of apple, the soaring aroma of mint, and the subtle saltiness of seagreens are an amazing combination. Get the sweetest apple you can find, such as Fuji or Braeburn.

Olive oil	6 tablespoons
Red wine vinegar	2 tablespoons
Whole grain or Dijon mustard	2 tablespoons
Salt	1 teaspoon
Arugula	1 pound
Fresh or frozen kelp, cut into bite-size pieces, or 2 ounces rehydrated dried kelp	1 pound
Fuji or Braeburn apples, very thinly sliced	4 each
Mint	15 sprigs, julienned
Black pepper, fresh cracked	as needed

1. In a large bowl whisk together the olive oil, vinegar, mustard and salt.

2. Add the arugula, seagreens, apple and mint and toss until well coated. Serve immediately with fresh cracked pepper.

Per Serving

Calories	150		Cholesterol	0	mg
Fat	9	g	Sodium	310	mg
Saturated Fat	1	g	Carbohydrates	16	mg
Trans Fat	0	g	Dietary Fiber	3	mg
Sugar	9	g	Protein	2	g

From Barton Seaver's *Superfood Seagreens: A Guide to Cooking with Power-Packed Seaweed,* Sterling 2016.

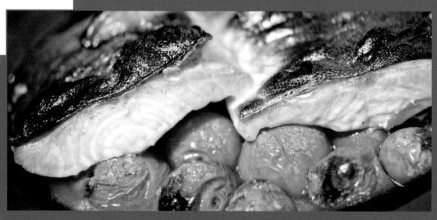

An Alliance of Taste and Health

Taste and health have been jockeying for position for years. Many believed you had to choose one over the other. Was "good" food tasty or healthful? Why not both? While many chefs ate and served healthful foods, and many in the nutrition community valued artfully prepared, flavorful dishes, advice on healthful eating tended to be very restrictive for many years. Eventually, Julia Child, one of the founders of The American Institute of Wine & Food (AIWF), became concerned about a growing "fear of food" in America. In October 1990, AIWF held a groundbreaking conference, *Resetting the American Table: Creating a New Alliance of Taste and Health*, to address this issue.

At this conference, 50 culinary and nutrition leaders – including co-author of this book Mary Abbott Hess, LHD, MS, RD, LDN, FAND, who was president of The American Dietetic Association (now The Academy of Nutrition and Dietetics) at the time – sought to build an alliance or at least achieve peaceful coexistence. A consensus document, *Standards for Food and Diet Quality*, was created under the umbrella tenet, "In matters of taste, consider nutrition. In matters of nutrition, consider taste. And in all cases, consider individual needs and preferences." The intent was to move Americans toward a more healthful diet without giving up the pleasures of the table. The document, with statements on nutrition, physical activity, food availability, quality and preparation, food safety, and education, was compiled and released by AIWF in 1993 as part of a national campaign. Twenty-five years later, many of its components have been incorporated into public policy and many of its core concepts have become the foundation of healthful cooking.

It just makes good sense for dietitians and chefs to work together. We are all concerned about proper eating habits. If we join and work together, we can help each other in reaching our common goal – healthful, good-tasting food.

Julia Child
The American Dietetic Association 1991 Annual Meeting

Attitudes Toward Healthful Eating

Until about ten years ago, lowering dietary fat (especially trans fat and saturated fat) was the primary focus of health advice. Today, the focus is on what we are getting in our foods, rather than what we are not. In other words, today we focus on the nutrients contained in foods, rather than the fat and sugar that was removed. While moderating fat and sugar remains important, today's healthful diet should include getting plenty of the vitamins, minerals, antioxidants, phytochemicals and fiber from a variety of fruits, vegetables and whole grain. With 70% of American adults and as many as a third of American children either overweight or obese, calories are also a major issue. [1, 2] Reflecting these concerns, the healthy diet paradigm has shifted from restriction to balance – seeking positive nutrients and balancing the number of calories consumed with the number burned. Contemporary menus reflecting this shift feature less processed and more fresh, whole foods, healthful cooking techniques and portion control. This is even taking place in fast food outlets. Most offer a selection of side and main course salads. In addition many restaurants are reducing portion sizes, which has the dual benefit of reducing food costs while promoting healthful eating. Think an espresso versus a "venti latte."

Today's attitudes toward healthy eating are more balanced, yet more extreme at the same time. Fewer Americans say they want to lose weight, according to a Gallup's annual Health and Healthcare poll (conducted November 2015). Only 49% of Americans are actively trying to lose weight, compared to 62% in 2004. This is the first time in at least 25 years that less than half of Americans want to lose weight. Only 24% of adults reported they are "seriously trying to lose weight. Yet many are following low carbohydrate, gluten-free and high protein diets. [3]

Health Risks

In 1902, human nutrition pioneer W. O. Atwater predicted: "The evils of overeating may not be felt at once, but sooner or later they are sure to appear – perhaps in an excessive amount of fatty tissue, perhaps in general debility, perhaps in actual disease." [4] In fact, within the last century, changes in diet and level of physical activity have been profound and have led to an increase in lifestyle diseases like heart disease, obesity and diabetes – to name a few. His predictions came true.

Today, chronic diseases are the leading causes of death and disability in the United States. Heart disease, cancer and stroke account for more than 50% of all deaths each year. About one-fourth of people with chronic conditions have one or more daily activity limitations. Four modifiable health risk behaviors – lack of physical activity, poor nutrition, tobacco use and excessive alcohol consumption – are responsible for much of the illness, suffering and early death related to chronic diseases and accidents. [**5**]

The obesity epidemic in America is one of the greatest public health threats of this century and has contributed to the increase in chronic diseases. According to the *Dietary Guidelines for Americans 2015-2020*, about half of all Americans have one or more preventable chronic diseases, many related to poor eating habits and lack of physical activity. [**6**] Eight or more different types of cancer are associated with being over-weight or obese. [**7**] Although a single nutrient is often tagged as the cause of a chronic disease -- for example, saturated fat and heart disease or salt and high blood pressure -- research over the past three decades shows that a cluster of dietary elements is usually at the root of the problem. [**8**]

Historically, people from nations that consume plant-based diets have lower incidences of diet-related diseases and disorders than Americans. Many of these diets are based on rice, grains, beans, legumes, nuts, fruits and vegetables. Foods are minimally processed with greater emphasis on seasonal and local produce. Immigrants living in the United States, however, typically adopt Western food practices – such as eating more processed foods – that lead to increasing the risk of developing diseases.

Probably, the most succinct way of summing up what to eat to be healthy was stated by Michael Pollan in his book, *Defense of Food: an Eater's Manifesto*: "eat food, not too much, mostly plants."

casebycase | Making Connections

We've come a long way from the old-fashioned salad bar. With the increasing popularity of fast-casual dining and the cultural trend toward healthy fresh fruits and vegetables, salad chains like Sweetgreen and Honey-grow are making their mark while also demonstrating the power of food.

While earning their undergraduate business degrees at Georgetown University, friends Jonathan Neman, Nathaniel Ru and Nicolas Jammet could not find the healthy, seasonal, affordable food they wanted near campus. So they raised $350,000, and in 2007, opened the first Sweetgreen with an emphasis on connecting people to real food, sustainability and a transparent supply chain. Now, 12 years later, Los Angeles-based Sweetgreen has 3,500 employees in more than 80 locations serving salads and grain bowls made from scratch with ingredients delivered from more than 500 local farmers daily.

Sweetgreen's "Food Ethos" connects all the dots: "We believe the choices we make about what we eat, where it comes from and how it's prepared have a direct and powerful impact on the health of individuals, communities and the environment.

"We're always looking for ways to source smarter, to make better decisions and to help Sweetgreen and its customers be a positive force in the world and on the food system. We feel a great sense of responsibil-ity and pride to change what it means to be in the business of feeding people."

Justin Rosenberg launched Honeygrow in Philadelphia in 2012 with a dream to fill the dining-out gap he experienced after going vegan. Today, Honeygrow has more than 25 locations serving customizable salads and stir-fries as well as cold-pressed juices in the eastern U.S. As with Sweetgreen, Honeygrow's food sources differ from location to location. Each restaurant posts a local list of local produce sources every month.

Honeygrow's commitment to "growing local" extends to its civic-minded partnerships with local businesses and its commitment to nurturing creativity and inno-vation in its employees, patrons and communities.

It's True: You Are What You Eat

What people consume as infants, toddlers, young children and teens builds the body they take into adulthood. In fact, five of the 10 leading causes of death are related to lifelong dietary choices (bolded in the list below). And although not in the top 10, cirrhosis of the liver and osteoporosis are also triggered by food choices made over time. The good news is that it's never too late to improve food choices.

Leading Causes of Death in the U.S.

1. **Heart disease**
2. **Cancer**
3. Chronic lower respiratory disease
4. Accidents
5. **Stroke**
6. Alzheimer's disease
7. **Diabetes**
8. Influenza and pneumonia
9. **Kidney disease**
10. Suicide

Source: National Center for Health Statistics, Centers for Disease Control and Prevention, U.S. Department of Health and Human Services. National Vital Statistics Report. Deaths: Final Data for 2015. Published November 27, 2017. https://www.cdc.gov/nchs/data/nvsr/nvsr66/nvsr66_06.pdf

Why We Eat What We Eat

At the most basic level, the purpose of food is to provide the nutrients and energy the body needs to grow and function. But many variables influence food choice.

Taste, Cost and Convenience

According to The International Food Information Council (IFIC) *The Food & Health Survey 2017* taste, price and healthfulness continue to be the biggest drivers of food purchasing decisions. Taste remains the main driver behind purchasing foods and beverages with 84% of consumers surveyed listing taste as their priority in choosing foods, down from the high of 90% in 2014. Consumers are not willing, nor should they have to, sacrifice taste for nutrition. Healthful foods can taste great too. [9]

Price continues as a significant factor also, ranking second in terms of priorities. Contrary to the beliefs of some, however, preparing healthier food does not have to cost more. For example, whole grains

and legumes are relatively inexpensive. Fruits and vegetables served in season are often less expensive than imported, out-of-season produce. The most expensive part of the meal, the animal protein source, can be served in a smaller portion. Shifting the balance of the plate to include more grains, fruits and vegetables, and less animal protein, helps control food costs while providing healthful options. And, of course, with the rise of farmer's markets, buying in-season, local foods can be very economical.

Healthfulness fell from 71% in 2014 to 63% in 2017, ranking it third in terms of importance. Eating more fruits and vegetables is the most common effort Americans take to improve their diets, followed by drinking water instead of soda, and eating more whole grains. The young and old are equally concerned about the healthfulness of their diets, making foodservice for teens and those over 65 equally important. This is obvious with the popular restaurant chain, Chipotle, and the emergence of fresh juice bars and various salad concepts.

That convenience plays a significant role in food selections is evidenced by the prevalence of not only quick-service restaurants, but carryout and meal delivery. Today there are an increasing number of grocery delivery services, most regional, such as Green Bean Delivery, Peapod, Spud and Amazon Fresh. Many of these delivery services are now focusing on fresh, local ingredients. In addition to groceries, there are also a growing number of services delivering ingredients ready to be assembled into meals, as well as completely prepared meals ready to pop in the oven. Most of these also focus on fresh, and often locally-sourced ingredients, such as the national companies, Hello Fresh, Blue Apron, BistroMD and Plated, as well as many local companies. For many consumers, the time available for home meal preparation and consumption is limited – and so are cooking skills. This combination of circumstances creates many opportunities for the foodservice industry to provide convenient and healthful meals.

In recent years IFIC surveys have indicated that regional and ethnic preferences play an important role in food selection. For example, rice and beans are served across the United States but in many different ways with different seasonings. In Louisiana, red beans and rice is a staple. In the South, Hoppin' John (black-eyed peas and rice) rules. In the Southwest, pinto beans and rice are a favorite. The popularity of ethnic cuisines has emboldened consumers to try new seasonings and flavors. This curiosity has brought greater diversity to the American diet and introduced many new options to replace fats and salt for flavor. Ethnicity and religion can dictate food selections on a daily basis, on specific holidays or during certain seasons. Chefs should understand the food practices, customs and holiday food traditions of the populations they serve and meet these expectations in creative yet healthful ways.

Sustainability

According to the 2015 IFIC survey, 38% of Americans say that sustainability is important to them. [9] Americans see "ensuring a sufficient food supply" as the most important aspect of sustainability. Reducing the amount of pesticides used to produce food, maximizing food output with minimal use of natural resources, optimal land and water use and efficiency, and less food and energy waste are important concerns as well. The increased awareness of global climate change and the desire to obtain food from local sources has spawned the growth of CSA's, Community Supported Agriculture, programs. These are farms or groups of farms that, for a yearly fee, provide a "share" of freshly harvested produce for members to pick up or have delivered. This is a way to support local farmers, share in their harvest and reduce the carbon footprint of foods shipped miles across the country

or world.

Food hubs are another system that facilitates the connection between food producers and the foodservice industry. Food hubs will provide a single point of aggregation for local and regional producers and manage the distribution of local products to many segments of the food and foodservice industry. Unlike farmers markets that sell directly to consumers, food hubs typically support wholesale customers like restaurants, schools and healthcare operations.

Marketing

Marketing also influences food selections. Food choices are influenced by the description of menu items on signage or printed menus. Gluten-free banana muffins might be off-putting to some, whereas almond banana streusel muffins, with the exact same ingredients, less so. Even the location of an item on the menu can affect selection. Comments made by servers also can influence guests' choices. An enthusiastic description of a dish, knowledge of ingredients and preparation methods, and helping the customer make a food selection (especially when the guest has food restrictions) makes the server a partner in the customer's successful dining experience and influences the patron to form a positive impression

The 2017 Food & Health Survey: Consumer Attitudes toward Food Safety, Nutrition & Health

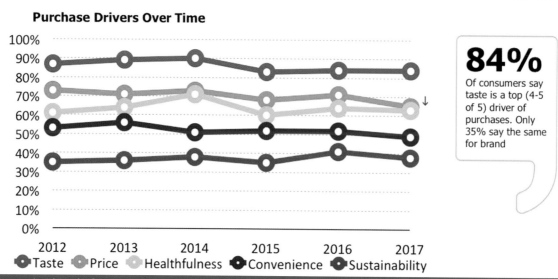

Taste, price, healthfulness reign supreme

Convenience relatively steady with half of consumers stating it as a top driver

Purchase Drivers Over Time

84%
Of consumers say taste is a top (4-5 of 5) driver of purchases. Only 35% say the same for brand

● Taste ● Price ● Healthfulness ● Convenience ● Sustainability

and become a repeat customer.

Customers are seeking higher quality foods and higher quality is characterized by better ingredients. Highlighting quality producers of key ingredients, farmers, or local sourcing of ingredients adds to the marketing message.

Social Interaction

Remember that people also use mealtime for social interaction. Dining with others offers many benefits beyond meeting nutrient needs. Eating together enhances quality of life and creates a time for sharing cultural values. Research provides clear evidence that family meals and shared meals are associated with better dietary intake and that these findings apply across the lifespan. [10] Youths who enjoyed family dinner on most days in a week had significantly higher intakes of protein, fiber, calcium, iron and other nutrients than those eating dinner with their family less often. [11] Additionally, increased frequency of family meals is associated with decreased intakes of low nutrient density foods and beverages. [12]

Marketing Food to Children

Marketing high-calorie, low-nutrient foods to children has garnered much attention and criticism over the last decade. In 2005, the Institute of Medicine (IOM) released *Food Marketing to Children and Youth: Threat or Opportunity?* The study, which was requested by Congress and sponsored by the U.S. Centers for Disease Control and Prevention, provided a comprehensive review of the scientific evidence on the influence of food marketing on diets and the diet-related health of children and youth. The report found that food and beverage marketing practices place children's long-term health at risk. If America's children and youth are to develop eating habits that help them avoid early onset of diet-related chronic diseases, they have to reduce their intake of high-calorie, low-nutrient snacks, fast foods and sweetened drinks.

The IOM report found that more than $10 billion is spent each year for marketing food and beverages to children and youth in America, and that the majority of products marketed are processed foods – high in calories, sugars, salt and fat, and low in many key nutrients.

The report's recommendations for the foodservice industry include:

- Use creativity, resources, and the full range of marketing practices to promote healthful meals for children and youth.
- Expand and actively promote healthier food, beverage, and meal options for children and youth.

- Provide calorie content and other key nutrition information, as possible, on menus and packaging that is prominently visible at the point of choice and use.

Since the release of the IOM recommendations the federal government, industry, and nutrition advocates have worked to improve the nutrition criteria of the foods and beverages marketed to children. Specifically, various organizations have taken the following steps.

- In 2013, food and beverage companies, as part of the Council of Better Business Bureaus' Children's Food and Beverage Advertising Initiative (CFBAI) established a uniform set of voluntary category-specific nutrition standards for participating companies, which took effect in January 2014.
- The National Restaurant Association's Kids LiveWell has established nutrition criteria for restaurants.
- The federal Interagency Working Group (IWG) on Food Marketed to Children has developed voluntary guidelines.
- The Center for Science in the Public Interest has developed guidelines for Responsible Food Marketing to Children.

Source: Food Marketing to Children and Youth: Threat or Opportunity? www.iom.edu/Reports/2005/Food-Marketing-to- Children-and-Youth-Threat-or-Opportunity.aspx

Restaurants today are popular because they are intense food-sharing enterprises necessary now that the home is losing its traditional importance as a place where food is prepared and served to a group.

Lionel Tiger
The Pursuit of Pleasure

Choosing Healthful Foods

People usually think they eat less than they really do. In fact, it is very difficult to determine what is actually eaten. Even when food records are kept, perception seldom precisely matches consumption, especially when snacks and alcohol are involved. What people say they want is often not what they choose. Many customers say they want healthful choices but don't select these items when they are offered, often because they believe the healthful or low-calorie options will not taste as good. Some restaurants are integrating healthful choices throughout the menu, rather than calling them out as healthy options. Food manufacturers use this "stealth health" approach, too, quietly reducing (but not eliminating) fat, salt and sugar in processed foods. Restaurants like Subway, however, have increased sales by highlighting and heavily advertising specific healthful or low-calorie choices. As restaurant food labeling is implemented, perceptions may change. Faced with the facts on calories, will customers make different choices? Some observers say that consumers do not want to be "confronted" with nutrition information when they eat out because it detracts from full enjoyment and celebration; others opine that consumers appreciate and use the information to make more healthful, lower-calorie choices.

The Academy of Nutrition and Dietetics and others in the world of food and nutrition have supported the idea that "all foods fit." While all foods **can** fit, moderation and balance present a challenge. For even a few foods high in fat, salt, sugar and calories to "fit" in the daily diet, plenty of healthful nutrient dense, fairly low-calorie foods are needed to offset them. While the concept that there are no good or bad foods and that what really counts is the total diet sounds good, it is not that useful – unless, of course, you are making a case for including "bad foods." One has to make many excellent choices in order to fit in a daily soft drink or French fries.

The reality of weight control and disease prevention is simple: It basically boils down to calories. Providing balance and moderation are among the chef's greatest challenges.

While it is ultimately the guests' choice, there should be a variety of healthful options that are appealing and interesting making it easier to choose healthful items. Offering smaller portions and downsizing portions of high-fat and high-sugar options make moderation far easier.

Nutrients in Foods

It is becoming increasingly important that chefs know what is in the food they make and serve. That does not mean that everything must fit a healthful profile, but knowing calorie count and some information about nutritional benefits and risks enables the chef to create balance and moderation across the total menu. Knowledge provides power – the power to make informed choices and to create positive change.

Foods provide a vast array of substances that are necessary to sustain life and health. There are six classes of **essential nutrients**:

- Carbohydrates
- Fats
- Proteins
- Vitamins
- Minerals
- Water

To be an essential nutrient, a substance must meet three criteria:

1. It must be needed by the human body.
2. It cannot be made by the body (or made in sufficient quantity) to meet bodily needs; thus, it must be provide by food sources.
3. If absent, it will create a deficiency disease or medical problem.

Essential nutrients are discussed in greater detail in later chapters.

All calories – the body's fuel – come from carbohydrates, proteins, fats and alcohol. Water and the many vitamins and minerals, each with specific functions, are vital to life and health but do not provide calories. Alcohol also provides calories but is not a nutrient.

Typical American Diet Compared to Recommended Intake Levels or Limits

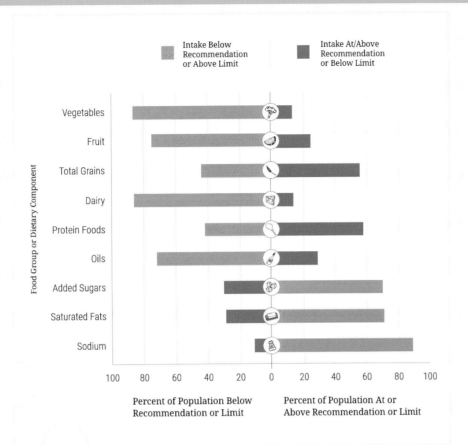

Source: *Dietary Guidelines for Americans, 2015-2020*. Based on data from *What We Eat in America*, NHANES 2007-2010 for average intakes by age-sex group. Healthy U.S.-Style Food Patterns, which vary based on age, sex, and activity level, for recommended intakes and limits.

Essential Nutrients

Carbohydrates	Fats	Protein	Vitamins	Minerals	Water
Fiber	Linoleic acid	Essential amino acids:	B_6	Calcium	Water
Glucose	Linolenic acid	Histidine	B_{12}	Chloride	
		Isoleucine	Biotin	Chromium	
		Leucine	Folate	Copper	
		Lysine	Niacin	Fluoride	
		Methionine	Pantothenic acid	Iodine	
		Phenylalanine	Riboflavin	Iron	
		Threonine	Thiamin	Magnesium	
		Tryptophan	Vitamin A	Manganese	
		Valine	Vitamin D	Molybdenum	
			Vitamin E	Phosphorus	
			Vitamin K	Potassium	
			Vitamin C	Selenium	
				Sodium	
				Sulfur	
				Zinc	

Energy Balance

Energy is measured in calories. Teens and adults need about 2,000 to 3,000 calories from food each day. Calorie needs are dependent on activity level, age, height, physical health and body composition. Calories are used to fuel physical activity, basic body functions and digestion.

Energy is needed to make and fuel cells of the body that are necessary for all life-sustaining activities – blood circulation, breathing, temperature maintenance, nerve activity and hormone secretion. These activities, taken together at the cellular level, are called **basal metabolism**. Age, gender, genetics, body composition and size affect basal metabolic energy needs, which account for 50% to 65% of total calorie needs.

In addition, energy supports activities such as walking, working the line, serving guests, running, cycling, rock climbing, skating, etc. Depending on the individual, this activity may account for 25% to 50% of total energy needs. Sedentary people need fewer calories because they burn fewer to support daily activities.

Energy is also needed to break food down into the small components that go into the bloodstream and later to cells. This process is called the **thermic effect** of food and accounts for 5% to 10% of total energy needs.

If you consume more calories than you need to maintain current weight, you gain weight. If you consume fewer than you need, you lose weight. Because total calorie needs decline after early adulthood, even maintaining the same eating habits and levels of calories consumed will cause weight gain each decade. Many people need fewer calories than they think they do, and most underestimate the number of calories that they eat. This combination results in weight gain over time.

Calculating Calories from Foods

Calories are the unit used to measure the energy in food. The energy-yielding nutrients in food (protein, fats and carbohydrates) are measured in grams. Foods are usually a mixture of protein, fat, carbohydrates and water. Few foods contain just one nutrient.

Nutrient	Calories per Gram
Carbohydrate	4
Fat	9
Protein	4
Alcohol	7

A teaspoon of oil weighs about 5 grams and contains approximately 5 grams of fat and 45 calories:

5 grams fat x 9 calories per gram = 45 calories

A cup of low-fat milk weighs about 245 grams and contains approximately 8 grams of protein, 12 grams of carbohydrates and 2.5 grams of fat. The balance of milk's weight comes from water (220 grams). One cup of low-fat milk will have:

8 grams protein x 4 calories/gram = 32 calories from protein

12 grams carbohydrate x 4 calories/gram = 48 calories from carbohydrate

2.5 grams fat x 9 calories/gram = 22.5 calories from fat

Total calories = 102.5

Factors Affecting the Basal Metabolic Rate (BMR)

Your BMR is influenced by a number of factors working in combination, including:

- Body size: larger adult bodies have more metabolizing tissue(biologically active cells) and a higher BMR.
- Age: metabolism slows with age due to a loss in muscle tissue and hormonal and neurological changes. BMR declines about 2% per decade after age 30.
- Gender: generally, men have faster metabolisms than women because they tend to have more muscle tissue and muscle tissue burns more calories.
- Amount of body fat: fat cells are sluggish and burn far fewer calories than most other tissues.
- Infection or illness: BMR increases because the body has to work harder to build new tissues and to create an immune response.

Crash dieting, starving or fasting - eating too few calories encourages the body to slow down the metabolism to conserve energy; BMR can drop by up to 15%. Lean muscle tissue is burned for energy and lost, which further reduces the BMR. Illnesses, especially those with fever, also can alter metabolic rate.

Estimated Calorie Needs per Day by Age, Sex and Physical Activity Level

Estimated amounts of calories a needed to maintain calorie balance for various gender and age groups at three different levels of physical activity. The estimates are rounded to the nearest 200 calories. An individual's calorie needs may be higher or lower than these average estimates. Calories needed are influenced by height, weight, amount of lean muscle, personal genetic factors and activity.

	Male			Female[d]		
	Activity Level					
Age (years)	Sedentary[a]	Moderately Active[b]	Active[c]	Sedentary	Moderately Active	Active
2	1,000	1,000	1,000	1,000	1,000	1,000
3	1,200	1,400	1,400	1,000	1,200	1,400
4	1,200	1,400	1,600	1,200	1,400	1,400
5	1,200	1,400	1,600	1,200	1,400	1,600
6	1,400	1,600	1,800	1,200	1,400	1,600
7	1,400	1,600	1,800	1,200	1,600	1,800
8	1,400	1,600	2,000	1,400	1,600	1,800
9	1,600	1,800	2,000	1,400	1,600	1,800
10	1,600	1,800	2,200	1,400	1,800	2,000
11	1,800	2,000	2,200	1,600	1,800	2,000
12	1,800	2,200	2,400	1,600	2,000	2,200
13	2,000	2,200	2,600	1,600	2,000	2,200
14	2,000	2,400	2,800	1,800	2,000	2,400
15	2,200	2,600	3,000	1,800	2,000	2,400
16-18	2,400	2,800	3,200	1,800	2,000	2,400
19–20	2,600	2,800	3,000	2,000	2,200	2,400
21–25	2,400	2,800	3,000	2,000	2,200	2,400
26–30	2,400	2,600	3,000	1,800	2,000	2,400
31–35	2,400	2,600	3,000	1,800	2,000	2,200
36–40	2,400	2,600	2,800	1,800	2,000	2,200
41–45	2,200	2,600	2,800	1,800	2,000	2,200
46–50	2,200	2,400	2,800	1,800	2,000	2,200
51–55	2,200	2,400	2,800	1,600	1,800	2,200
56–60	2,200	2,400	2,600	1,600	1,800	2,200
61–65	2,000	2,400	2,600	1,600	1,800	2,000
66–75	2,000	2,200	2,600	1,600	1,800	2,000
76+	2,000	2,200	2,400	1,600	1,800	2,000

Notes: These estimates are based on the Estimated Energy Requirements (EER) equations, using reference heights (average) and reference weights (healthy) for each age-sex group. For children and adolescents, reference height and weight vary. For adults, the reference man is 5 feet 10 inches tall and weighs 154 pounds. The reference woman is 5 feet 4 inches tall and weighs 126 pounds.

Estimates range from 1,600 to 2,400 calories per day for adult women and 2,000 to 3,000 calories per day for adult men. Within each age and sex category, the low end of the range is for sedentary individuals; the high end of the range is for active individuals. Due to reductions in basal metabolic rate that occur with aging, calorie needs generally decrease for adults as they age. Estimated needs for young children range from 1,000 to 2,000 calories per day, and the range for older children and adolescents varies substantially from 1,400 to 3,200 calories per day, with boys generally having higher calorie needs than girls. These are only estimates, and approximations of individual calorie needs can be aided with online tools such as those available at www.supertracker.usda.gov.

[a] Sedentary means a lifestyle that includes only the physical activity of independent living.

[b] Moderately Active means a lifestyle that includes physical activity equivalent to walking about 1.5 to 3 miles per day at 3 to 4 miles per hour, in addition to the activities of independent living.

[c] Active means a lifestyle that includes physical activity equivalent to walking more than 3 miles per day at 3 to 4 miles per hour, in addition to the activities of independent living.

[d] Estimates for females do not include women who are pregnant or breastfeeding.

Source: Institute of Medicine. Dietary Reference Intakes for Energy, Carbohydrate, Fiber, Fat, Fatty Acids, Cholesterol, Protein, and Amino Acids. Washington (DC): The National Academies Press; 2002.

Nutrient Density

Nutrient density is a measure of positive nutrients to calories. Nutrient dense foods pack a lot of essential nutrients into relatively few calories. In other words, they are particularly healthful food choices and ingredients. Vegetables, fruits, whole grains, fish, eggs, low-fat milk, lean meat, beans and poultry prepared without added solid fats or sugars are nutrient dense. Nutrient dense foods are often described as **nutrient rich**. The *Dietary Guidelines for Americans* suggest getting the most nutrition from calories consumed and eating a variety of nutrient dense foods and beverages within and among the basic food groups. Foods that have low nutrient density supply calories but relatively small amounts of vitamins and minerals. For example, whole-wheat bread provides fiber and vitamins from the whole grain for a minimum of calories (approximately 80 per slice) so it is **nutrient dense**, while a croissant, made from refined white flour, has little fiber and vitamins, and a hefty calorie tag of 300, therefore it has a low nutrient density.

Numerous researchers and organizations have developed approaches based on nutrient density that can be used as tools to help consumers improve their dietary patterns by selecting more nutritious food items. This approach, called **nutrient profiling**, is the process of ranking foods based on their nutrient content. Some of the models developed focus on nutrients to limit (giving higher scores to foods low in fat, sugar and salt); others have factored in nutrients known to be beneficial to health (giving higher scores to foods rich in vitamins, minerals and fiber). Some models are a combination of both (with a calculation that adds points for essential nutrients and removes points for those substances that should be limited). Several nutrient profiling approaches are described in the next chapter.

What's in a Name: Some Surprises

Location, location, location may be the mantra in real estate, but marketing and packaging is important with food. According to the *IFIC Food & Health Survey 2015*, 40% of those surveyed regularly purchase foods because they are labeled "natural," and 30% purchase foods because they are labeled with "no added hormones or steroids" or "organic." No doubt the sustainability of food has come into the mainstream, with seven out of ten Americans (71%) giving thought to the production of their foods. [13] As taste is the main driver behind what we choose to eat, the tastier a food sounds, (regardless of the ingredients), the more likely it is to sell—on the supermarket shelf as well as on menus. This is where things can get tricky.

A best-selling book by David Zinczenko with Matt Goulding called *Eat This, Not That!* (Rodale Books, 2010) lists the nutrition numbers of brand-name foods and restaurant dishes, showing how many seemingly healthy sounding dishes are anything but. Here are a few examples:

- Applebee's Grilled Shrimp 'N Spinach Salad sounds healthy, but weighs in at 1,000 calories, 66 grams of fat and 50 grams of sugar.
- Sonic's Blackberry Green Iced Tea contains 55 grams of sugar, more than a similar quantity of soda.
- Olive Garden's Strawberry Smoothie contains no fiber, 330 calories and 65 grams of sugar.

The *Eat This, Not That!* series of books on supermarket, restaurant and other choices is full of shocking values, but everyone can compare foods using food labels and menu declarations where calories, fat and sugar levels are disclosed.

Portion Distortion

Many chefs are very interested in nutrition and believe they are serving (mostly) healthful food. A survey conducted by Clemson University has reported that although chefs recognize the importance of nutrition in menu planning, they are serving meals that are inconsistent with the current *Dietary Guidelines for Americans*. A key area of concern is portion size. A survey of 300 chefs attending culinary and research chef meetings revealed that 76% thought they served "regular" portions, but they actually served portions two to four times larger than recommended serving sizes. Although chefs say they know that large portions pose problems for weight management, many believe that customers expect large portions and see it as better value. Some restaurant patrons expect to take home part of a meal and save enough for another meal. Many customers, however, have a "clean plate" mindset that drives them to eat everything on the plate regardless of portion size. [14]

Over the past two decades, portion sizes of individually packaged foods have grown, too. Consequently, customers now think large portions are normal. The small soft drink in a fast food restaurant is a good example, and most casual restaurants add free refills. This "**portion distortion**" can hinder efforts to control

weight and improve health. [15] One of the goals of this book is to help chefs understand appropriate portions and provide food that is satisfying, yet healthful. Later chapters will explore portions and strategies for focusing on food quality rather than excessive quantity. Every chef wants to make customers happy and improve the dining experience. Helping customers (and themselves) stay healthy is a bonus. Keep in mind that you are selling one meal, not two. Plus, the carry-out container adds to your costs.

However, recently there has been an increase in small plates in fine dining restaurants. Small plates are intended to let patrons get a taste of many items and/or to share among a table of friends. Tapas, dim sum, sushi and sliders have all become popular in recent years. Eight-ounce cans of soda are again available in supermarkets. Other restaurants offer half-portions, especially of pasta and sandwiches. Maybe it is time to rethink the oversized restaurant plates and bowls that have added to the problem. Smaller plates, bowls and glasses assist in serving more normal portions.

Portion sizes and corresponding calories have increased over the last 20 years. Here are some examples.

Portions and Calories - 20 Years Later

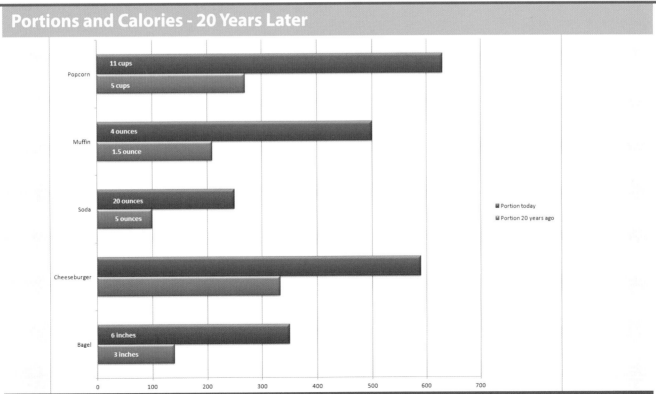

Source: Portion Distortion Quiz, Dept. of Health & Human Services, National Institutes of Health, and National Heart, Lung, and Blood Institute. Available at http://hp2010.nhlbihin.net/portion.

A Place for Healthful Food in Foodservice

After years of courtship, culinary professionals and nutritionists have come together in a way that will benefit both – as well as the people they serve. There is agreement: Healthy foods can taste good, and tasty foods can be healthful. In fact, all types of foodservice operations are incorporating healthful items across their menus. College students demand it and onsite dining facilities, fast casual and quick-service restaurants, chains, and full-service and fine dining restaurants are offering healthier foods. Some establishments that were once concerned only with taste are now mindful of nutrition and health as well and are preparing foods that nourish the body as much as they feed the senses.

Traditional providers of healthful meals – schools, colleges and universities, hospitals, and long-term care (or senior care) facilities – are very aware that healthful meals also must taste good and look good. When a person eats all or most meals in one foodservice venue, consistently healthful food is particularly important. Fine dining establishments often have health-conscious diners, but nutrition is of less concern for the occasional celebratory meal.

Operational Implications

Preparing and serving healthier foods requires some changes in labor and training, equipment, and purchasing. Changing menus seasonally and using local products demands more menu planning time. In some situations – for example, in a hospital – developing specific seasonal menus may be challenging. Featuring "seasonal green vegetables" provides some wiggle room. Healthier menu items may require nutrient data calculation and seeking new ingredients with lower levels of sodium, sugar or fat. Buying local, seasonal products may necessitate a larger vendor list. Creating standardized recipes, and following them exactly, will ensure that customers are served the calories listed on the menu. But flexibility is important, too. If a school lists fresh peaches on the menu for August, but the local crop is late, a menu substitution will be needed.

Preparing healthier foods may also entail equipment changes. For example, baking or roasting rather than deep-frying (think oven-baked sweet potato strips or roasted vegetables) will take more time and certainly requires more oven space. Fresh or frozen vegetables require more refrigeration or freezer space than canned varieties as well as different equipment for pre-prep. Steamers or grills may be needed, and healthier food preparation may mean more a la minute cooking.

Staffing changes also may be necessary. More labor may be needed to pre-prep fruits and vegetables. On the other hand, using items such as pre-shredded carrots and cabbage or diced red peppers or onions that already have the labor cost built in makes it easier to define costs. Kitchen staff may need additional training in using standardized recipes and in measuring procedures, especially if calories and grams of fat are posted for customers.

Even though adding healthier items to the menu may require some operational realignment in the kitchen, the change can be good for business. According to research from the Mintel Group, consumers are demanding greater transparency from restaurants in terms of ingredients, processes and preparation. These expectations have been driven in part by a greater awareness and understanding of healthy eating. Operators have responded with a slew of healthy offerings in terms of ingredients, preparations, portion sizing and menuing to meet varying definitions of "healthy." [16] This change demonstrates an important attitude adjustment among consumers. The notion of food deprivation is giving way to feelings of enjoyment and eating to feel fit and well.

"Shipping is a terrible thing to do to vegetables. They probably get jet-lagged, just like people."

Elizabeth Berry Sebastian
Food writer

Nutrition Isn't an Afterthought

"Nutrition is an important part of what we teach students," notes William Reynolds, retired provost, Chicago's Washburne Culinary Institute. Established in 1937, Washburne is the nations' oldest culinary program. "Nutrition is not what most students are thinking about when registering," Bill continues, "but by graduation, nutrition should be as much a consideration as ingredient quality, preparation method and flavor."

Bill, who is an honorary member of the Academy of Nutrition and Dietetics and an active member of the Academy's Food & Culinary Professionals Dietetic Practice Group, believes that most chefs don't give nutrition the priority it deserves: "We need to get away from 'taking stuff out' after the fact to make a recipe more healthful. Nutrition should be a consideration from the beginning of the process. You don't make the food and then remake it to be more nutritious," he explains. "From the outset, choose key ingredients that are nutrient rich and cooking methods that enhance taste and texture."

The Alliance of Taste and Health Moves Forward

Taste and health, together, can lead to better, healthier foods for all. We continue to move forward, incorporating healthful food choices in all aspects of our lives and culture. The foodservice industry is an important participant in the effort to help America become a healthier nation. Here are some recent changes that have moved us in a positive direction.

- Nutrition education and healthful cooking techniques are included in culinary school curricula.
- Chef certification now requires knowledge of nutrition.
- Chefs, restaurateurs and dietitians collaborate in many work settings.
- Healthful cooking and baking classes are growing in popularity for professional chefs as well as home cooks.
- Food and culinary expertise has grown within the profession of dietetics.
- Food and culinary topics are increasingly popular continuing education topics for maintaining the registered dietitian credential.
- Nutrition advice has become more taste-conscious, moving away from prohibitive, restrictive diets and toward more emphasis on positive food components.
- Improved technology allows more exact nutrient calculation and evaluation of recipes.
- Readership of magazines such as *Eating Well*, *Clean Eating, Better Nutrition, Food and Nutrition* magazine from the Academy of Nutrition and Dietetics, and of books on flavorful, healthful cooking has increased.
- Schools and youth organizations are planting gardens and teaching children to enjoy a wider range of produce.
- Specialty cookbooks focusing on ancient grains, specific vegetables and other healthful ingredients.
- Many excellent cookbooks feature plant-based diets and cuisines that are mainly plant-based.
- Customers in schools, colleges and universities, and other foodservice settings are demanding healthful foods.
- Farmers markets, organic farming, seasonal foods and "eating local" continue to grow in popularity. The Edible Communities', Edible magazine which focus on sustainability and fresh local foods are now in more than 85 markets.
- José Andrés, Ann Cooper, Jamie Oliver, Rachael Ray, Alice Waters, Art Smith and other celebrity chefs have become advocates for healthful foods in schools and communities.
- Media interest in healthy foods and cooking has grown as evidenced by documentaries and books that expose unhealthy food choices and/or food production practices.
- More companies are introducing single-portion packaging and 100-calorie snacks.
- Beverages are available in smaller single-serve containers.
- Many major food companies are voluntarily reducing sodium across their product lines and offering more reduced-sodium ingredients.
- The *Dietary Guidelines for Americans* encourage restaurants and the food industry to offer health-promoting foods that are low in sodium; limited in added sugar, refined grains and solid fat; and served in small portions.
- Flavored and mineral waters are replacing many sweetened drinks as beverages of choice.

What Is a Registered Dietitian Nutritionist?

A *registered dietitian nutritionist (RDN)* is a food and nutrition expert who has met established academic and professional requirements and has passed a comprehensive national examination to qualify for the RDN credential. The academic and professional requirements are set by the Academy of Nutrition and Dietetics (AND) - formerly The American Dietetic Association - and the examination is administered by the Commission on Dietetic Registration. Ongoing continuing education is required for recertification every five years to ensure competency. Some states also offer a licensed dietitian (LD) or licensed dietitian nutritionist (LDN) credential. Registration and licensure ensure maintaining science-based expertise and professional ethics and were created to protect the public from charlatans.

Because anyone can use the unregulated title "nutritionist" (without the registered or licensed designation), many calling themselves nutritionists have minimal true nutrition expertise and are promoting products, services or diets without the benefit of education in foods and nutrition at accredited universities. Some advice (even if well-meaning) can endanger health, some encourage use of unnecessary and/or expensive products or recommend unbalanced diets. Like infomercials and advertising, be cautious of whose information and products you trust.

Partnering with a Registered Dietitian

Many RDN's work in the treatment or prevention of diseases, including medical nutrition therapy, in healthcare facilities. Others work in community settings, public health, private practice counseling, academia and research. A growing number of RDN's work in the food industry, schools and college foodservice, business, sports nutrition, journalism, corporate wellness and other settings.

The culinary professional or chef and the registered dietitian (RD) or nutritionist have an opportunity to work as partners in planning, preparing and serving healthier foods to consumers across the country in a variety of foodservice venues. A culinary registered dietitian can be a valuable resource when a chef has questions about nutrition or needs nutrient calculation for a recipe. A culinary RD also can review menus and help fine-tune menu offerings with an eye toward nutritional health. Some dietitians are trained as chefs and some own restaurants or food businesses, often with a health focus. Chefs can request assistance finding a local RD with the needed expertise from the Academy of Nutrition and Dietetics Food & Culinary Professionals Dietetic Practice Group (FCP) by simply contacting the group's administrator (**www.foodculinaryprofs.org**/) and asking to post a query on the FCP website.

Three chefs have been granted honorary membership by the Academy of Nutrition and Dietetics, thereby recognizing their commitment to healthful cooking. They include celebrity chef Graham Kerr; president emeritus of the Culinary Institute of America, Ferdinand Metz; and retired provost from Chicago's Washburne Culinary Institute, William Reynolds.

Opportunities for Chefs

Nutrition should never be an afterthought for the chef. Rather, it should be an integral part of the menu development process. Food professionals have an opportunity to help change the way consumers eat and to have a positive effect on the overall health of people.

The focus on nutritional health has shifted from restriction to balance – that is, seeking positive nutrients and balancing the number of calories consumed with the number burned. Food can taste good and be healthful – especially when the focus is on what you can eat, not on what you should avoid. Contemporary menus reflecting this shift feature less processed foods and more whole grains, vegetables, fruits, legumes, low-fat dairy products and lean protein foods, healthful cooking techniques and portion control. The chef who can make healthful food with great taste and texture, as well as provide a good dining experience, is positioned well for the changing times.

Learning Activities

1. Select a menu from a foodservice operation that you work in or visit frequently. Identify the nutrient-dense menu items.

2. Based on your age, gender and activity level, identify the calorie level that will maintain your healthy weight.

For More Information

- Academy of Nutrition and Dietetics, **www.eatright.org**
- Duyff RL, Academy of Nutrition and Dietetics Complete Food & Nutrition Guide. Boston: Houghton Mifflin Harcourt; 2017.
- Food & Culinary Professionals, a dietetic practice group of the Academy of Nutrition and Dietetics, **www.foodculinaryprofs.org**
- *Gastronomica: The Journal of Food and Culture*, **www.gastronomica.org**
- Hess MA. *Resetting the American Table.* J Am Diet Assoc. 1991;91(2):228-30.
- International Food Information Council, **www.ific.org**
- National Restaurant Association, **www.restaurant.org**
- Pollan M, *In Defense of Food: An Eater's Manifesto*. New York: Penguin Books; 2008.
- U.S. Department of Agriculture Food Composition Tables, **www.nal.usda.gov/fnic/foodcomp/search**

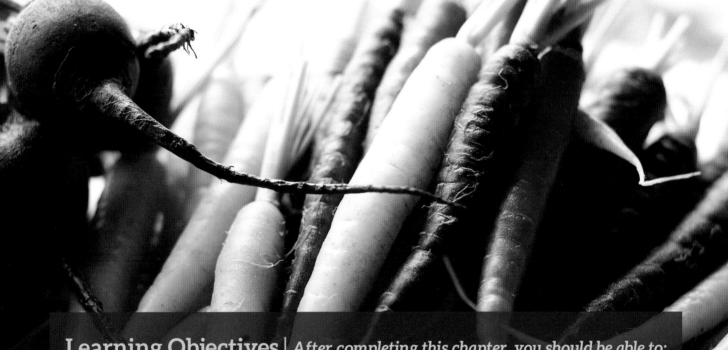

Chapter Two

Nutrition Standards and Tools

Learning Objectives | *After completing this chapter, you should be able to:*

- Explain the function of the recommended Dietary Reference Intakes
- Describe and discuss the *Dietary Guidelines for Americans* and identify challenges for chefs
- List the food groups found in *MyPlate* and recommended servings from each group
- Explain how *MyPlate* encourages variety, proportionality and moderation
- Read and analyze food labels, nutrient claims and health claims
- Discuss the attributes and limitations of various food rating systems

This chapter explores the various U.S. government standards and tools developed for the greater good – that is, to promote the health of Americans as a population. Keep in mind that each person has unique nutrition needs based on history, environment, personal taste, ethnicity and cultural values and beliefs. This chapter also looks at various tools and food label terminology that help chefs and consumers make informed food choices.

Some nutrition standards refer to adequacy and recommend levels of intake based on research; some identify actions that promote moderation; others describe components of a healthful diet. All of the commonly used standards and tools are based on four cornerstones:

- **Adequacy** means providing or eating foods that supply all of the essential nutrients needed for life and health. For those with severe dietary restrictions or intolerances, dietary supplements can fill nutrient gaps.

- **Balance** means that the whole diet should provide enough, but not too much, of each of the essential nutrients. Balance also means including foods from all of the food groups, which requires considerable planning.

- **Moderation** means serving and eating adequate, appropriate portions. In light of today's tendency toward over-consumption, moderation is critical to a healthy diet and menu planning. It often requires recalibrating the menu to reduce portions of meat and high-fat, high-sugar, highly salted foods while still meeting the consumer's desire for value.

- **Variety** means serving different foods within each food group to increase the likelihood of a nutritionally adequate diet. Different food groups provide different essential nutrients as do a range of foods within each group. Variety also refers to incorporating different cooking methods, flavors, colors and temperatures to create attractive and enjoyable meals.

Dietary Reference Intakes

The **Dietary Reference Intakes** (DRIs), developed by the Food and Nutrition Board of the Institute of Medicine, National Academy of Sciences, are based on medical research and food intake surveys. DRIs refer to minimum recommended and maximum safe levels of many nutrients by age and gender. DRIs aim to prevent chronic diseases and promote optimal health. They are used primarily by dietitians and other health professionals to assess and plan diets for healthy individuals and groups. Each DRI category (minimum, recommended and maximum) refers to average daily intake over time – at least one week for most nutrients. The concept of "nutrient intake adequacy over time" means that a specific level does not have to be met each and every day.

Programs such as school nutrition must meet a certain percentage of the DRIs at each meal. Correctional and long-term care facilities, however, must develop menus that meet the total nutrient needs of residents. Most chefs do not need to be particularly concerned about DRI levels other than to know their intended use. Generally, planning menus using the *Dietary Guidelines for Americans* and *MyPlate* will meet DRI requirements. (See Appendix B for a DRI chart.)

Daily Values

Daily Values (DVs), which are used on all food and supplement labels, are derived from recommended levels of nutrients in the DRIs based on a 2,000-calorie diet. The DV amounts for total fat, saturated fat, cholesterol and sodium are maximum amounts per day. The DVs for total carbohydrate and dietary fiber are minimum amounts per day. (See Appendix C.) A food that has 20% of a DV is an excellent source of that stated nutrient; a food that has 10% to 19% of a DV is a good source of that nutrient; while a food that has 0% to 5% DV of a nutrient is a poor source of that nutrient.

Interactive DRI for Healthcare Professionals

A web-based tool and mobile app can be used to calculate daily nutrient recommendations for dietary planning based on the Dietary Reference Intakes (DRIs). This tool can be found at **http://fnic.nal.usda.gov/fnic/interactiveDRI/**. It can also be downloaded from the Apple iTunes App Store or from the Google Play Store.

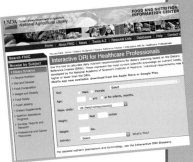

Dietary Guidelines for Americans 2015-2020

The **Dietary Guidelines for Americans** (www.dietary-guidelines.gov), which are targeted to those over 2 years of age living in the United States, identify actions that will help the public meet the Dietary Reference Intakes. They provide science-based advice to promote health and reduce risk for chronic disease through diet and physical activity. The U.S. Departments of Agriculture (USDA) and Health and Human Services (HHS) have published revised guidelines every five years since 1980. Because of their focus on health promotion and risk reduction, the *Dietary Guidelines* form the basis of federal food, nutrition education and information programs. They also set some nutrition standards used by the food industry such as specifications for foods served in federally funded feeding programs. Although many of the recommendations have remained relatively consistent over time, the *Dietary Guidelines* have evolved with scientific knowledge. For example, recent research has examined the relationship between overall eating patterns and health. Consequently, eating patterns (rather than specific nutrient levels) are a main focus of the *2015-2020 Dietary Guidelines*.

The current edition of the *Guidelines* includes recommendations for the general population as well as specific recommendations for certain populations such as racial/ethnic groups, vegetarians and others with special dietary needs. The *Dietary Guidelines* also recognize that in recent years nearly 49 million Americans face food insecurity and have been unable to obtain enough food to meet their needs. The guidelines can help these people maximize the nutritional content of their meals even with limited resources.

The *Dietary Guidelines* are developed from the Report of the *Dietary Guidelines Advisory Committee* (www.health.gov/dietaryguidelines/2015-scientific-report/), a document based on a review of the scientific literature and evidence-based research. This publication also acknowledges that the majority of Americans, although overweight or obese, are also undernourished in several key nutrients.

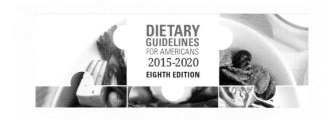

The *Dietary Guidelines for Americans 2015-2020* provide five overarching guidelines:

The Guidelines

1. **Follow a healthy eating pattern across the lifespan**. All food and beverage choices matter. Choose a healthy eating pattern at an appropriate calorie level to help achieve and maintain a healthy body weight, support nutrient adequacy, and reduce the risk of chronic disease.

2. **Focus on variety, nutrient density and amount**. To meet nutrient needs within calorie limits, choose a variety of nutrient-dense foods across and within all food groups in recommended amounts.

3. **Limit calories from added sugars and saturated fats and reduce sodium intake**. Consume an eating pattern low in added sugars, saturated fats and sodium. Cut back on foods and beverages higher in these components to amounts that fit within healthy eating patterns.

4. **Shift to healthier food and beverage choices**. Choose nutrient-dense foods and beverages across and within all food groups in place of less healthy choices. Consider cultural and personal preferences to make these shifts easier to accomplish and maintain.

5. **Support healthy eating patterns for all**. Everyone has a role in helping to create and support healthy eating patterns in multiple settings nationwide, from home to school to work to communities.

Key Recommendations

The *Dietary Guidelines'* Key Recommendations for healthy eating patterns should be applied in their entirety, given the interconnected relationship that each dietary component can have with others.

The goal is to consume a healthy eating pattern that accounts for all foods and beverages within an appropriate calorie level.

A healthy eating pattern includes:

- A variety of vegetables from all of the subgroups — dark green, red and orange, legumes (beans and peas), starchy and other
- Fruits, especially whole fruits
- Grains, at least half of which are whole grains
- Fat-free or low-fat dairy, including milk, yogurt, cheese and/or fortified soy beverages
- A variety of protein foods, including seafood, lean meats and poultry, eggs, legumes (beans and peas), and nuts, seeds and soy products
- Oils

A healthy eating pattern limits:

- Saturated fats and trans fats, added sugars and sodium

Key recommendations that are quantitative (expressed as numbers or percentages) are provided for several components of the diet that should be limited. These components are of particular public health concern in the United States, and the specified limits can help individuals achieve healthy eating patterns within calorie limits:

- Consume less than 10 percent of calories per day from added sugars.
- Consume less than 10 percent of calories per day from saturated fats.
- Consume less than 2,300 milligrams (mg) per day of sodium.
- If alcohol is consumed, it should be consumed in moderation—up to one drink per day for women and up to two drinks per day for men—and only by adults of legal drinking age.

In tandem with the recommendations above, Americans of all ages—children, adolescents, adult, and older adults—should meet the *Physical Activity Guidelines for Americans* to help promote health and reduce the risk of chronic disease. Americans should

aim to achieve and maintain a healthy body weight. Diet and physical activity together contribute to managing body weight.

Key Elements of Healthy Eating Patterns

A premise of the *Dietary Guidelines* is that nutritional needs should be met primarily from foods. All forms of foods – fresh, canned, dried and frozen – can be included in healthy eating patterns. Importantly, foods should be in the most nutrient-dense form possible. These foods contain essential vitamins and minerals, dietary fiber, and other naturally occurring substances that generally have positive health effects. Nutrient-dense foods include all vegetables, fruits, whole grains, seafood, eggs, beans and peas, nuts and seeds, fat-free and low-fat dairy products and lean meats and poultry, when purchased, prepared, served and eaten with little to no added saturated fats, sugars, refined starches and salt.

Shifts Needed to Align with Healthy Eating Patterns

Unfortunately the typical eating patterns currently followed by most individuals do not align with the *Dietary Guidelines* recommendations.

- About three-fourths of the population has an eating pattern that is low in fruit, vegetables and dairy.
- More than half of the population is meeting or exceeding total grain and total protein foods intake, but would benefit from increasing the variety of foods consumed within these food groups, to improve nutrient intake and adequacy.
- Most Americans exceed the recommendations for added sugars, saturated fats and sodium.
- Most Americans are consuming too many calories.

To stay within calorie needs while consuming a nutritionally adequate diet, most individuals would benefit from selecting healthier options, both across and within each food group, to choices that are more nutrient dense. In many food groups, foods as they are typically eaten are not nutrient dense— they often contain additional calories from added sugars and/or saturated fats, and many are also high in sodium. In simpler words, serve fewer refined grains such as white bread and pasta and fewer high-fat meat and dairy products. Prepare all foods with less added fats, sugar and salt. Limit frequency and portion size of fried foods.

casebycase | SPE Certification: Health Through Food

The New York-based nutrition consultancy SPE Certified (http://specertified.com/) works to enhance the nutritional quality of meals without compromising taste. SPE stands for Sanitas Per Escam – Latin for Health Through Food. The company's registered dietitian nutritionists follow SPE's 90-page charter, which documents culinary, nutrition and sustainability best practices.

The brainchild of Belgian entrépreneur Emmanuel Verstraeten, SPE combines cutting-edge research with international health standards with guidance from a committee of world-renowned nutrition scientists and experts. SPE guidelines focus on three key elements:

- **Sourcing**: selecting ingredients seasonally, locally, and with a focus on nutritional characteristics
- **Preparation**: using specific cooking techniques that preserve the integrity and nutritional qualities of the ingredient
- **Enhancement**: optimizing nutritional value by the synergy of product combination and menu diversity

The SPE philosophy originated in 2001 at Verstraeten's Rouge Tomate restaurant in Brussels. In 2008, the model debuted in the United States at the Michelin-starred Rouge Tomate in New York City, first located on the Upper East Side and followed by a more casual concept in Chelsea.

SPE menus emphasize food synergies in which ingredients eaten in certain combinations are more nutritionally powerful than when eaten separately. Early SPE always featured whole grains, fatty fish, cruciferous vegetables and legumes, as well as animal proteins including pastured poultry, sustainably-sourced seafood, grass-fed beef and lean game meats. No butter or cream was used in entrées and appetizers and was used only in limited amounts in desserts.

Today, SPE Certified continues to carry out its mission to improve the health and well-being of all people through food across all levels of food service. Culinary Nutritionist Kristy Del Coro, MS, RDN, CDN, explains the process at a recipe-level. "For us, it's not about what you can't use; it's thinking about what you can use - about balance, portions and preparation. We look at produce for our inspiration, and then we consider what else to put on the plate to boost nutrient density and maximize flavor."

For operations wanting to understand how they measure up against best-practices and dietary guidelines and standards, SPE Certified offers a comprehensive nutrition and sustainability evaluation and one-to-three-star certification program.

MyPlate

Over the years there have been many guides to healthful eating. Since 1943, government guidance for healthful eating has evolved from the Basic 7, to the Basic 4, to the Food Guide Pyramid, to *MyPyramid* and now to **MyPlate**, which uses a familiar image – a place setting for a meal – to illustrate the five food groups that are the building blocks for a healthy diet.

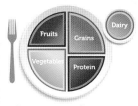

Choose**MyPlate**.gov

MyPlate Emphasizes Building a Healthy Eating Style

All food and beverage choices matter – focus on variety, amount and nutrition.

- Focus on making healthful food and beverage choices from all five food groups to get the nutrients you need.

- Eat the right amount of calories for you based on your age, sex, height, weight and physical activity level.
- Building a healthier eating style can help you avoid overweight and obesity and reduce your risk of diseases such as heart disease, diabetes and cancer.

Choose an eating style low in saturated fat, sodium and added sugars.

Make small changes to create a healthier eating style.

- Make half your plate fruits and vegetables. Focus on whole fruits rather than juices. Vary your veggies.
- Make half your grains whole grains.
- Move to low-fat and fat-free dairy.
- Vary your protein routine.
- Eat and drink the right amount for you.

MyPlate Portions

Fruits

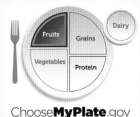

ChooseMyPlate.gov

What Is in the Fruits Group?

Any fruit or 100% fruit juice counts as part of the Fruits Group. Fruits may be fresh, canned, frozen or dried and may be whole, cut-up or pureed.

How Much Is Needed?

The amount of fruit needed depends on age, sex and level of physical activity. Amounts range from 1 to 2 cups.

What Counts as a Cup?

In general, 1 cup of fruit or 100% fruit juice, or ½ cup of dried fruit can be considered 1 cup from the Fruits Group. One small apple, orange, pear or banana also equals 1 cup.

Nutrients and Health Benefits of Fruit

- Most fruits are naturally low in fat, sodium and calories. None contains cholesterol.

- Fruits contain essential nutrients that are lacking in the diets of many Americans, including potassium, dietary fiber, vitamin C and folate (folic acid).

- Diets rich in potassium may help maintain healthy blood pressure levels. Fruit sources of potassium include bananas, prunes and prune juice, dried peaches and apricots, cantaloupe, honeydew melon and orange juice.

- Dietary fiber from fruits, as part of an overall healthy diet, helps reduce blood cholesterol levels and may lower risk of heart disease. Fiber is important for proper bowel function. It helps reduce constipation and diverticulosis. Fiber-containing foods help provide a feeling of fullness with fewer calories. Whole or cut-up fruits are sources of dietary fiber; fruit juices contain little or no fiber.

- Vitamin C is important for growth and repair of all body tissues, helps heal cuts and wounds and keeps teeth and gums healthy. Citrus fruits and strawberries are particularly rich in this vitamin.

- Folate (folic acid) helps the body form red blood cells. Women of childbearing age who may become pregnant should consume adequate folate from foods and in addition take folate supplements (often in the form of a prenatal vitamin) to reduce the risk of many types of birth defects in fetal development.

Grains

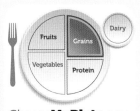

ChooseMyPlate.gov

What Is in the Grains Group?

Any food made from wheat, rice, oats, cornmeal, barley or other cereal grain is a grain product. Bread, pasta, oatmeal, breakfast cereals, tortillas and grits are examples of grain products.

Grains are divided into two subgroups: whole grains and refined grains.

Whole grains contain the entire grain kernel — the bran, germ and endosperm.

Examples include:

Brown rice, wild rice	Oatmeal
Whole cornmeal	Whole-wheat flour
Bulgur (cracked wheat)	Whole-grain breakfast cereal

Refined grains have been milled, a process that removes the bran and germ to give grains a finer texture and improve shelf life. Refining also removes dietary fiber, iron and many B vitamins. Many refined grains are enriched, meaning certain B vitamins (thiamin, riboflavin, niacin and folic acid) and iron are added after processing. Fiber is not added back to enriched grains. Check the ingredient list on refined-grain products to make sure that the word "enriched" is included in the grain name. Some food products are made from mixtures of whole grains and refined grains.

Examples of refined-grain products include:

Cornflakes (and other breakfast cereals made from refined grains)

De-germed cornmeal

White breads and crackers

Most pasta

White flour

White rice

Couscous

How Much Is Needed?

The amount of grain needed depends on age, sex and level of physical activity. Amounts range from 3 to 8 ounce equivalents. Most Americans consume plenty of grains, but not enough whole grains. At least half of all the grains eaten should be whole grains.

What Counts as a 1 Ounce Equivalent?

In general, 1 slice of bread, ½ of a small sandwich bun, bagel or English muffin, 1 cup of ready-to-eat cereal, or ½ cup of cooked rice, cooked pasta, or cooked cereal or grain, or 1 small slice of pizza (crust is bread equivalent) can be considered a 1 ounce equivalent from the Grains Group. Many sandwich buns, rolls and pizza slices are quite large and count as 3 or 4 ounce equivalents. Bread loaves have slices of different sizes, with some being 1 ounce and others are 2 ounces.

Health Benefits of Whole Grains

- Consuming whole grains as part of a healthy diet may reduce the risk of heart disease.
- Consuming foods containing fiber, such as whole grains, as part of a healthy diet, can reduce constipation.
- Eating whole grains may help with weight management.

- Eating grain products fortified with folate before and during pregnancy helps prevent neural tube defects during fetal development.

Nutrients and Health Benefits of Whole Grains

Grains are important sources of many nutrients, including dietary fiber, several B vitamins (thiamin, riboflavin, niacin and folate) and minerals (iron, magnesium and selenium).

Dietary fiber from whole grains or other foods may help reduce blood cholesterol levels and may lower risk of heart disease, obesity and type 2 diabetes. Fiber is important for proper bowel function; it helps reduce constipation and diverticulosis. Fiber-containing foods such as whole grains help provide a feeling of fullness with fewer calories.

The B vitamins (thiamin, riboflavin and niacin) play a key role in metabolism, helping the body release energy from protein, fat and carbohydrates. B vitamins are also essential for a healthy nervous system. Many refined grains are enriched with B vitamins.

Folate (folic acid) helps the body form red blood cells. Women of childbearing age who may become pregnant should consume adequate folate from foods and in addition take folate supplements (often in the form of a prenatal vitamin) to reduce the risk of neural tube defects, spina bifida and anencephaly during fetal development.

Iron is used to carry oxygen in the blood. Many teenage girls and women in their childbearing years have iron-deficiency anemia and should eat more foods high in heme-iron (meats) or other iron-containing foods along with foods rich in vitamin C, which can improve absorption of non-heme iron. Whole and enriched refined-grain products are major sources of non-heme iron in American diets. Since many fruits and vegetables contain Vitamin C, simply adding tomatoes to sandwiches or serving citrus fruits or melon with a sandwich improves the absorption of iron from the bread.

Whole grains contain magnesium and selenium. Magnesium is a mineral used in building bones and releasing energy from muscles. Selenium protects cells from oxidation and is important for a healthy immune system that resists infections.

Vegetables

What Is in the Vegetables Group?

Any vegetable or 100% vegetable juice counts as a part of the Vegetables Group. Vegetables may be raw or cooked; fresh, frozen, canned or dried/dehydrated; and whole, cut-up or mashed.

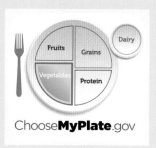

ChooseMyPlate.gov

Vegetables fall into five subgroups based on their nutrient content: dark green vegetables, orange vegetables, beans and peas, starchy vegetables and other vegetables.

Dark Green Vegetables

Arugula

Bok choy (and other Asian deep green leafy vegetables)

Beet greens

Broccoli and broccoli rabe

Collard greens

Dark green leafy lettuces

Kale

Mesclun

Mustard greens

Romaine lettuce

Spinach

Swiss chard

Turnip greens

Watercress

Orange Vegetables

Acorn squash

Butternut squash

Carrots

Hubbard squash

Pumpkin

Red and orange peppers

Sweet potatoes

Tomatoes

Tomato juice

Beans and Peas

Black beans

Black-eyed peas

Garbanzo beans (chickpeas)

Kidney beans

Lentils

Lima beans (dried or white)

Navy beans

Pinto beans

Soybeans

Split peas

White beans, cannellini beans

Starchy Vegetables

Cassava

Corn

Green bananas, plantains

Green peas

Lima beans (green)

Potatoes

Taro

Water chestnuts

Other Vegetables

Artichokes

Asparagus

Avocado

Bean sprouts

Beets

Brussels sprouts

Cabbage

Cauliflower

Celery

Cucumbers

Eggplant

Green beans

Green peppers

Iceberg (head) lettuce

Leeks

Mushrooms

Okra

Onions

Parsnips

Peapods

Rutabagas

Sugar snap peas

Summer squash

Turnips

Wax beans

Zucchini

How Much Is Needed?

The amount of vegetables needed depends on age, sex and level of physical activity. Amounts range from 1 to 3 cups daily. Most adults should have 3 cups of vegetables every day. While potatoes count as a starchy vegetable and have some nutrients, deep green and orange vegetables have far more nutrients and fewer calories, especially when compared to potatoes that are fried or made with a lot of butter or cream.

What Counts as a Cup?

In general, 1 cup of raw or cooked vegetables or vegetable juice, or 2 cups of raw leafy greens can be considered 1 cup from the Vegetable Group.

Nutrients and Health Benefits of Vegetables

Most vegetables are naturally low in fat and calories. None contains cholesterol. (Sauces, butter or oils used in cooking, however, add fat, calories and/or cholesterol.)

Vegetables are important sources of many nutrients, particularly potassium, dietary fiber, folate (folic acid), vitamin A and vitamin C.

Diets rich in potassium may help to maintain healthy blood pressure and reduce risk of developing kidney stones. Vegetable sources of potassium include sweet potatoes, white potatoes, white beans, tomato products (paste, sauce and juice), beet greens, soybeans, lima beans, spinach, lentils and kidney beans.

Dietary fiber from vegetables helps reduce blood cholesterol levels and may lower risk of heart disease and type 2 diabetes. Fiber is important for proper bowel function. It helps reduce constipation and diverticulosis. Fiber-containing foods such as vegetables help provide a feeling of fullness with fewer calories.

Eating a diet rich in vegetables as part of an overall healthy diet may reduce risk for heart disease, including heart attack and stroke and may protect against colon and other types of cancers.

Folate (folic acid) helps the body form red blood cells. Women of childbearing age who may become pregnant should consume adequate folate to reduce the risk of birth defects. Leafy greens are the richest source of folate.

Vitamin A keeps eyes and skin healthy and helps to protect against infections.

Vitamin C is important for growth and repair of all body tissues, helps heal cuts and wounds, and keeps teeth and gums healthy. Broccoli, cauliflower, greens, red peppers and cabbage are excellent sources of this vitamin.

More about Beans and Peas

Beans and peas are the mature forms of **legumes**. They include kidney beans, pinto beans, black beans, lima beans, black-eyed peas, garbanzo beans (chick-peas), split peas and lentils. Available in dry, canned, refrigerated and frozen forms, beans and peas are excellent sources of plant protein and provide other nutrients such as iron and zinc. Because they are similar to meats, poultry and fish in their nutrient composition, legumes are considered part of the Protein Foods Group. Many people use beans and peas as vegetarian alternatives to meat, poultry or seafood. They are also considered part of the Vegetable Group because they are excellent sources of dietary fiber and nutrients such as folate and potassium, which are often low in the diets of many Americans. With many people being vegetarians and vegans, offering a variety of menu items with peas and beans, prepared with no animal products, increases menu appeal.

Despite their names, green peas, green lima beans, wax beans, sugar snap peas, peapods and green (string) beans are not considered part of the beans and peas subgroup, as they do not have much protein. Green peas and green lima beans are grouped with other starchy vegetables. Green beans, wax beans and peapods are grouped with other vegetables such as onions, lettuce, celery and cabbage.

Protein Foods

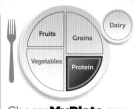

What Is in the Protein Foods Group?

All foods that come from meat, poultry, seafood, beans and peas, eggs, processed soy products, and nuts and seeds are considered part of the Protein Foods Group. Beans and peas are also part of the Vegetables Group. Select a variety of protein foods to improve nutrient intake and health benefits, including at least 8 ounces of cooked seafood per week. Young children need less, depending on their age and calorie needs. The advice to consume seafood does not apply to vegetarians. Vegetarian options in the Protein Foods Group include beans and peas, processed soy products, and nuts and seeds. Most meat and poultry choices should be lean or low-fat. Some commonly eaten choices in the meat and beans group are:

Meats
Lean Cuts
- Beef
- Ham
- Lamb
- Pork
- Veal

Lean Luncheon/Deli Meats
- Beef
- Chicken
- Ham
- Pork
- Turkey

Game Meats
- Bison
- Buffalo
- Rabbit
- Venison

Organ Meats
- Giblets
- Liver

Poultry
- Chicken
- Duck
- Goose
- Turkey

Beans and Peas
- Bean burgers
- Black beans
- Black-eyed peas
- Chickpeas (garbanzo beans)
- Edamame (young soybeans)
- Falafel (spiced, mashed chickpeas)
- Fava beans (broad beans)
- Hummus (chickpea spread)
- Kidney beans
- Lentils
- Lima beans (mature)
- Navy beans
- Pinto beans
- Soybeans
- Split peas
- White beans

Soy Products
- Tempeh
- Texturized vegetable protein (TVP)
- Tofu (made from soybeans)
- Veggie burgers
- Soy meat replacements

Eggs
- Chicken eggs
- Duck eggs

Nuts and Seeds
- Almonds and almond butter
- Cashews
- Chia seeds
- Hazelnuts (filberts)
- Mixed nuts
- Peanuts and peanut butter
- Pecans
- Pistachios
- Pumpkin seeds
- Sesame seeds and tahini
- Sunflower seeds
- Walnuts

Seafood

Finfish	**Shellfish**
Catfish	Clams
Cod	Crab
Flounder	Crayfish
Grouper	Lobster
Haddock	Mussels
Halibut	Octopus
Herring	Oysters
Mackerel	Scallops
Pollock	Shrimp
Porgy	Squid (calamari)
Rockfish	
Salmon	**Canned Fish**
Sea bass	Anchovies
Snapper	Clams
Sole	Mackerel
Sushi	Salmon
Swordfish	Sardines
Tilapia	Tuna
Trout	
Tuna	

How Much Is Needed?

The amount of food from the Protein Foods Group needed depends on age, sex and level of physical activity. Most Americans eat more than enough food from this group but need to make leaner and more varied selections. Needs range from 5 to 7 ounce equivalents per day for those over 8 years of age.

What Counts as a 1 Ounce Equivalent?

In general, 1 ounce of cooked meat, poultry or fish, ¼ cup cooked beans, 1 egg, 1 tablespoon of peanut butter, or ½ ounce of nuts or seeds can be considered a 1 ounce equivalent from the Protein Foods Group.

Nutrients and Health Benefits of Protein Foods

Meat, poultry, fish, beans and peas, eggs, and nuts and seeds supply protein, B vitamins (niacin, thiamin, riboflavin, and B6), vitamin E, iron, zinc and magnesium.

Proteins function as building blocks for bones, muscles, cartilage, skin, blood, enzymes, hormones and vitamins. Proteins are one of three nutrients that provide calories (the others are fat and carbohydrates).

B vitamins help the body release energy, play a vital role in the function of the nervous system, aid in the formation of red blood cells and help build tissues.

Iron is used to carry oxygen in the blood. Teenage girls and women in their childbearing years who have iron-deficiency anemia should eat foods high in heme-iron (meats) or eat other iron-containing foods along with a food rich in vitamin C, which can improve absorption of non-heme iron. Iron from red meats is particularly well absorbed and useful in maintaining adequate iron levels.

Magnesium helps build bones and release energy from muscles.

Zinc is necessary for biochemical reactions and helps the immune system function properly resist infection.

Docosahexaenoic acid (DHA) and eicosapentaenoic acid (EPA) are omega-3 fatty acids found in seafood. Eating 8 ounces per week of seafood may help reduce the risk for heart disease. Eating seafood each week is recommended for heart-healthy eating.

Diets that are high in saturated fats are thought to raise "bad" cholesterol – LDL (low-density lipoprotein) – levels in the blood, which increases the risk for coronary heart disease. Some food choices in this group are high in saturated fat, including fatty cuts of beef, pork and lamb; regular (75% to 85% lean) ground beef; regular sausages, hot dogs and bacon; some luncheon meats, such as regular bologna and salami; and some poultry, such as duck served with skin.

Including large portions of high-fat meats makes it difficult to avoid eating more calories than are needed and provides too much saturated fat..

Benefits of Eating 8 Ounces of Seafood per Week

Seafood contains a range of nutrients beyond protein, including the omega-3 fatty acids EPA and DHA. Eating about 8 ounces per week from a variety of seafood contributes to the prevention of heart disease. Smaller amounts of seafood are recommended for young children. Tuna canned in oil and then drained provides more of the desirable fatty acids than water-packed albacore tuna.

The health benefits of seafood outweigh the health risk associated with consuming small amounts of mercury, a heavy metal found in varying levels in some seafood such as swordfish and other higher-fat fish and albacore tuna.

The seafood varieties commonly consumed in the United States that are higher in EPA and DHA and low in mercury include salmon, anchovies, herring, sardines, Pacific oysters, trout, and Atlantic and Pacific mackerel (but not king mackerel, which is high in mercury).

Shrimp, tuna and salmon are among the most popular seafood choices of both adults and children in America.

Benefits of Eating Nuts and Seeds

Eating peanuts and certain tree nuts (such as walnuts, almonds and pistachios) may reduce the risk of heart disease as part of a diet that is nutritionally adequate and within calorie needs. Peanut and other nut butters should be "natural" or made without hydrogenation. Nuts and seeds are high in calories and should be consumed in small portions. They can replace other protein foods in the diet, such as meat or poultry. Unsalted nuts and seeds help reduce sodium intake. Adding some nuts to a salad, dessert or vegetarian main dish adds flavor, texture and protein.

Dairy

What Is in the Dairy Group?

All fluid milk products and many foods made from milk are considered part of this food group. Most Dairy Group choices should be fat-free or low-fat. Foods made from milk products that retain their calcium content are part of this group; foods made from milk that have little to no calcium, such as cream cheese, cream and butter, are not. Calcium-fortified soymilk (soy beverage) is part of the Dairy Group, which also includes:

All fluid milk

    Fat-free (skim)

    Low-fat (1%)

    Reduced-fat (2%)

    Whole milk

    Buttermilk

Flavored milks

    Chocolate

    Strawberry

Kefir

Lactose-reduced or lactose-free milks

Milk-based desserts

    Puddings made with milk

    Ice milk

    Frozen yogurt

    Ice cream

Hard natural cheese, such as:

    Cheddar

    Mozzarella

    Swiss

    Parmesan

Soft cheeses, such as:

    Ricotta

    Cottage cheese

All yogurts

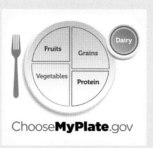

ChooseMyPlate.gov

How Much Is Needed?

The amount of food needed from the Dairy Group depends on age. Amounts range from 2 to 3 cups of liquid milk or the equivalent each day.

What Counts as a Cup?

In general, 1 cup of milk, yogurt or soymilk (soy beverage), 1-½ ounces of natural cheese, 2 ounces of processed cheese, ½ cup ricotta cheese, 2 cups cottage cheese, 1 cup pudding made from milk or 1 cup frozen yogurt can be considered 1 cup from the Dairy Group.

Nutrients and Health Benefits of Dairy Foods

Dairy products are linked to improved bone health and may reduce the risk of osteoporosis.

Dairy products are important to bone health throughout life but especially during childhood and adolescence, when bone mass is being built. It is also important to protect the bones of pregnant women and the development of healthy babies.

Dairy products are associated with a reduced risk of cardiovascular disease and type 2 diabetes and with lower blood pressure in adults.

Calcium is used for building bones and teeth and maintaining bone mass. Dairy products are the primary source of calcium in American diets. Diets that provide 3 cups or the equivalent of dairy products per day may improve bone mass.

Fermented dairy products, with live active cultures, are probiotic. These help the body resist infections and improve digestion along with other positive health effects.

Diets rich in potassium help to maintain healthy blood pressure. Dairy products, especially yogurt, fluid milk and soymilk (soy beverage), provide potassium. Greek yogurt has some liquid removed and is a more concentrated source of protein and calcium than milk or regular yogurt. Using Greek yogurt is as an ingredient boosts nutrient values and is a good substitute for cream or sour cream in some recipes.

Vitamin D helps the body maintain proper levels of calcium and phosphorous needed to build and maintain bones. Milk and soymilk (soy beverage) that are fortified with vitamin D are good sources of this nutrient. Other sources include vitamin D-fortified yogurt and vitamin D-fortified ready-to-eat breakfast cereals.

Hard cheeses, like Parmesan and Cheddar, are concentrated sources of protein, calcium and other nutrients. Small amounts used in cooking or atop salads can boost dairy intake for those who do not drink milk regularly.

Many cheeses, whole milk and products made from them are high in total fat and saturated fat. Diets high in saturated fat raise LDL (low-density lipoprotein) or "bad" cholesterol levels in the blood. High LDL cholesterol increases the risk for coronary heart disease. Read labels and choose lower-fat cheeses and other dairy products most of the time.

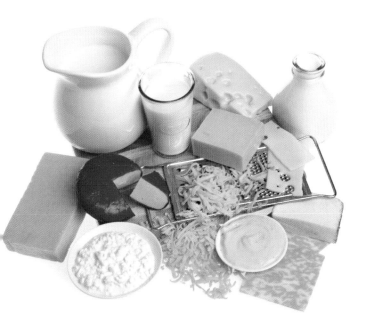

Oils

Although oils are not a food group, they do provide essential nutrients and thus are included in USDA's food patterns. Oils are fats that are liquid at room temperature – for example, the vegetable oils used in cooking. Oils come from many different plants and also from fish. Some commonly eaten oils include:

Canola oil

Corn oil

Cottonseed oil

Olive oil

Safflower oil

Soybean oil

Sunflower oil

Some oils are used mainly as flavorings, such as walnut oil and sesame oil. Foods naturally high in oils include:

Nuts

Olives

Some fish

Avocados

A person's allowance for oils depends on age, sex and level of physical activity. Amounts range from 3 to 7 teaspoons per day; most Americans eat far more than that. This total includes all oils used in cooking, in salad dressings and in prepared foods.

Chefs will surely notice that certain foods such as cream, butter, bacon, processed meats, charcuterie, sugar, sweetened beverages, most baked desserts, jams, and other foods and ingredients are not found on *MyPlate*. The *Dietary Guidelines for Americans* recommend limiting these foods and substituting more healthful options. The authors of this book take a more liberal approach and recommend using high-fat, high-saturated fat and high-sugar foods ingredients sparingly and only as necessary to make delicious food. Serve small to moderate portions of foods containing such ingredients and enjoy them. For most chefs this means fewer fried foods, smaller portions of desserts, meat and rich sauces. Offset these changes with more colorful vegetables, fruits and whole grains and use smaller plates to enhance visual presentations. Strive for better rather than more!

Daily Amounts of Food from Each Group in *MyPlate*

These amounts are appropriate for individuals who get less than 30 minutes per day of moderate physical activity, beyond normal daily activities. Those who are more physically active may be able to consume more while staying within calorie needs.

	Age	Fruit	Vegetable	Grains	Protein Food	Dairy	Oils Allowance
Children	2-3 years	1 cup	1 cup	3 ounce equivalents	2 ounce equivalents	2 cups	3 teaspoons
	4-8 years	1-1 ½ cups	1½ cups	5 ounce equivalents	4 ounce equivalents	2 ½ cups	4 teaspoons
Girls	9-13 years	1 ½ cups	2 cups	5 ounce equivalents	5 ounce equivalents	3 cups	5 teaspoons
	14-18 years	1 ½ cups	2½ cups	6 ounce equivalents	5 ounce equivalents	3 cups	5 teaspoons
Boys	9-13 years	1 ½ cups	2½ cups	6 ounce equivalents	5 ounce equivalents	3 cups	5 teaspoons
	14-18 years	2 cups	3 cups	8 ounce equivalents	6 ½ ounce equivalents	3 cups	6 teaspoons
Women	19-30 years	2 cups	2½ cups	6 ounce equivalents	5 ½ ounce equivalents	3 cups	6 teaspoons
	31-50 years	1 ½ cups	2½ cups	6 ounce equivalents	5 ounce equivalents	3 cups	5 teaspoons
	51+ years	1 ½ cups	2 cups	5 ounce equivalents	5 ounce equivalents	3 cups	5 teaspoons
Men	19-30 years	2 cups	3 cups	8 ounce equivalents	6 ½ ounce equivalents	3 cups	7 teaspoons
	31-50 years	2 cups	3 cups	7 ounce equivalents	6 ounce equivalents	3 cups	6 teaspoons
	51+ years	2 cups	2½ cups	6 ounce equivalents	5 ½ ounce equivalents	3 cups	6 teaspoons

Healthy Eating Plate (an alternative view)

Nutrition experts at Harvard School of Public Health (HSPH) have developed the Healthy Eating Plate, a visual guide similar to *MyPlate*. Healthy Eating Plate addresses concerns HSPH has with *MyPlate*. Although at first glance, the plate illustration looks like *MyPlate*, it: promotes half the plate containing vegetables and fruits; the specific inclusion of whole grains; it stresses heart-healthy oils and specific protein sources; significantly limits potatoes, fruit juices, red meat, refined grains, butter, milk and dairy products; and advises avoidance of processed meats, trans fats, and sugary drinks. The intent of both plates is similar but the HSPH plate is a more aggressive plan for disease prevention with more dietary restrictions.

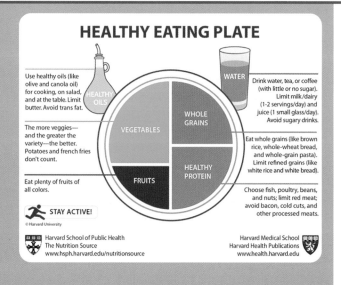

Food Pyramids

As mentioned previously, *MyPlate* was preceded by *MyPyramid*. Various groups developed alternative pyramids to reflect special needs. The **Mediterranean Diet Pyramid** illustrated the healthy traditional food and dietary patterns of the Mediterranean region. Other globally influenced dietary pyramids include the Latin American and the Asian Diet pyramids, which represent the traditional food models of populations with historically low incidences of chronic, diet-related diseases. Remember, however, that other areas of the world have lifestyle patterns, including more physical activity and far less processed food, that may impact disease prevention. Pyramids also have been developed for children and other age groups and for specific health concerns. Oldways Preservation Trust developed a series of Heritage Pyramids that can be viewed at oldwayspt.org/resources/ heritage-pyramids.

Food Labels

Although fresh ingredients used in preparing menu items in foodservice do not carry a package label, processed and packaged products are required to have a label with useful information. All food labels must include the common or usual name of the product; the name and address of the manufacturer, packer or distributor; net contents in weight, measure or count; the Nutrition Facts panel; and the ingredients listed in descending order of predominance by weight. The label also might feature health claims, allergy warnings, nutrient claims, organic designation and/or country of origin.

Nutrition Facts Label

The **Nutrition Labeling and Education Act of 1990** (NLEA: Public Law 101-535) created the **Nutrition Facts panel** and initiated education to help consumers use the label to make better food choices. The list required on the Nutrition Facts panel focuses on the nutrients and food components of greatest public health concern as determined by the *Dietary Guidelines for Americans* at that time. There have been some changes in the food labeling law over time, such as the addition of information on trans fats, sugars and labeling for common allergens.

Changes to the Nutrition Facts Panel

The FDA has updated the Nutrition Facts label to reflect changes based on new nutrition science, the amount of food people are actually eating and drinking (which was more than 20 years ago) and a new design. Changes are being phased in with all new labels required by 2021 so you may see "old" and "new" label formats on products.

Changes based on new nutrition science

- Requires the declaration of "added sugars" on the label. Currently, "sugars" include both "added sugars" and sugars that are naturally occurring in food. Americans on average eat 16% of their total calories from added sugars, with the major sources being soda, energy and sports drinks, grain-based desserts, sugar-sweetened fruit drinks, dairy-based desserts and candy.

- Removes the requirement for declaring "calories from fat." Research shows that the total fat in the diet is less important than the type of fat. FDA continues to require "total fat," "saturated fat," and "trans fat" on the label.

- Revises the nutrients of public health significance that must be declared on the label. These are nutrients for which the U.S. population is consuming inadequate amounts and are associated with the risk of chronic disease. FDA has determined that calcium, vitamin D, potassium, and iron should be mandatory. Calcium and iron were already required; vitamin D and potassium are newly required. Mandatory labeling no longer requires vitamin C or vitamin A because current data indicate that deficiencies are not common; these vitamins would still be allowed to be declared on labels voluntarily.

- Revises Daily Values for certain nutrients that are either mandatory or voluntary on the label. Examples include calcium, sodium, dietary fiber and vitamin D. Some Daily Values are intended to guide consumers about maximum intake—saturated fat, for example—while others are intended to help consumer meet a nutrient requirement—iron, for example.

Updated serving size requirements and labeling for certain packages

By law, serving sizes must be based on amounts of food and drink that people customarily consume, not on what people should be eating. People are generally eating larger portions today than 20 years ago.Therefore, FDA is updating the reference values used by manufacturers to set serving sizes to make them more realistic, reflecting what people really eat and drink.

FDA set the current reference values (Reference Amounts Customarily Consumed, or RACCs) in 1994. More recent food consumption data show RACCs should be changed for different food categories. Additionally, FDA now requires that some food products previously labeled as more than one serving be labeled as a single serving, because people typically eat or drink them in one sitting. All packages containing between 150% and 200% of the RACCs can no longer be labeled as more than one serving. Examples would be a 20-ounce can of soda or a 15-ounce can of soup. Certain larger packages that could be consumed in one sitting or in multiple sittings are required to be labeled per serving and per package.

Refreshed design

The look of the label would remain, but FDA has made several changes to highlight key parts of the label that are important in addressing current public health problems like obesity. The new format will:

- Highlight the caloric content of foods by increasing the type size and placing in bold type the number of calories and servings per container.

- Shift to the left of the label % Daily Value (DV). The %DV is intended to help consumers place nutrient information in the context of a total daily diet.

- Declare the actual amount, in addition to %DV, for all vitamins and minerals when they are declared.

- Change "Amount Per Serving" to "Amount per ___", with the blank filled in with the serving size in common household measures, such as "Amount per 1 cup."

- Replace the listing of "Total Carbohydrate" with "Total Carbs" and indenting "Added Sugars" directly beneath the listing for "Sugars." This makes clearer that some foods have naturally occurring sugars.

- Remove the prior footnote that describes the Daily Values for 2,000 and 2,500 calories to provide more space to better explain the percent dietary value. This part of the nutrition label is often misunderstood by consumers, and FDA is conducting an experimental study to help determine how the footnote can help consumers to better understand the %DV.

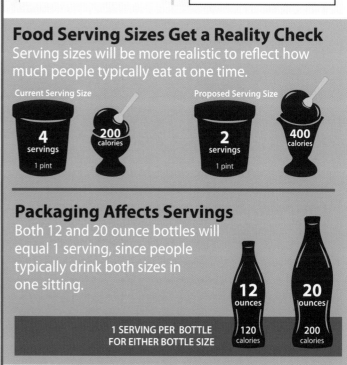

Nutrient Content Claims

"Fat-free," "reduced-sugar" and "low-sodium" are not just catch phrases on packages. They have legal definitions. The chart below describes the criteria used. A **reference food** is the common form of that food used as a base-point for comparison. For example, mayonnaise would be the reference food for low-fat mayonnaise.

	Free Other terms: zero, no, without, trivial source of, negligible source of or dietary insignificant source of	**Low** Other terms: little, few, contains a small amount of or low source of	**Reduced/Less** Other terms: lower or fewer
Calories	Less than 5 calories per serving	40 calories or less per serving Meals and main dishes: 120 calories or less per 100 grams	At least 25% fewer calories than the reference food Meals and main dishes: at least 25% fewer calories per 100 grams
Total Fat	Less than 0.5 gram per serving	3 grams or less per serving of most foods Meals and main dishes: 3 grams or less per 100 grams and not more than 30% of calories from fat	At least 25% less fat per serving than an appropriate reference food
Saturated Fat	Less than 0.5 gram saturated fat and less than 0.5 gram trans fatty acids per serving	1 gram or less per serving and 15% or less of calories from saturated fat Meals and main dishes: 1 gram or less per 100 grams and less than 10% of calories from saturated fat	At least 25% less saturated fat per serving than an appropriate reference food
Cholesterol	Less than 2 milligrams per serving	20 milligrams or less per serving Meals and main dishes: 20 milligrams or less per 100 grams	At least 25% less cholesterol per serving than an appropriate reference food Meals and main dishes: at least 25% less cholesterol per 100 grams
Sodium	Less than 5 milligrams per serving; contains no ingredient that is sodium chloride or generally understood to contain sodium "Salt Free" must meet criterion for "Sodium Free"	140 milligrams or less per serving (and per 50 grams if reference serving is small) Meals and main dishes: 140 milligrams or less per 100 grams "Very Low Sodium": 35 milligrams or less per reference serving (and per 50 grams if reference serving is small) Meals and main dishes: 35 milligrams or less per 100 grams	At least 25% less sodium per serving than an appropriate reference food Meals and main dishes: at least 25% less sodium per 100 grams
Sugar	Less than 0.5 gram sugars per reference serving and per labeled serving Meals and main dishes: less than 0.5 gram per labeled serving Contains no ingredient that is a sugar or generally understood to contain sugar	Not defined	At least 25% less sugar per reference serving than an appropriate reference food Meals and main dishes: at least 25% less sugar per 100 grams

Other Nutrient-Content Claims

Claims such as "Lean ground beef," "excellent source of vitamin C" or "extra fiber" relate to the nutrient content of foods.

Claim	Requirement
High, rich in or excellent source of	Contains 20% or more of the Daily Value
Good source, contains or provides	10% – 19% of the Daily Value
More, fortified, enriched, added, extra or plus	10% or more of the Daily Value; used for vitamins, minerals, protein, dietary fiber and potassium
Lean	On meat, poultry and fish products that contain less than 10 grams total fat, 4.5 grams or less saturated fat and less than 95 milligrams cholesterol per serving
Extra lean	On meat, poultry, and fish products that contain less than 5 grams total fat, less than 2 grams saturated fat and less than 95 milligrams cholesterol per serving
Contains antioxidant(s)	• A Recommended Dietary Intake (RDI) must be established for each of the nutrients that are the subject of the claim. • Each nutrient must have existing scientific evidence of antioxidant activity. • The level of each nutrient must be sufficient to meet the definition for "high," "good source" or "more." • Beta-carotene may be the subject of an antioxidant claim when the level of vitamin A present as beta-carotene in the food is sufficient to qualify for the claim.

Health Claims

Health claims describe a relationship between a food, food component or dietary supplement ingredient and reducing the risk of a disease or health-related condition. The Food and Drug Administration (FDA) approves health claims, which must be supported by significant scientific evidence and undergo a lengthy approval process. Claims change from time to time as scientific consensus validates the relationship of a substance in food to its effect on health. In addition, wording varies on different products.

FDA currently permits **qualified health claims**, each of which is considered on an individual basis. These claims do not meet the "significant scientific" standard. Rather, they are based on emerging, but not conclusive, evidence for a relationship between a food, food component or dietary supplement and reduced risk of disease or health-related condition. These claims require a disclaimer, such as "scientific evidence suggests but does not prove that . . . ."

For example, a qualified health claim might say, "Green tea may reduce your risk of cancer*." The disclaimer might say, "*Very limited and preliminary scientific research suggests green tea reduces risk of cancer. The FDA concludes that there is little scientific evidence supporting this claim."

Health Claims Report Card

The following four-tiered ranking system is used to categorize the quality and strength of scientific evidence for qualified health claims.

Grade	Level of Confidence in Health Claim	Label Disclaimers Required by the FDA
A	High: significant scientific agreement	The health claims do not require disclaimers.
B	Moderate: evidence not entirely conclusive	"Although there is scientific evidence supporting this claim, the evidence is not conclusive."
C	Low: evidence limited and inconclusive	"Some scientific evidence suggests [health claim]. However, the FDA has determined that this evidence is limited and not conclusive."
D	Extremely low: little scientific evidence	"Very limited and preliminary scientific research suggests [health claim]. The FDA concludes that there is little scientific evidence supporting this claim."

Health claims based on authoritative statements allow certain health claims to be used on foods based on an authoritative statement from a scientific body of the government or the National Academy of Sciences. ***Structure/function*** claims may be used without FDA permission. Claims such as "fiber maintains bowel regularity" or "calcium builds strong bones" are examples of this type of claim.

FDA has approved 12 health claims and four health claims based on authoritative statements for use on food labels. Each claim must meet specific guidelines for the amount of the specific nutrient mentioned. Additional claims are being evaluated. (**www.fda.gov/Food/LabelingNutrition/LabelClaims/default.htm**)

Health Claims - Supported by science and generally accepted by health experts.

Approved Claims	Requirements for Food	Model Claim/Statement
Calcium and osteoporosis	High in calcium	Regular exercise and a healthy diet with enough calcium help teens and young adult white and Asian women maintain good bone health and may reduce their high risk of osteoporosis later in life.
Sodium and hypertension	Low sodium	Diets low in sodium may reduce the risk of high blood pressure, a disease associated with many factors.
Dietary fat and cancer	Low fat or extra lean	Development of cancer depends on many factors. A diet low in total fat may reduce the risk of some cancers.
Dietary saturated fat and cholesterol and risk of coronary heart disease	Low fat or extra lean, low saturated fat, and low cholesterol	While many factors affect heart disease, diets low in saturated fat and cholesterol may reduce the risk of this disease.
Fiber-containing grain products, fruits, and vegetables and cancer	Grain product, fruit or vegetable that contains dietary fiber; low fat and good source of dietary fiber (without fortification)	Low fat diets rich in fiber-containing grain products, fruits, and vegetables may reduce the risk of some types of cancer, a disease associated with many factors.

Health Claims - Supported by science and generally accepted by health experts *continued*

Approved Claims	Requirements for Food	Model Claim/Statement
Fruits, vegetables and grain products that contain fiber, particularly soluble fiber, and risk of coronary heart disease	Fruit, vegetable or grain product that contains fiber; low fat, low saturated fat, low cholesterol	Diets low in saturated fat and cholesterol and rich in fruits, vegetables, and grain products that contain some types of dietary fiber, particularly soluble fiber, may reduce the risk of heart disease, a disease associated with many factors.
Fruits and vegetables and cancer	Fruit or vegetable that is low fat and a good source (without fortification) of at least one of the following: vitamin A or C or dietary fiber	Low fat diets rich in fruits and vegetables (foods that are low in fat and may contain dietary fiber, vitamin A or vitamin C) may reduce the risk of some types of cancer, a disease associated with many factors. Broccoli is high in vitamin A and C, and it is a good source of dietary fiber.
Folate and neural tube defects	At least 40 micrograms of folate per serving	Healthful diets with adequate folate may reduce a woman's risk of having a child with a brain or spinal cord defect.
Dietary non-carcinogenic carbohydrate sweeteners and dental caries	Sugar free	Frequent between-meal consumption of foods high in sugars and starches promotes tooth decay. The sugar alcohols in [name food] do not promote tooth decay.
Soluble fiber from certain foods and risk of coronary heart disease	Low saturated fat and cholesterol; must contain one of more of following: oat bran, rolled oats, whole oat flour, whole-grain barley or dried millet barley	Soluble fiber from foods such as [name of soluble fiber source and, if desired, name of food product], as part of a diet low in saturated fat and cholesterol, may reduce the risk of heart disease. A serving of [name food] supplies __ grams of the [necessary daily dietary intake for the benefit] soluble flour from [name of soluble fiber source] necessary per day to have the effect.
Soy protein and risk of coronary heart disease	At least 6.25 grams of soy protein per serving; low fat, saturated fat and cholesterol	• 25 grams of soy protein a day, as part of a diet low in saturated fat and cholesterol, may reduce the risk of heart disease. A serving of [name food] supplies __ grams of soy protein. • Diets low in saturated fat and cholesterol that include 25 grams of soy protein a day may reduce the risk of heart disease. One serving of [name food] provides __ grams of soy protein.

Health Claims - Supported by science and generally accepted by health experts *continued*

Approved Claims	Requirements for Food	Model Claim/Statement
Plant sterol/stanol esters and risk of coronary heart disease	At least 0.65 gram of plant sterol esters per serving of spread and salad dressings; at least 1.7 grams of plant stanol esters per serving of salad dressings, snack bars and dietary supplements; low saturated fat and cholesterol	• Foods containing at least 0.65 gram of vegetable oil sterile esters, eaten twice a day with meals for a daily total intake of at least 1.3 grams, as part of a diet low in saturated fat and cholesterol, may reduce the risk of heart disease. A serving of [name food] supplies __ grams of vegetable oil sterol esters. • Diets low in saturated fat and cholesterol that include two servings of foods that provide a daily total of at least 3.4 grams of plant stanol esters in two meals may reduce the risk of heart disease. A serving of [name food] supplies __ grams of plant stanol esters.
Whole-grain foods and risk of heart disease and certain cancers (based on authoritative claims)	51% or more whole-grain ingredients by weight per serving; low fat; dietary fiber	Diets rich in whole grain foods and other plant foods and low in total fat, saturated fat, and cholesterol, may reduce the risk of heart disease and some cancers.
Potassium and the risk of high blood pressure and stroke (based on authoritative claims)	Good source of potassium; low sodium, total fat, saturated fat and cholesterol	Diets containing foods that are a good source of potassium and that are low in sodium may reduce the risk of high blood pressure and stroke
Fluoridated water and reduced risk of dental caries (based on authoritative claims)	Bottled water meeting all general requirements for health claims with the exception of minimum nutrient contribution; fluoride	Drinking fluoridated water may reduce the risk of dental caries or tooth decay.
Saturated fat, cholesterol and trans fat, and reduced risk of heart disease (based on authoritative claims)	Low saturated fat and cholesterol; quantitative trans fat labeling; limits on trans fat and total fat	Diets low in saturated fat and cholesterol, and as low as possible in trans fat, may reduce the risk of heart disease.

Labeling Exemptions

The following foods are currently exempt from label requirements:

- Packages with less than 12 square inches for labeling (must have address or phone number, but not full labeling)
- Foods produced by small businesses – for example, businesses with food sales of less than $50,000/year and businesses with fewer than 100 full-time equivalent employees that have sales of fewer than 100,00 units annually
- Restaurant food, unless a health claim is made
- Food served for immediate consumption (vending machines, hospital cafeterias, airplanes, shopping malls and sidewalk vendors)
- Ready-to-eat food that is not for immediate consumption but is prepared primarily on site (bakery, deli and candy store items)
- Foods shipped in bulk but not for sale in that form to consumers
- Medical foods
- Plain tea, coffee, spices and foods with no significant amount of any nutrient
- Nutrient supplements, herbs and related products

What Puts the 'Whole' in Whole-Wheat Bread?

Bread labeled "whole-wheat" must contain whole-wheat flour in greater quantity than any other ingredient, which also means that it will be first on the ingredient list. If flour or enriched flour is listed first, and whole wheat is the second or lower, the bread is not whole-wheat bread. Recently white whole wheat flour has come to market. It is a grain variety that grinds to a white colored flour but does contain the whole grain.

Ingredient List

A food label must include a list of ingredients in descending order by weight. The ingredient that weighs the most is listed first, and the ingredient that weighs the least is listed last. Ingredients are always listed by their common or usual name – for example, sugar versus sucrose. The ingredient list also includes, when appropriate, identification of Food and Drug Administration certified food additives, sources of protein hydrolysates used as flavors or enhancers, a declaration that casein is a milk derivative and the total percentage of juice in juice beverages.

Allergen Labeling

The **Food Allergen Labeling and Consumer Protection Act (FALCPA) of 2004** is an amendment to the Federal Food, Drug, and Cosmetic Act. It requires that the label of a food that contains an ingredient that is or contains protein from a major food allergen declare the presence of that allergen. This act was passed to make it easier for people with food allergies to identify and avoid the eight major food allergens that account for 90% of food allergic reactions and are the sources from which many other ingredients are derived. While other allergens are being considered for labeling, the eight foods originally identified by the law are:

- Milk
- Eggs
- Fish (e.g., bass, flounder, cod)
- Crustacean shellfish (e.g., crab, lobster, shrimp)
- Tree nuts (e.g., almonds, walnuts, pecans)
- Peanuts
- Wheat
- Soybeans

Ingredients Most Likely to Be of Concern to Customers

Vegetable sources of saturated fat
Although coconut oil has come into vogue for cooking and baking, it is a source of saturated fat. The question is if that specific configuration of fatty acids in coconut oil raises or lowers fat levels in human blood. There are both positive and negative research studies. Coconut oil, palm kernel oil, palm oil, some hydrogenated oils, vegetable shortenings, stick margarines are sources of trans fatty acids

Animal sources of saturated fat
Lard, beef fat, bacon fat, salt pork, butterfat, milk-fat, cheese, cream cheese, dried or frozen liquid whole eggs, and egg yolks (not egg whites)

Primary sources of sweeteners
Glucose (glucose, dextrose, corn syrup); fructose (fructose, fruit sugar, fructose corn syrup, levulose); honey (honey, raw honey, unpasteurized honey, invert sugar, invert sugar syrup, tupelo honey); maltose (maltose, malted syrup, maltodextrin, dextrins); sorghum (sorghum molasses, grain sorghum syrup); lactose (milk sugar, whey); sugar alcohols (sorbitol, manitol, xylitol).

Primary sources of sodium
Sodium chloride (salt), monosodium glutamate (MSG), calcium disodium phosphate, EDTA, whey, dried buttermilk powder, cheeses, Dutch-processed cocoa, soy sauce, baking powder, baking soda, Worcestershire sauce, barbecue sauce, sauerkraut, pickles and pickled foods.

Primary sources of gluten
Found in wheat, rye, and barley, gluten can be hard to avoid as many foods are made with components of these ingredients. Wheat based ingredients include white and whole-wheat flour, graham flour, kamut, semolina, spelt, wheat germ and bran. Please see Chapter 13 for more information on gluten and gluten-free diets.

Potential allergens
Milk, eggs, fish, shellfish, peanuts, tree nuts, wheat and soy in all forms, tartrazine and other artificial colors, monosodium glutamate (MSG), sulfites, casein and nitrites.

FALCPA has designated these eight foods and any ingredient that contains protein derived from one or more of them as major food allergens. Even small amounts of these foods – as whole foods, ingredients or contaminants – can be dangerous to a person with a food allergy. (For more on food allergies see Chapter 13.)

The law requires that food labels identify source names of all major food allergens used to make the product. This requirement is met if the common or usual name of an ingredient (e.g., buttermilk) already identifies the name of the allergen's food source – in this case, milk. Otherwise, the allergen's food source name must be declared at least once on the food label in one of two ways.

1. In parentheses following the name of the ingredient.

   Examples: "lecithin (soy)," "flour (wheat)" and "whey (milk)"

2. Immediately after or next to the list of ingredients in a "contains" statement.

3. Example: "contains wheat, milk and soy."

Organic and Natural Labeling

USDA's National Organic Program (NOP) (www.ams.usda.gov/nop) regulates standards for any farm, wild crop harvesting or handling operation that wants to sell an agricultural product as organically produced. NOP also accredits certifying agents (foreign and domestic) who inspect organic production and handling operations to ensure that they meet USDA standards.

The Organic Foods Production Act, which was included in the 1990 Farm Bill, and the National Organic Program assure consumers that the organic agricultural products they purchase are produced, processed and certified to consistent national organic standards. Except for operations whose gross income from organic sales totals $5,000 or less, farm and processing operations that grow and process organic agricultural products must be certified by USDA-accredited certifying agents.

Organic is a labeling term that indicates that the food or other agricultural product has been produced through approved methods that integrate cultural, biological and mechanical practices that foster cycling of resources, promote ecological balance and conserve biodiversity. The USDA organic seal verifies that:

In crops: Irradiation, sewage sludge, synthetic fertilizers, prohibited pesticides and genetically modified organisms were not used.

In livestock: Producers met animal health and welfare standards, did not use antibiotics or growth hormones, used 100% organic feed and provided animals with access to the outdoors.

In multi-food ingredients: The product has 95% or more certified organic content by weight.

Organic labeling requirements apply to raw, fresh and processed products that contain organic agricultural ingredients. Labeling requirements are based on the percentage of organic ingredients in a product.

- Products labeled ***100% organic*** must contain only organically produced ingredients and processing aids (excluding water and salt). The USDA Organic Seal may be used on the product package.

- Products labeled ***organic*** must consist of at least 95% organically produced ingredients (excluding water and salt). Any remaining product ingredients must consist of nonagricultural substances approved on the national list including specific non-organically produced agricultural products that are not commercially available in organic form. The USDA Organic Seal may be used on the product package.

- Processed products that contain at least 70% organic ingredients can use the phrase ***made with organic ingredients*** and list up to three of the organic ingredients or food groups on the principal display panel. For example, soup made with at least 70% organic ingredients and only organic vegetables may be labeled either "soup made with organic peas, potatoes and carrots" or "soup made with organic vegetables." The USDA Organic Seal may not be used on the product package.

- Processed products that contain less than 70% organic ingredients cannot use the term organic anywhere on the principal display panel; however, they may identify the specific ingredients that are organically produced on the ingredients statement on the information panel.

Natural

USDA has defined "**natural**" for meat and poultry only. Meat and poultry products that contain no artificial ingredients or added color and that are minimally processed (the raw product not fundamentally altered) may be labeled natural. The label must explain the use of the term natural – for example, "no added colorings or artificial ingredients" or "minimally processed."

For all other food products and processed products, there is no legal definition of the term natural. It is left to the producer or manufacturer to create its own definition. The term often suggests that a food is healthful, but it may not be. Many fried, sweet and salty snacks are marketed as natural.

When purchasing food and ingredients, remember that the "organic" label is not an indicator of a food being more nutritious – it simply signifies a type of food production. The current body of research shows no significant difference in the nutritional content or safety between organic and conventionally produced foods. Organic production protects land and the environment but generally carries a higher price tag. If food budgets are very limited, more vegetables and fruits are probably a better choice then a smaller quantity of organically produced ones.

Today with the emphasis on farm-to-table, many restaurants are sourcing ingredients straight from the farmer. And many farmers, especially small ones, do not have the systems in place to be labeled organic. However their products are likely to have been produced naturally, raised on grass, free range, and grown without pesticides or fertilizers. In most instances, local trumps "organic," as local is more likely fresh picked and transported a limited distance.

Front-of-Package (FOP) Nutrition Labeling

In response to public interest in identifying healthier foods, some manufacturers have voluntarily added nutrition information and ratings to the front of food packages. The large number of different FOP approaches and messages, however, confuses consumers and is ultimately counterproductive. FOP labeling systems are linked to differing sets of nutritional criteria developed by manufacturers, supermarket chains,

trade organizations or health organizations. Many FOP programs are regional or specific to a particular chain of stores.

Some manufacturers that make high-fat products use labels to promote low sugar content, while some manufacturers of high-sugar products promote them as being fat-free – but neither type of product is a truly healthful choice. In addition to confusing consumers, this selective FOP labeling may give an impression of healthfulness that can encourage overconsumption of products for which nutritional quality is mediocre at best.

In addition, FDA has found when a product has FOP or shelf labeling, consumers are less likely to check the more complete Nutrition Facts panel on the back or side of the package. FDA is on the lookout for FOP labels that appear to be misleading and for symbols that imply nutrient content claims.

The Institute of Medicine (IOM) along with the Centers for Disease Control and Prevention, the FDA, and USDA's Center for Nutrition Policy and Promotion formed a committee in 2010 to study and report on FOP labeling. The committee concluded that it is time to move to one system "that encourages healthful food choice through simplicity, visual clarity and the ability to convey meaning without written information." [1]

The IOM committee recommended that FDA and USDA develop a standard FOP system for use on all food products. Suggested characteristics include:

- Calories in common household measure serving sizes. For example, xx calories per cup.
- A symbol system that shows saturated and trans fats, sodium and added sugars.
- Information integrated with the Nutrition Facts panel so that they reinforce each other.
- Similar labeling on all grocery products to allow consumers to compare food products across and within food categories.

FDA is developing a proposed regulation to develop standardized, science-based nutrition criteria that must be met by manufacturers making broad FOP or shelf-label nutrition claims in text or via symbols. [2]

Various Front-of-Package Label Systems Currently Used

- *Symbols that broadly suggest that a food is "healthy," "good for you," or "a better choice."* The American Heart Association's Heart-Check Mark is an example.

- *Shelf-label symbols used by supermarkets that give foods a "grade."* Examples include Guiding Stars (the more stars, the "healthier" the food) and NuVal, which gives a numerical score based on several factors associated with the food.

- *Symbols that provide both specific nutrition information and gradations about positive or negative nutrient levels.* The British voluntary "traffic light" system is an example. Great Britain has neither mandatory nutrition labeling nor a mandatory format for nutrition labeling; however, if a claim is made, nutrition labeling is required.

- *Federal dietary guidance symbols that are intended to provide advice on how to construct a healthy diet.* The presence of logos such as *MyPlate* is not determined by the specific nutrient profile of a food. Questions have been raised about whether or not using such a logo implies that a food has healthy attributes, even if the total fat, saturated fat content, cholesterol and/or sodium content are high.

- *Symbols that list key nutrients found in the food on the front of the package.* Facts Up Front was developed by the Grocery Manufacturers Association and the Food Marketing Institute and is a nutrient-based labeling system that summarizes important information from the Nutrition Facts Panel in a simple and easy-to-use format on the front of food and beverage packages.

The *Facts Up Front* icons (numbers on colored tabs) are designed to allow consumers to quickly see, understand and use key nutrient information as they peruse store shelves and navigate aisles. The basic *Facts Up Front* label lists calories and information about saturated fat, sodium and sugar – nutrients the *Dietary Guidelines for Americans* recommend limiting. The four nutrient facts are always presented together as a consistent set.

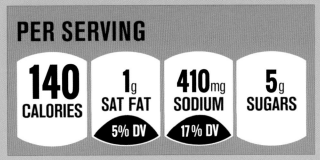

PER SERVING — 140 CALORIES | 1g SAT FAT (5% DV) | 410mg SODIUM (17% DV) | 5g SUGARS

Manufacturers may also choose to include information on up to two "nutrients to encourage." These nutrients – potassium, fiber, protein, vitamin A, vitamin C, vitamin D, calcium and iron – are needed to build a "nutrient-dense" diet, according to the *Dietary Guidelines for Americans*. These "nutrients to encourage" can only be placed on a package when it meets the FDA requirements for a "good source" nutrient content claim.

From the Kitchen
Shawn Weed
Chef/Owner,
The Acre,
Albuquerque,
New Mexico

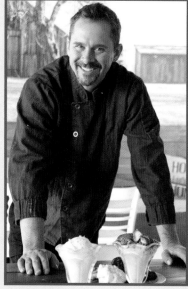

We live in a culture that has enthusiastically accepted preservatives, pesticides, genetically modified ingredients, giant portions, grease-laden fast-food, and meat with every meal. The idea of food as medicine is something that I not only accept but embrace. When we nourish our bodies thoughtfully and well, it is remarkable how well our body can cure itself of what ails it.

I consider myself a Flexitarian. At home, my family eats clean, seasonal food with an emphasis on non-meat dishes that incorporate bright flavors and spices. At the restaurant, our menu features local, seasonal, often organic produce, and eliminates meat altogether. We emphasize scratch-cooking and pay a lot of attention to portion control. Instead of huge portion sizes and platters, we plate an appropriate and satisfying amount of food. My goal is to feed people great food made with real ingredients while giving them a nurturing environment to dine in.

Shawn Weed is Chef and Owner of The Acre, a comfort vegetarian restaurant in Albuquerque where farm-to-fork intersects with food favorites. The restaurant prides itself on local, seasonal, organic ingredients while serving dishes that are approachable and affordable. From burgers and "comfort" dogs to meat(less)loaf, pot pie, and homemade ice cream, diners are offered a whimsical vegetarian spin on American classics. The Acre also serves wine from sustainable vineyards and local craft beer.

Growing up in Indiana around his grandparents' farm, Shawn was exposed to fresh ingredients and seasonal dining. He developed a deep appreciation for where food comes from and how it's used to nourish our bodies while nurturing the family. Some chefs cook for the art. Some, like Shawn, cook for the people. This means paying attention not only to what people love to eat, but how it makes them feel, including what effect it has on their health.

Spicy Vegetarian Loaf
10 servings

Shawn Weed,
The Acre, Albuquerque, New Mexico

We recommend serving this vegetarian loaf with good, old-fashioned mashed potatoes or cheesy grits and sautéed seasonal vegetables.

Cremini mushrooms, chopped	8	cups
Red onion, chopped	1	each
Olive oil	4	tablespoons
Zucchini, chopped	2	each
Chickpeas, drained	8	cups
Cumin	2	tablespoons
Paprika	2	tablespoons
Red chile powder	1	tablespoon
Salt	1	teaspoon
Panko breadcrumbs	4	cups
Spicy ketchup	3	tablespoons

1. Heat oven to 400 °F.
2. Pulse mushrooms and onions in a food processor until they are pea-sized pieces. Toss mushroom/onion mixture in olive oil. Place the mixture on a sheet tray and roast for 20 minutes. Remove the mushroom and onion mixture from the oven. Allow it to cool enough to handle. Stir the mushroom mixture. Roast an additional 10 minutes.
3. Place zucchini in a food processor, pulse to roughly chop. Set aside.
4. Puree the chickpeas with the cumin, paprika, chile powder, salt and pepper.
5. Combine the chickpea mixture with the mushroom mixture. Add zucchini and breadcrumbs. The mixture should be damp but not wet.
6. Form the mixture into a loaf and place on parchment paper on a hotel pan. Top the mixture generously with spicy ketchup and bake for 40 minutes. The mixture should be quite firm and the texture of meatloaf. Let rest 10 minutes before slicing or blast chill if using later.

Per Serving

Calories	410		Cholesterol	0	mg
Fat	11	g	Sodium	1230	mg
Saturated Fat	1	g	Carbohydrates	66	mg
Trans Fat	0	g	Dietary Fiber	9.5	mg
Sugar	7	g	Protein	14	g

Opportunities for Chefs

The cornerstones of a healthy diet are adequacy, balance, moderation and variety. Various nutrition standards, such as the *Dietary Guidelines for Americans* and *MyPlate*, are built on that foundation. The *Dietary Guidelines* and *MyPlate* should be used for the basis of menu planning and recipe development for healthful meals. Nutrition tools such as food labeling and food rating systems based on nutrient density are used to communicate healthy diet principles to consumers. While it is not necessary for chefs to know the specific amounts needed for every nutrient, it is helpful to understand the tools developed to implement national health policy and to consider how menus and recipes might better fulfill nutrition recommendations. As people seek more healthful food in restaurants and other foodservice settings, the chef who understands how the cornerstones of nutrition are reflected in current standards and tools will have a head start in meeting consumer demands.

Learning Activities

- Choose food labels from two similar items (cereal, condiments, etc.) and compare the Nutrition Facts panel of each food item.

- Visit *MyPlate* at www.choosemyplate.gov and create your personalized plan. Use your *MyPlate* plan to design a healthful menu.

- Find food labels that make different legal health claims.

- From each food group, identify a core, healthful option and a food from that same group that is a high-fat or high-sugar choice. Compare calories and nutrient contributions of each pair.

For More Information

- Claims That Can Be Made for Conventional Foods and Dietary Supplements, **https://www.fda.gov/Food/LabelingNutrition/ucm111447.htm**

- Dietary Reference Intakes, **https://www.nal.usda.gov/fnic/dietary-reference-intakes**

- How to Understand and Use the Food Label, **https://www.fda.gov/food/nutrition-education-resources-materials/how-understand-and-use-nutrition-facts-label**

- *MyPlate*, **www.choosemyplate.gov**

- *Dietary Guidelines for Americans 2015-2020*, **www.dietaryguidelines.gov**

Chapter Three

Carbohydrates

Learning Objectives | *After completing this chapter, you should be able to:*

- Describe how the body uses carbohydrates

- Distinguish between simple carbohydrates and complex carbohydrates and list examples of the foods that contain them

- Explain the importance of fiber in the diet and identify the differences between insoluble and soluble fiber

- List the recommendations of *Dietary Guidelines for Americans* related to sugar, refined grains and fiber

- Identify common and uncommon whole grains and give examples of how to increase their use in menu planning

- Explain the functions of sugar in food preparation and discuss how to decrease the amount of sugar used while maintaining texture and flavor

- Compare and contrast caloric sweeteners (sugars) with non-nutritive sweeteners (sugar substitutes)

Carbohydrates, often called the "ideal fuel," provide energy for the body. The *Dietary Guidelines for Americans* suggest eating plenty of whole-grain complex carbohydrates, which are high in vitamins, minerals and fiber, along with lots of nutrient-rich fruits and vegetables. The guidelines recommend limiting added sugars, which provide little more than calories, and avoiding refined grains.

Carbohydrates are typically grouped as starches, which are complex carbohydrates, and simple sugars which are simple carbohydrates. Complex carbohydrates are made of long chains of simple sugar units. They are found in grains, breads, cereals, pasta, dried peas and beans and starchy vegetables like potatoes and corn. Naturally occurring simple sugars (one or two sugar units) are found in fruit, milk, honey and syrups. Simple sugars are added in food preparation and processing in the form of table sugar, corn syrup, high-fructose corn syrup and other sugars.

Many carbohydrates also contain fiber, which is chemically similar to starch. **Fiber** is an indigestible carbohydrate that contains chemical bonds that cannot be broken down by enzymes in the human digestive tract.

A common misconception about carbohydrates is that they are fattening. Some carbohydrate intake is necessary for basic bodily functions, but too many calories from any energy source will convert to body fat and cause weight gain. One gram of carbohydrate, simple or complex, contains 4 calories – the same number of calories as 1 gram of protein and fewer calories than a gram of either alcohol (7 calories per gram) or fat (9 calories per gram). Carbohydrates become calorically heavy when they are eaten in combination with fat – for example, bread laden with butter, French fries cooked in oil, and potatoes and pastas with rich sauces. Cutting carbohydrates often results in cutting fat calories, too. It is important to read labels to identify calories, fat and carbohydrate. Some low-fat foods, such as salad dressings, remove fat and add sugar with little reduction in calories.

More complex carbohydrate-based dishes and whole grains with reasonable amounts of healthy fat used in preparation or plating would be a great improvement in the typical person's diet.

Nutrition Science

How the Body Uses Carbohydrates

Carbohydrates have three main functions in the body: to provide energy, assist in fat metabolism and spare protein.

Providing energy. Red blood cells, the brain and the nervous system use carbohydrates as their essential fuel. During digestion, the body breaks down or converts all sugars and starches from foods into glucose, the smallest sugar unit and the major source of energy for the body's cells.

After digestion, glucose enters the bloodstream ("blood glucose", often known as "blood sugar") providing fuel for cells throughout the body. Some glucose is stored in the liver as glycogen to be used when blood sugar gets too low and body cells need fuel. The amount of glycogen is relatively small when compared to stored fat and muscle protein. An adult carries about a half-day's supply of energy as glycogen. In addition, some glycogen is stored in the muscles to be used during exercise. Once glycogen stores are full, the body will convert excess glucose into fat, which is stored as body fat.

Fat metabolism. Breaking down body fat requires a small amount of carbohydrates for the chemical reaction to produce energy. If carbohydrates are not available, fat is broken down incompletely, resulting in the accumulation of by-products called ketones that can have toxic effects on the body.

Protein sparing. When carbohydrates from food are low, the body next uses protein from food for energy. When that protein is gone, the body uses protein from lean body tissues (muscle and organ tissue) to produce glucose for brain and nerve functions and for metabolic processes. A minimum of 100 grams, or 400 calories, of carbohydrate is necessary daily to prevent protein from being used as an energy source. Carbohydrates provide quick energy for physical activity and athletes generally need more than others so that muscle tissue is not used as an energy source.

Carbohydrates in Foods

There are two types of carbohydrates – simple (sugars) and complex (starches). Carbohydrate-rich foods also provide varying amounts of fiber as well as essential vitamins and minerals.

Sugars

Simple carbohydrates include naturally occurring sugars in fruits, vegetables, milk and honey as well as added and processed sugars in soft drinks, candy, baked goods, jams, jellies, syrups, etc. All simple carbohydrates contain small sugar units – ***monosaccharides*** (one sugar) and ***disaccharides*** (two sugars) – that are easily broken down and converted to glucose. Fruits contain simple sugars and also contribute fiber, vitamins, minerals and protective phytochemicals. Milk and other dairy products that contain simple carbohydrates also provide calcium, phosphorus, riboflavin, vitamin D and protein. Other simple carbohydrate foods, however, such as table sugar, soft drinks, honey, jams and jellies, are often considered ***empty-calorie*** foods because they provide few nutrients except carbohydrates. Some call these nutrient-poor foods (or junk) as opposed to nutrient-rich carbohydrate foods.

The human body cannot tell the difference between natural and refined sugar. By the time they are digested and absorbed, they are identical. Most natural sugars, however, are in foods that also carry essential protective nutrients. Table sugar, on the other hand, is 99% pure sugar and provides 16 calories per teaspoon (4 grams) with virtually no other nutrients.

The U. S. Department of Agriculture estimates that Americans consumed about 74.5 pounds of caloric sweeteners (primarily cane and beet sugars and high-fructose corn syrup sweeteners in soft drinks) per person in 2016. [1] This number represents about 370 calories per day! The 2015-2020 *Dietary Guidelines for Americans* recommends limiting added sugars to no more than 10% of calories; however, Americans get 13-17% of calories from added sugar, primarily from sugar sweetened beverages, snacks and sweets. [2]

Types of Sugar and Their Sources

All the chemical names of sugars end in "ose." Glucose and fructose are monosaccharides. Sucrose, maltose and lactose are dissacharides.

Sugars	Common Names	Sources
Glucose	Blood sugar or blood glucose, dextrose	Corn syrup, sugar, fruits, and vegetables such as carrots and beets
Fructose	Fruit sugar	Fruits and juices, honey, table sugar, high fructose corn syrup
Sucrose (glucose+fructose)	Sugar, table sugar or granulated sugar	Sugar, brown sugar, molasses, turbinado, raw sugar, cane sugar, powdered sugar, fruits
Maltose (glucose+glucose)	Malt sugar	Molasses, bread
Lactose (glucose+galactose)	Milk sugar	Milk, dairy products, whey

Sources of Added Sugars on Ingredient Lists

Sugars are added to many foods during processing. The sugar content and type are listed on food labels. Below are various names for sugars commonly seen on ingredient lists:

Brown sugar

Corn sweetener

Corn syrup

Dextrose

Fructose

Fruit juice concentrates

Glucose

High-fructose corn syrup

Honey

Invert sugar

Lactose

Maltose

Malt syrup

Molasses

Raw sugar

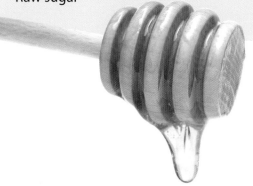

Natural sugars, such as the lactose found in milk and fructose found in fruits, are not limited because the foods they are in typically provide many other nutrients. ***Added sugars***, which are incorporated into foods and beverages during processing and production, provide calories with few nutrients. Major sources of added sugar include candy, soft drinks, fruit drinks, pastries, cookies, sweetened cereals and desserts. Nutrition Facts labels state the number of grams of added sugar and the total carbohydrates.

Research has shown that the one health problem caused specifically by eating too much sugar is dental caries, also called tooth decay. [3] Cavities are formed when bacteria in the mouth mix with carbohydrates to produce acid, which eats away at teeth and leads to tooth decay. All types of sugars, both naturally occurring and refined, can promote tooth decay, particularly if consumed in sticky foods. Sugary foods eaten between meals are more likely to cause tooth decay than those eaten at mealtime. Starches also may promote tooth decay if they remain in the mouth and on the teeth for a long enough time.

While the scientific evidence does not support the popular belief that sugar causes hyperactivity in children, there is evidence that eating sweetened foods influences the brain to seek more sugar, which can lead to a habit of eating many sweet foods that are usually not nutrient-rich and can cause weight gain. [4, 5] Some studies connect the growing rate of childhood obesity to high levels of intake caused by the advertising and promotion of sweet foods to America's children. [6] Limiting the amount of soft drinks, sweetened beverages, candy, sugary desserts and highly sweetened breakfast cereals and snacks, especially for children, makes good sense. Although parents and caregivers have the primary role in controlling the diets of children, chefs and the food industry can play an important role by providing healthier options.

Some sugar added to nutrient-dense foods, such as breakfast cereals and reduced-fat dairy products, often increase intake by enhancing palatability and thus improving nutrient intake without contributing excessive calories or sugars.

Starches

Starches – complex carbohydrates or polysaccharides (many linked sugar units) – are long strands of thousands of glucose units. Because of their length, "complex" starches take longer to break down during digestion. As a result, they enter the bloodstream more slowly than simple sugars.

Starch, which is a plant's form of glucose storage, is found in grains, breads, legumes, cereals and vegetables. Popular examples include pasta, baked beans, polenta, carrots, bagels, tortillas, oatmeal, rice and potatoes. Many complex carbohydrates, particularly whole grains and legumes, also provide fiber, vitamins, minerals and protective phytochemicals. Research has shown that whole grains reduce the risk of heart disease, stroke, cancers of the digestive tract and obesity.

Glycemic Index

Dividing carbohydrates into simple and complex makes sense on a chemical level, but it doesn't do much to explain what happens to different kinds of carbohydrates inside the body. The **glycemic index** is a scale that ranks carbohydrates by how much and how high they raise blood glucose levels compared to pure glucose. The index is sometimes used to evaluate carbohydrate quality. Foods with a high glycemic index, like white bread, cause rapid spikes in blood sugar. Foods with a low glycemic index, like whole oats, are digested more slowly, causing a lower and gentler change in blood sugar.

Some research has linked diets rich in high-glycemic-index foods, which cause quick and strong increases in blood sugar levels, to an increased risk for diabetes, heart disease and obesity. Foods with a low glycemic index have been linked to controlling type 2 diabetes and improved weight loss.

Some guests may be using the glycemic index to control their diets; so chefs should know what it is, but are not expected to plan menus using these values.

The index is difficult to use because individual foods have differing scores and effects, thus making a mixed diet almost impossible to evaluate. But eating whole grains, beans, fruits and vegetables – foods with a low glycemic index – is good for many aspects of health.

What Health Authorities Say about Added Sugar

One of the key recommendations of the *2015-2020 Dietary Guidelines for Americans* is to reduce the intake of calories from added sugars to lower the calorie content of the diet without compromising nutrient adequacy. Specifically, the *Guidelines* recommend that less than 10 percent of the calories consumed per day come from added sugars.

The American Heart Association (AHA) recommends a drastic reduction in the consumption of added sugars. AHA suggests that a prudent upper limit of intake is half of the discretionary calorie allowance, which for most American women is no more than 100 calories per day (25 grams) from added sugars and for most American men, no more than 150 calories per day (about 38 grams). Recent evidence suggests that eating excessive amounts of added sugar boosts triglyceride levels, increasing risk of heart disease.

The World Health Organization recommends that less than 10% of calories come from added sugars, which are sometimes called "free sugars."

These guidelines mean that there is little or no room in a healthful diet for highly sweetened beverages, cereals, candy or desserts.

Sources: 2015-2020 *Dietary Guidelines for Americans*, www.dietary-guidelines.gov, American Heart Association; www.heart.org; and World Health Organization and the Food Agriculture Organization of the United Nations, http://www.who.int/nutrition/publications/guidelines/sugars_intake/en/

Glycemic Index Levels

Low	0 – 55
Moderate	56 – 69
High	70 or more

Fiber

Dietary fiber is a form of carbohydrate in plant foods that is edible but not digested. While fiber adds no calories to the diet, it performs many vital functions important to health. Fiber is a mixture of several components including cellulose, hemicellulose and lignin. These substances, which act as the structural building materials in the cell walls of plants, are chains of glucose units connected by chemical bonds that human digestive enzymes cannot break down. Other components of fiber – pectins and gums – are part of plant cell structure and metabolism. The proportion of these fiber components varies considerably from food to food. Factors such as plant species, stage of plant maturity and parts of the plant have a strong influence on a food's fiber composition.

The fiber in food is divided into two basic types: soluble and insoluble. Each type has different and important functions in the body. For optimal health, it is best to eat foods that provide both types. It is better to eat a wide variety of foods rather than focus on any single food as a source of fiber in the diet.

- *Soluble fibers* dissolve in water and are found in beans (such as kidney or black beans), some fruits and vegetables, and oats and barley. These fibers play a role in lowering blood cholesterol by binding with bile acids in the intestinal tract. Cholesterol is then excreted from the body along with the bile acid molecules. Reduced blood cholesterol levels are associated with the prevention of heart disease. In addition, some soluble fibers, such as those found in vegetables of the cabbage (brassica) family, may reduce the incidence of some forms of cancer. Soluble fibers, such as those in oatmeal, also help regulate the body's use of sugars, slowing their digestion and absorption and delaying the sensation of hunger. This function helps control blood glucose levels in people with diabetes.

- *Insoluble fibers* do not dissolve in water. Instead, they absorb water and provide bulk in the diet, thus adding to the feeling of fullness after a meal, helping the body remove waste and lessening constipation. Adequate intake of insoluble fiber has been found to decrease risk of colon cancer. Foods such as wheat bran, whole grains, fruits with many small seeds, and vegetables also contain this type of fiber. Eating fruits and vegetables with their skins, such as apples, eggplant, pears, potatoes, etc., adds valuable fiber to the diet.

The roles of fiber in promoting health and reducing risk of several diseases has become a more important part of advice for healthful eating in recent years. Food labels are generally the best source of current fiber values of foods. A food may be labeled "high fiber" if it contains more than 5 grams or more per serving. Most dried and canned beans and other legumes are at this level. A "good source of fiber" has 2.5 to 4.9 grams of fiber per serving. Nutrient data-bases are updating fiber values as the technology for measuring fiber in foods improves. Nutrient calculations are discussed in Chapter 11.

Fiber is Lost in Processing

When foods are processed, fiber is sometimes lost. This table shows the effect of processing on select foods, comparing 100 gram portions.

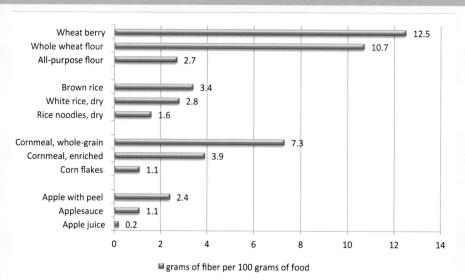

grams of fiber per 100 grams of food

Fiber Content in Select Grains, Beans, Nuts, Fruit and Vegetables

Grains (per 1 cup, cooked)	Fiber (grams)
Wheat, bulgur	8.2
Wheat berries	8.0
Kamut	6.7
Barley, pearled	6.0
Teff	5.5
Quinoa	5.2
Amaranth (a seed)	5.2
Oatmeal	4.0
Rice, brown	3.5
Rice, wild	3.0
Millet	2.3
Rice, white	0.6

Beans (per 1 cup, cooked)	Fiber (grams)
Navy	19.1
Split peas	16.3
Lentils	15.6
Pinto beans	15.4
Black beans	15.0
Lima beans	14.0
Garbanzo beans	12.5
Kidney beans	11.3
Black-eyed peas	11.2
Chickpeas	8.0
Soybeans	7.6

Seeds (per 1 ounce)	Fiber (grams)
Flax	7.7
Sesame	3.3
Sunflower	2.4
Pumpkin	1.7

Cereal (per 1 cup)	Fiber (grams)
100% bran cereal	17.2
Bran flakes	7.0
Raisin bran	5.2-6.8
Shredded wheat squares	5.7
Oatmeal	4.0
Wheat flakes	3.5
Wheat squares	3.2
Oat circles	3.0

Nuts (per 1 ounce)	Fiber (grams)
Almonds	3.5
Pistachios	2.8
Filberts, hazelnuts	2.7
Pecans	2.7
Macadamia	2.4
Peanuts	2.4
Brazil	2.1
Walnuts	1.9
Pine nuts, pignolia	1.1
Cashews	0.9

Fruit (per 1 cup)	Fiber (grams)
Prunes	12.4
Dates	11.8
Apricots, dried	9.5
Raspberries	8.0
Raisins, seedless	5.8
Banana	3.9
Strawberries	3.0
Apples	3.0

Vegetables (per 1 cup, cooked)	Fiber (grams)
Peas	8.8
Artichokes	7.7
Brussels sprouts	6.4
Winter squash	5.7
Broccoli	5.2
Sweet potatoes	3.2
Potatoes	1.8

Source: U.S. Department of Agriculture, Agricultural Research Service. 2015. USDA National Database for Standard Reference, Release 28. Nutrient Data Laboratory, http://www.ars.usda.gov/services/docs.htm?docid=8964

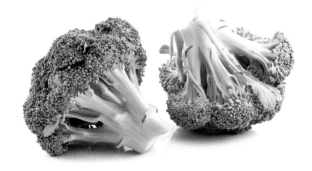

Recommendations for Carbohydrates

The following recommendations are made in the *2015-2020 Dietary Guidelines for Americans*:

- Consume less than 10 percent of calories per day from added sugars.

- Limit the consumption of foods that contain refined grains, especially refined grains that contain solid fats, added sugars and sodium.

- Consume at least half of all grains as whole grains. Increase whole grains by replacing refined grains with whole grains.

- When refined grains are eaten, they should be enriched.

- Eat more fruits, vegetables, and dried peas and beans to get vitamins, minerals and fiber.

- The majority of fruit recommended should come from whole fruits rather than from juice. When juice is consumed, 100% juice should be encouraged. Fruit canned in 100% juice is encouraged over fruit canned in syrup.

- Drink water instead of sugary drinks.

The *Dietary Guidelines* suggest that 45% to 65% of total calories should come from carbohydrates. This range of intake for 2,000 calories translates to 225 to 325 grams of carbohydrate per day. Some popular diets advise severely restricting carbohydrates. Most nutrition experts do not agree with this strategy. On a low-carb diet, protein, fat and alcohol are the only remaining sources of calories. High amounts of any of these nutrients can create health risks. Most healthful weight-loss regimens are designed to provide fewer calories than needed to maintain weight while consuming carbohydrates, protein and fat in reasonable amounts, plus increasing activity to burn calories, raise metabolic rate and build or retain muscle mass.

Few Americans eat the recommended amount of fiber. Men age 50 should consume 38 grams and women 25 grams of total dietary fiber, while men and women over age 50 should get 30 and 21 grams, respectively, of fiber daily. These recommendations are based on an estimated need for 14 grams of fiber for every 1,000 calories consumed. [4]

Carbohydrate Calories and Grams at 45% and 65% of Calories

Calories/day	% Carbohydrate	Carbohydrate Calories	Carbohydrate Grams
2000 calorie diet	45% carbohydrate	900 calories from carbohydrate	225 grams of carbohydrate
2000 calorie diet	65% carbohydrate	1300 calories from carbohydrate	325 grams of carbohydrate

Serving vs. Portion

"Serving," as used in *MyPlate*, is not necessarily the same as servings used for nutrition labeling on food packages. Food label serving sizes are based on data from food consumption studies. *MyPlate* servings are recommended healthful portion sizes for foods within each group. In addition, the sizes of servings used in these tools are quite different from portions served at home or in restaurants. For example, a restaurant portion of 2 cups of pasta is equal to 4 servings; each serving in *MyPlate* is only ½ cup of pasta or 1 ounce of bread per serving. Many rolls and buns are equal to 3 or 4 servings based on weight. While 6 servings of grains sounds abundant, it is quite modest for a daily total.

Standard Servings

MyPlate suggests that Americans need to increase their consumption of foods high in carbohydrates – specifically, fruits, vegetables and whole grains. *MyPlate* recommends amounts of food from each group based on caloric needs. For a 2,000-calorie diet, this advice translates into 6 ounces of grains, 3 cups milk, 2½ cups of vegetables and 2 cups of fruit daily. One serving of each group can be added if more than 2,000 calories per day are needed.

Carbohydrate Counting

Many people on diets for control of diabetes or weight use **carbohydrate counting**, also called carb counting. In carb counting, each carb unit is 15 grams of carbohydrate. In this system, the person carefully regulates carbohydrates with less attention to calories, protein or fat. The individual is allotted a specific number of units (sometimes called points or servings) each meal or day. Note that carb counting has different serving sizes for various foods from either *MyPlate* amounts or serving sizes used for food labeling. **Appendix G** is a list of foods and amounts used in carb counting.

Culinary Science

Ingredients

Menu planning often focuses on the main course or the meat portion of a meal; but fruit, vegetables and whole grains are an important component of menu planning too. Remember, foods high in complex carbohydrates – fruits, vegetables and whole grains – should play a major role in a meal; they should never be an afterthought. Generally, the meat or protein should cover one-quarter of the plate, with grains, fruits and vegetables providing the rest of the meal. While this philosophy may cause some chefs to hesitate, creating high-quality, plant-focused menu items offers an excellent creative opportunity.

A good strategy for increasing the use of fruit, vegetables and whole grains is to incorporate them throughout the meal – appetizers, soups, salads, breads, sauces and desserts. In the main course, chefs often treat vegetables as an obligation or garnish, rather than integrating them as an important part of the dish and including them in the menu description: for example, "Quinoa-crusted diver scallops perched on wilted spinach and mashed parsnips."

Grains

Any food made from wheat, rice, oats, cornmeal, barley or another cereal grain is a grain product. Bread, pasta, oatmeal, breakfast cereals, tortillas and grits are examples of grain products.

Grains are divided into two groups:

- **Whole grains** contain all essential parts of the grain seed—the bran, germ and endosperm. In addition to fiber, whole grains provide protein, vitamins and minerals, as well as protective antioxidants in surprisingly large amounts — similar to levels in fruits and vegetables. An unprocessed grain in its whole, natural form in which all parts of the kernel remain is called an **intact grain** (Examples include: barley, quinoa, and wheat berries).

- **Refined grains** have been milled, a process that removes the bran and germ. Milling gives grains a finer texture and improves their shelf life but also removes dietary fiber, iron and many B vitamins. Most refined grains are enriched. This means certain B vitamins (thiamin, riboflavin, niacin and folic acid) plus iron are added back after processing. Fiber is not added back to enriched grains. Check the ingredient list on refined-grain products to make sure that the word "enriched" is included in the grain name.

Many food products are made from mixtures of whole grains and refined grains. Read labels carefully; "made with whole grain" is not the same as "whole-grain" bread. The ingredient list on the food label lists ingredients in order of weight, so it is easy to determine if there is more refined or whole grain in a product. Some brown breads have caramel color added. Breads and rolls with seeds (sesame, poppy, caraway, flax or millet) on top or within generally have more fiber.

An easy way to find whole grain is to look for a stamp from the Whole Grain Council that indicates the product is 100% whole grain. A list of foodservice products is also available from **www.wholegrainscouncil.org**.

Whole Grains	Refined Grains
Amaranth	All-purpose flour
Barley	Cake and pastry flour
Brown rice	Corn flour
Buckwheat	Couscous
Bulgur (cracked wheat)	Degermed cornmeal
Corn, whole cornmeal	Most ready-to-eat cereals
Emmer	Rice flour
Farro	Rice noodles or wraps
Freekeh	White bread
Kamut	White pasta, noodles
Kasha	White rice
Millet	
Oats, oatmeal	
Popcorn	
Quinoa	
Rye	
Spelt	
Sorghum (milo)	
Teff	
Wheat	
Wheat berries	
Whole wheat flour	
Wild rice	

The amount of grains a person should eat depends on age, sex and level of physical activity. Recommended daily amounts range from 6- to 8-ounce equivalents for adults. Most Americans consume enough grains, but not enough whole grains. At least half of all grains eaten should be whole grains. Serving whole-grain breads, rolls and crackers is a start; whole-grain pastas, pancakes and pizza dough, brown rice, oatmeal and barley are excellent menu additions. The *Dietary Guidelines* suggest that we lower our intake of refined grains and substitute whole grains for them when possible.

A Serving of Grain Is . . .

- ½ cup cooked rice or other grain
- ½ cup cooked pasta
- 1 ounce uncooked pasta, rice or grain
- 1 ounce bread slice
- 1 very small muffin
- 1 ounce ready-to-eat cereal
- ½ cup cooked hot cereal
- 1 4½-inch pancake
- 7 small round or square crackers
- 1 small tortilla

Source: www.choosemyplate.gov

casebycase | Going with the Grain

InHarvest began in 1978 as small family company in the northern climes of Bemidji, Minnesota, where wild rice grows abundantly in shallow lakes and rivers. Soon California grew to be a major wild rice producer as well. By 1987, InHarvest had grown to include a variety of grains and legumes and had built a major processing and packaging plant in the Golden State.

As it has grown, InHarvest has created some of the industry's strictest quality control standards. Products go through three separate cleaning methods as well as a meticulous quality review. As part of its mission to pursue agro-diversity and provide innovative products, InHarvest began working with seed banks in the early 1980s to find heritage varieties of grains that hold the flavor and nutritional profile lost in many of today's modified versions. In addition, the company continues to search the globe for new rice, grain and legumes to introduce to customers.

InHarvest works across the food service spectrum to provide unique, high-quality products to its customers around the country, including school food service. One of the company's chefs, Coleen Donnelly, a Culinary Institute of America graduate, has worked for InHarvest since 2011 and has special expertise in the K-12 market. All of the grain-based blend recipes she and her colleagues develop include a nutritional analysis and meal component calculation.

Coleen has worked closely with CIA alumna and renowned foodservice guru Chef Ann Cooper on fresh, healthy, sustainable food preparation. "In 2005, Ann sent me a stack of recipes and a computer and told me to use them to create meal plans that met federal Child Nutrition Program guidelines at that time," Coleen explains. "It was then that I really began to understand the principles of balance in school meal planning."

When Coleen is not developing recipes at her San Francisco office, she travels around the country to meet school food service directors, menu planners, and workers to teach them about whole and intact grains in general and InHarvest's blends in particular. She demonstrates working whole grains into menus using cooking equipment typically found in school kitchens, and she shares preparation tips to make dishes more appealing and flavorful for the various ages and ethnicities within the K-12 system. "It's the best part of my job," she says. "We like giving people solutions, and it's a lot harder to win over the staff than it is the kids."

Coleen occasionally crosses over from school food-service to work with other InHarvest clients. "Markets like the military and corporate food have strict guide-lines, too," she notes. "Sometimes I can adapt school recipes to meet those markets and vice versa." Even cruise ships have recipe cross over potential. "We developed a mushroom-grain-lentil burger for a cruise line," Coleen says. "With a few tweaks to meet guidelines, it just might make its way into schools, too."

FDA Statement on Whole-Grain Label Claims

The Food and Drug Administration (FDA) is responsible for regulations and activities dealing with the proper labeling of foods, including ingredient statements, nutrient content and health claims. FDA also offers guidance to help manufacturers understand what the agency considers appropriate for statements on food labels, including those related to whole-grain content.

According to the FDA, whole grains are cereal grains that consist of the intact, ground, cracked or flaked kernel, which includes the bran, the germ and the inner most part of the kernel (the endosperm). Some examples of whole grains include whole wheat, oatmeal, whole-grain cornmeal, brown rice, whole-grain barley, whole rye and buckwheat. Spelt, often thought of as a unique whole grain, is actually a member of the wheat family.

When trying to select products that contain whole grains, look for those that show whole grains listed first on the ingredient list. The ingredient list on a food label shows ingredients in the order of the most abundant by weight. For products such as bread or pasta to be labeled whole grain, the grain can be ground, cracked or flaked, but it must retain the same proportions of bran, germ and endosperm as the intact grain.

Vegetables

Any vegetable or 100% vegetable juice counts as a serving from the vegetable group. Vegetables may be raw or cooked; fresh, frozen, canned, or dried/dehydrated; and whole, cut-up or mashed. It is best to use healthful cooking techniques to maximize the health benefits of vegetables. Deep-fried vegetables should be limited or used in small amounts as crispy garnishes. Aside from all too common deep-fried vegetables, an abundance of vegetables in the diet will enrich the nutritional quality of a meal.

The amount of vegetables a person should eat depends on age, gender and level of physical activity. Recommended total daily intake ranges from 2 ½ to 3 cups for adults. It is wise to eat a wide selection of vegetables regularly; including plenty of dark green and orange varieties as well as dried peas and beans. These vegetables are richest in vitamins, minerals, fiber and protective phytochemicals.

Fruit

Any fruit or 100% fruit juice counts as part of the fruit group. Fruits may be fresh, canned, frozen or dried and may be whole, cut-up or pureed. The amount of fruit a person should eat depends on age, gender and physical activity. Recommended daily intake is 2 cups of fruit a day for adults.

Frozen, minimally processed fruits are equal in nutrients and calories to fresh fruits. Fruits canned or bottled in fruit juice or water are also equal to fresh fruit. Fruits canned in light or heavy syrup generally have at least twice the calories and sugar of fresh or frozen fruit.

Dried fruits are more concentrated sources of natural sugars and fiber than fresh varieties because much of the water has been removed. Fruit juices retain the carbohydrate, vitamins and minerals of the fruit, but the pressing or extraction process removes the fruit's fiber and many protective phytochemicals. Thus, from a nutrition perspective, eating a whole or sliced apple is far better than drinking apple juice. Fruit drinks do not count as fruit servings as they usually offer little fruit but lots of sugar.

An Equivalent of 1 Cup of Vegetable Is . . .

- 1 cup raw or cooked vegetable
- 1 cup vegetable juice
- 2 cups raw leafy greens

Source: www.choosemyplate.gov

An Equivalent of 1 Cup of Fruit Is . . .

- 1 cup fruit, raw or cooked
- 1 cup 100% fruit juice
- ½ cup dried fruit
- 1 apple, banana, orange, peach or similar size fruit
- 1 cup berries

Source: www.choosemyplate.gov

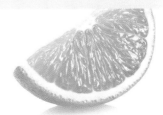

Culinary Applications: Sugar

In addition to adding sweetness and improving flavor and texture, sugars help retain moisture, act as a preservative and extend shelf life. As a preservative, sugar increases the firmness of canned fruit, discourages browning and retards flavor loss. Reducing the sugar content of an item causes it to dry out faster and spoil more quickly. When cooking with sugar, consider form (crystal, powder or syrup) as well as sweetening power in order to maximize taste and texture. Heating sugar, which causes caramelization, changes flavor and texture.

Types of sugar include:

- **Table sugar** (sucrose), which is produced by concentrating sugar cane or beet juice, is composed of joined molecules of fructose and glucose.

- **Confectioner's sugar** (powdered sugar), also a sucrose product, is finely ground to a powder and mixed with some cornstarch, which prevents it from caking and makes it easy to incorporate into cooking mixtures. A light sprinkling of confectioner's sugar (and perhaps a few berries) over a dessert makes an attractive garnish.

- **Superfine sugar**, another sucrose product, is ground fine but not powdered. It dissolves quickly and is useful in batters, meringues and for sweetening beverages.

- **Brown sugar** is the sugar crystals of molasses syrup.

- **Fructose** is light syrup or crystals made from cornstarch or the simple sugar found in fresh fruits. For most food applications, fructose provides 1.2 times the sweetness of table sugar.

- **Turbinado** sugar is raw sugar that has been partially refined and washed. Raw sugar is processed from cane sugar and retains some of the cane sugar molasses. It can also contain contaminants such as molds, fibers and waxes. Raw sugar should not be given to infants.

Sweeteners also come in the form of syrups. Syrups are useful in cooking when a smooth glaze is desired.

Flavor variations can be achieved by using a variety of syrups:

- **Honey** is a natural mixture of fructose and glucose. It is made by bees from nectar and stored in hives as food. Honey comes in different flavors based on the plant providing the nectar. Thus, chestnut honey will have a flavor different from orange blossom honey. Regardless of the source, honey is a more concentrated source of carbohydrate than sugar and has about 25% more calories than an equal measure of sugar. Both provide only calories and no other nutrient in significant amounts. Honey can carry bacteria and should not be given to babies or those with a poor immune response.

- **Molasses** is syrup produced when sugar is extracted from sugar cane. It is deep brown and has a distinctive flavor. Molasses is the only sweetener with some iron, calcium and potassium, but because the amount used in a serving of prepared food is usually very small, its nutrient value is not significant.

- **Maple syrup** is made from a reduction of the sap flow of sugar maple trees and is mainly composed of sucrose, fructose and glucose. Often maple syrup is replaced by pancake syrup, which is sugar syrup with maple flavoring.

- **Corn syrup**, a liquid made from cornstarch, is composed of maltose, fructose and glucose.

- **High-fructose corn syrup** (HFCS) is corn syrup treated with enzymes to change about half of the glucose into fructose, which makes it super-sweet.

- **Agave nectar** composition varies, but typically is primarily fructose. It has about the same amount of calories as sugar, but some say it has a sweeter flavor (up to 1.4 to 1.6 times sweeter than sugar). That means less is needed, saving calories. Agave nectar is often substituted for sugar or honey in recipes. Because agave is primarily fructose, it takes longer to influence blood sugar levels. Some people with diabetes use agave as a sweetener. Vegans commonly use agave nectar to replace honey in recipes.

High-Fructose Corn Syrup

High-fructose corn syrup (HFCS) is a group of corn syrups that have undergone enzymatic processing to convert some of their glucose into fructose. The fructose is then mixed with pure corn syrup (100% glucose). Because of traditional agricultural subsidies for corn and taxes on imported sugar, HFCS is less expensive than sugar and, as a liquid, is easier to blend and transport.

Use of HFCS has expanded greatly since the Food and Drug Administration granted it generally recognized as safe (GRAS) status in 1983. Soft drinks are a major source of high-fructose corn syrup in the diets of many Americans. The ingredient is also used in many other processed foods such as yogurt, cookies, salad dressing, cereals, jams, sauces, tomato soup, and even peanut butter and processed meats. Check the ingredient list on food labels.

Studies suggest that high rates of obesity parallel the rise in consumption of HFCS and that larger quantities of fructose stimulate the triglyceride formation and insulin resistance that contribute to diabetes. The Corn Refiners Association and other industry organizations have launched aggressive campaigns to position HFCS as natural and argue that it is safe and equal to sugar in health effects.

The bottom line is that most people eat too much added sugar, whatever the form. Nevertheless, many consumers prefer products that say "no high-fructose corn syrup" and prefer to purchase products with other sweeteners or no sweeteners.

Functions of Sugar in Cooking

- **Adds sweetness**. The main characteristic of most cakes and pastries is their sweetness; thus, sugar is the defining ingredient in most baked goods, especially desserts.

- **Aids in the creaming process**. The crystalline structure of granulated sugar makes it an effective agent for the incorporation of air into batters mixed by the creaming method. Fat, which is the other main ingredient in creaming, holds the air introduced by the sugar.

- **Creates softening of spreading action**. By interacting with the starch component of flour to delay its gelatinization, sugar causes batters and cookie dough to stay softer longer and spread out over a greater area before setting during baking.

- **Promotes good grain and texture**. Sugar has a denaturing effect on the gluten in flour. Along with the delay in gelatinization, this effect produces a softer crumb and finer grain in breads and cakes.

- **Retains moisture and prolongs freshness**. Sugar absorbs moisture from other ingredients as well as from the atmosphere, thus keeping a finished product moist.

- **Imparts crust color**. Sugar caramelizes and helps form a browner, firmer, crisper crust during baking.

- **Aids in fermentation of yeast**. Sugar supplies a source of food for yeast; the amount of sugar in a recipe can control the rate of fermentation.

- **Balances acidity**. Foods containing vinegar, tomatoes and other acidic ingredients have a more balanced and pleasing flavor profile if a small amount of sugar is added.

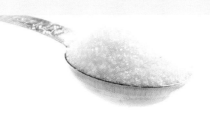

Sugar Substitutes

Sugar substitutes (sometimes referred to as non-nutritive sweeteners, artificial sweeteners or low-calorie sweeteners) are generally several hundred to several thousand times sweeter than sugar. They are used in foods and beverages to provide sweetness without adding a significant amount of calories. Many chefs do not use sugar substitutes (or other modified foods), preferring to limit the amount of sugar used instead. Studies show, however, that consumer demand for artificial sweeteners continues to grow. Many guests ask for reduced-calorie or sugar-free products because they enjoy sweetness but do not want extra calories. Individuals with diabetes are advised to avoid added sugars, and many rely on sugar substitutes for sweet flavors. Because chefs who work in healthcare settings and personal chefs may use sugar substitutes, we have included this information about their sources and use.

- ***Acesulfame-K*** is a high-intensity, non-caloric sweetener. It is approximately 200 times sweeter than sucrose. Acesulfame-K has a clean, quickly perceptible, sweet taste that does not linger or leave an aftertaste. It is not metabolized by the body and is excreted unchanged. Acesulfame-K currently is approved for use in foods and oral-hygiene products such as chewing gum, dry beverage mixes, instant coffee and tea, gelatins, puddings, non-dairy creamers and tabletop sweeteners. It remains stable under high temperatures and has an excellent shelf life. The sweet taste of acesulfame-K remains unchanged during baking.

- ***Advantame*** is the sixth highest-intensity sweetener that is stable at higher temperatures, making it useful (in place of sugar) in a wide variety of cooking applications. Advantame can be used as a general purpose sweetener or as a flavor enhancer and is safe to use in everything from baked goods and beverages, to chewing gum and jams and jellies.

- ***Allulose*** (also called psicose) is a low calorie sugar that has the taste and texture of sugar. It is not absorbed by the body as a carbohydrate and is not metabolized as energy so it has negligible calories. Allulose has received GRAS status from FDA. It is not available as a table top sweetener but is used in manufactured foods and beverages.

- ***Aspartame*** is about 180 times sweeter than sucrose and does not have a bitter aftertaste. Aspartame is made from two amino acids, L-phenylalanine and L-aspartic acid. People with phenylketonuria (PKU), who are not able to metabolize phenylalanine, should not use aspartame.

  Though aspartame is used extensively, it is not suitable in cooked foods because it loses its sweetness when heated. Aspartame also loses sweetness over time in liquids, so always check the date codes on diet soft drinks. Aspartame's taste is very similar to the taste of sugar. Aspartame has the ability to intensify and extend fruit flavors, such as cherry and orange, in foods and beverages. For example, aspartame makes chewing gum taste sweet and more flavorful longer than sugar-sweetened gum.

- ***Cyclamate*** is used widely in canned fruits, chewing gum, oral-hygiene products and diet soda in about 100 countries around the world. Cyclamate was taken off the market in the United States in 1970 when questions about its safety and cancer-causing potential surfaced. Cyclamate continues to be used in Canada and elsewhere.

- ***Monk fruit*** concentrate, marketed as Fruit-Sweetness™, has been granted GRAS status as a sweetener and flavor enhancer by the Food and Drug Administration (FDA). It is the first, and to date only all-natural zero-calorie fruit concentrate sweetener, to be GRAS certified by FDA. Sometimes you will see it listed on the ingredient label with its Chinese name "luo han guo" or "luo han fruit" (luo han translates as "monk" and guo is Chinese for "fruit").

- ***Neotame*** is a derivative of amino acid, aspartic acid and phenylalanine. It is approximately 7,000 to 8,000 times sweeter than sugar. Neotame is marketed both as a sweetener with a clean sweet taste without bitter, metallic or off flavors as well as an enhancer to other flavors for foods and beverages.

- ***Saccharin***, the oldest sugar substitute, is a sweetener containing no calories. It was used initially as an antiseptic and food preservative. Saccharin dominated the artificial sweetener market for more than 60 years but was replaced by cyclamate in the 1950s and 1960s. Dieters, people with diabetes and diet-soda drinkers make up a substantial portion of consumers currently using saccharin.

Although virtually all of the research on saccharin indicates it is safe for human consumption, controversy over its safety continues. Findings of bladder tumors in some male rats that were fed very high doses of saccharin led to a public outcry to ban saccharin's use as a sweetener. There is a requirement that foods containing saccharin include a warning label. It is important to note that while some people worry about saccharin, no human risk has ever been substantiated by medical research.

- **Stevia** is a leafy plant native to South America. Stevia sweeteners are highly purified steviol glycosides, which make up the sweetest part of the stevia plant. Stevia sweeteners are natural, contain zero calories, and are 200 to 300 times sweeter than sugar. Stevia is used in many food and beverage products, including some juice and tea beverages, as well as some tabletop sweeteners. For some people, stevia has a licorice-like flavor and aftertaste. Some chefs say it tastes bitter when combined with cocoa or chocolate.

- **Truvia**® is made from stevia leaf extract (listed as rebiana), erythritol, and natural flavors. It is up to 400 times sweeter than table sugar and has a similar granular texture, due to the high-content of erythritol (a sugar alcohol) which serves as a bulking agent. Behind Splenda®, Truvia® is the second best-selling non-nutritive sweetener

- **PureVia**™ is almost identical to Truvia® in chemical makeup, except that it includes isomaltase (sucrose-derived) in addition to the stevia leaf extract (listed as Reb A), erythritol, and natural flavors.

- **Sucralose**, sold under the brand name of Splenda®, is a non-caloric sweetener derived from sugar. It withstands heat and can be used in cooking and baking. The granular tabletop sweetener can be used as a spoon-for-spoon replacement for sugar. Splenda® is FDA approved for use in 18 food categories. Splenda® blend is a combination of granulated Splenda® and sugar, providing half the calories and carbohydrates of sugar.

The Center for Science in the Public Interest, an organization that has been a vocal opponent of artificial sweeteners for many years, has listed neotame and sucralose as the two safest artificial sweeteners (www.cspinet.org/nah/05_08/ chem_cuisine.pdf).

- The sugar alcohols **xylitol**, **erythritol**, **sorbitol**, **isomalt**, **maltitol**, **lactitol** and **mannitol** are sugar-like compounds that naturally occur in some fruits and vegetables. They provide 1.5 to 3 calories per gram, as opposed to sugar's 4 calories per gram. Sugar alcohols have long been used to sweeten sugar-free cookies, candies, chewing gum and toothpastes. They are not as sweet as sucrose and are absorbed more slowly; thus, the government has permitted foods that contain them to be labeled sugar-free. Sugar alcohols do not promote tooth decay, but large amounts can have laxative effects. They are used in some processed foods but are not a cooking ingredient.

Types of Sugar Substitutes

Sweetener	FDA Approved	Sweeter than Sugar	Main Brand Names
Acesulfame-K	1988	200x	Sunette®, Sweet One®
Aspartame	1981	180x	NutraSweet®, Equal®
Neotame	2002	7,000x	n/a
Saccharin	1958	300x	Sweet 'N Low®, Sweet Twin, Sugar Twin®, Necta Sweet
Stevia	2008	200 to 300x	Truvia®, PureVia™, Sweetleaf®, Sun Crystals®
Sucralose	1998	600x	Splenda®

Adapted from: Kroger M, Meister K, Kava R. Low calorie sweeteners and other sugar substitutes: A review of the safety issues. Comprehensive Reviews in Food Science and Food Safety. 2006;5:35-47

From the Kitchen
Susan E. Notter
former Program Co-coordinator
Pastry Arts
Pennsylvania School of Culinary Arts, a division of YTI Career Institute

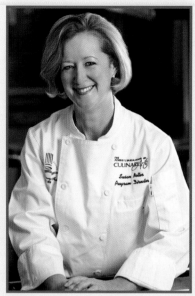

As a child I loved being let loose in the kitchen, baking birthday cakes for my three younger sisters. Given my creative nature and my love of preparing sweets for people, becoming a pastry chef was really a no-brainer, though of course it has its challenges. Being around pastries, chocolates, and creams all day certainly makes it harder to focus on eating a nutritionally balanced diet. In our program, we teach students to prepare desserts with fresh, good quality ingredients, following a European model where moderation is the key. Personally, I really enjoy cooking and eating good food. At home, I cook almost every day, making sure to include fresh fruits for breakfast and fresh vegetables for lunch and dinner—a gym membership helps as well. I think of myself as a person that "Lives to eat," not one that "Eats to live."

As for my favorite ingredients, I enjoy squash in the cooler months; I love the sweet acidity of kumquats, milk couverture from Switzerland and fresh butter lettuce. I'm fortunate to live in Amish country, with lots of local markets selling locally grown-produce, home-made yogurts, preserves, and grass-fed cattle. A perfect snack for me is a freshly baked baguette, a piece of sharp cheddar, tomatoes, and some English pickle.

As chefs, we have a responsibility to our customers to model healthy habits. We must practice what we preach and take the time to enjoy the experience of eating with others socially, rather than just grabbing a sandwich to eat at our desks. I was fortunate to spend time in Italy recently; in the restaurants, people did not have their phones out, they were interacting, having conversations—how novel! All of this—the experience of dining—is equally important to our health and well-being as the food.

Susan Notter grew up in the kitchen, baking cakes decorated like the English cottages of her Birmingham neighborhood. With a mother who didn't bake, this was often the only way she could get her hands on something sweet. She also happened to be good at it. As her interest in pastries blossomed, she left the more traditional dessert culture of England behind for Germany and Switzerland, where she learned about chocolate and spun-sugar while continuing to hone her talent for intricately designed creations.

Since then her career has flourished, and she has amassed a seemingly endless array of titles. She's a culinary Olympian, a top-10 pastry chef, an official Pastry Queen, and a Food Network Champion, to name a few. As Pastry Arts Program Coordinator for the Pennsylvania School of Culinary Arts, she now spends much of her time sharing her skills and knowledge with today's budding pastry chefs.

During the one-year program, three months of which are spent completing an out-of-house externship, Susan's students learn a wide-range of pastry competencies, from how to roll out a simple pie dough to the creation of a centerpiece for their final display. Though her own creations are often referred to as works of art, she understands the importance of a solid foundation—rolling out a crust, whipping up frosting; the artistry can come later.

As for the challenges of maintaining a healthy relationship with sweets when you've made a life out of sugar, Notter's philosophy is simple. She practices what she preaches, and what she preaches is that food is important: How it is grown, where it comes from, what it's treated with, and how it's prepared. No step in the chain is less crucial than another.

Roasted Pineapple Cake with Pina Colada Sorbet and Mango Passion Coulis

Serves: 8

Susan E. Notter,
Program Co-coordinator Pastry Arts, Pennsylvania School of Culinary Arts, a division of YTI Career Institute

This spectacular recipe won a gold medal at the regional ACF Pastry Chef of the Year tryouts.

Pina Colada Sorbet

Dextrose	17	grams
Sugar	80	grams
Stabilizer	2	grams
Water	131	grams
Glucose	25	grams
Pineapple puree	300	grams
Coconut puree	165	grams
White rum	22	grams

1. Combine the dextrose, sugar and stabilizer.
2. Warm the water and whisk in the dry ingredients; add the glucose. Allow to stand for 1 hour. Add the fruit puree and rum.
3. Freeze in a batch freezer.

Coconut Tuile

Butter	38	grams
Glucose	38	grams
Sugar	75	grams
Pectin	1.2	grams
Shredded coconut	65	grams

1. Melt the butter and glucose; whisk in the sugar and pectin and cook for 2 minutes. Stir in the coconut.
2. Spread on a Silpat and bake at 350 °F until golden brown.
3. Allow to cool. Grind into small pieces.

Roasted Pineapple

Butter	35	grams
Brown sugar	25	grams
Orange juice	50	grams
Vanilla bean	1	each
Fresh pineapple	350	grams
Dark rum	35	grams

1. Heat the butter, sugar, juice and vanilla.
2. Place trimmed pineapple in a roasting pan. Add the butter mixture and rum; cover and roast in oven until tender. Remove cover and allow to brown on the outside.

Mango Passion Coulis

Mango puree	100	grams
Passion fruit puree	20	grams
Sugar	5	grams
Gelespessa	1	gram

1. Mix all ingredients; blend with the immersion blender for 2 minutes.

Pineapple Cake

Cake flour	75	grams
Salt	1.5	grams
Nutmeg	1	grams
Cinnamon	1	grams
Baking soda	2	grams
Brown sugar	75	grams
Butter, melted	75	grams
Eggs, whole	65	grams
Dark rum	4	grams
Vanilla bean	1	piece
Fresh pineapple, chopped	40	grams

1. Sift flour, salt, spices and baking soda together in a bowl.
2. Add sugar, melted butter, eggs, rum and scraped vanilla bean.
3. Mix until blended. Fold in the chopped pineapple.
4. Bake at 350 °F for approximately 10 minutes.

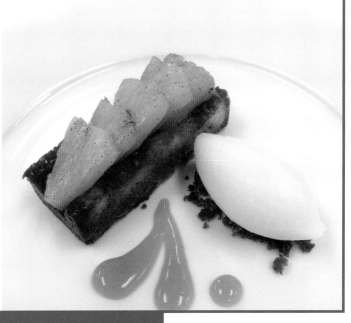

Per Serving

Calories	510	Cholesterol	70	mg
Fat	22 g	Sodium	170	mg
Saturated Fat	1.5 g	Carbohydrates	74	mg
Trans Fat	0.5 g	Dietary Fiber	3	mg
Sugar	62 g	Protein	3	g

Opportunities for Chefs

In addition to being the major source of calories in the diet, foods high in carbohydrates provide an abundance of fiber, vitamins and minerals. Not all carbohydrates, however, are created equal. Emphasis should be placed on preparing meals with foods rich in complex carbohydrates that provide fiber, vitamins and minerals, such as whole grains, vegetables, dried beans and peas, and simple sugars from fruits and dairy products. Care should be taken to limit products with added sugars that contribute few other nutrients to the diet.

Learning Activities

1. Compare the fiber content of equal servings of five different grains or grain products and five different legumes.

2. Compare the sugar content in a selection of 10 beverages: for example, orange juice, apple juice, milk, sweetened green tea beverage, 8-ounce soda, 20-ounce soda, iced coffee, latte, fruit punch, lemonade.

3. Research an uncommon grain and develop a recipe using that grain.

4. Using ingredient lists on food labels, find 10 different foods that contain high-fructose corn syrup.

5. Using nutritional information provided on-site or on the website of a fast food restaurant, plan three meals that provide 8 or more grams of fiber and identify the sources of soluble and insoluble fiber provided.

6. Select three ready-to-eat meals that are marketed to children. Using the label information, compare the grams of total carbohydrate, sugar and dietary fiber in each meal. Using the label information on grams of sugar, determine how many teaspoons of sugar are in each meal. Identify all forms of sugar in the meal from the ingredient list.

For More Information

- Calorie Control Council, **www.caloriecontrol.org**
- Facts about Low-Calorie Sweeteners, International Food Information Council, **www.ific.org/publications/factsheets/lcsfs.cfm**
- *MyPlate*, **www.choosemyplate.gov**
- Nutrition and Health Eating, Mayo Clinic, **www.mayoclinic.com/health/added-gugar/MY00845**
- Whole Grains Council, **www.wholegrainscouncil.org**

Chapter Four

Fats and Oils

Learning Objectives | *After completing this chapter, you should be able to:*

- Describe how the body uses fats
- Distinguish between saturated, monounsaturated, polyunsaturated and trans fats
- List the foods that contain various types of fat and cholesterol
- Explain the recommended daily range of intake for fats
- State the current *Dietary Guidelines for Americans* that relate to fat intake
- Explain the functions of fats in food preparation and discuss how to decrease the amounts used while maintaining texture and flavor
- Compare kinds of oils and fats and identify the best fats to use for various food preparations

Fat adds creaminess to soups, the crunch to a chip and the sizzle to a steak. It also can add excessive calories to the diet and inches to your waist as well as contribute to heart disease. A high fat intake – specifically saturated fats and trans fat – has been linked to a variety of life-threatening diseases, particularly cardiovascular disease and some types of cancer.

Fat is a nutrient. Fats in the diet are essential to life, supplying calories and essential fatty acids that help bodies absorb fat-soluble vitamins A, D, E and K. Our bodies need fat for the normal transmission of brain and nerve signals, to help keep skin smooth, to cushion body organs, to make hormones and to maintain body temperature. While some fat is essential, excessive intake of fats from foods leads to both weight gain and increased health risks. Fat is the body's primary form of stored energy and serves as an emergency fuel reserve in times of decreased food intake.

Fat is very useful in food. It enhances palatability through the senses of smell, sound, touch, taste and texture. Quite simply, fat makes food taste good. For example, while the aroma and sizzling sound of cooking bacon may stimulate the appetite, the crisp, chewy texture of bacon adds to eating enjoyment.

Excess calories from any source — fat, carbohydrate, protein or alcohol — are converted to body fat. Since all fats have 9 calories per gram, and carbohydrates and proteins only 4 calories per gram, fats add

calories more quickly than any other nutrient. Every teaspoon of fat or oil provides about 45 calories. Fats and oils are a concentrated source of calories and should be used carefully when limiting calories. Although individuals have different calorie needs to maintain a healthy weight, most Americans eat too many calories, which has resulted in very high rates of overweight and obesity in this country.

Foods rich in fat are valuable for people who need energy to survive in intensely cold weather or through long periods of physical exertion, such as hiking, hunting, long-distance running or biking. On the other hand, fat-rich foods may deliver too many calories to the person who is not physically active. Labor-saving devices and prolonged time looking at screens have made sedentary lifestyles more common, with weight gain as a frequent result.

Current thinking is that for good health, adults ages 19 and older should consume 20% to 35% of calories from dietary fat each day. [1] Those levels translate into 44 to 78 grams of fat, or 3 to 6 tablespoons of oil, per day for a 2000 calorie diet (see table below, Dietary Fat Guidelines). This range of total fat intake is associated with reduced risk of cardiovascular and other chronic diseases while providing adequate intakes of essential nutrients. These guidelines are not easy for most Americans to follow. The goal is to limit the amount of fat used and select the best types of fat.

Dietary Fat Guidelines

Calories/day	% calories from fat	Calories from fat	Total grams of fat
2000	20%	400	44 grams
2000	35%	700	78 grams

Calories/day	% calories from saturated fat	Calories from saturated fat	Total grams of saturated fat
2000	Less than 10%	200	Less than 22 grams

Fat Isn't All Bad

Many people think that they should eliminate all fat in their diets and that any amount of fat on their bodies is unhealthy. In fact, both dietary fat and body fat have many positive functions. It's important to maintain a sufficient amount of body fat as well as eat enough fat to make hormones, protect organs and help absorb other nutrients.

In addition to its health benefits, fat also plays an important role in the food experience. Fat in food provides crispy, tender and creamy textures. It makes food flaky, crunchy, chewy and sticky – not to mention rich and delicious. Fat also contributes to the flavor and aroma of food.

How do the chef, restaurateur and consumer learn to control fat and use different types of dietary fats to achieve a balance in the diet? Creativity and moderation are the keys.

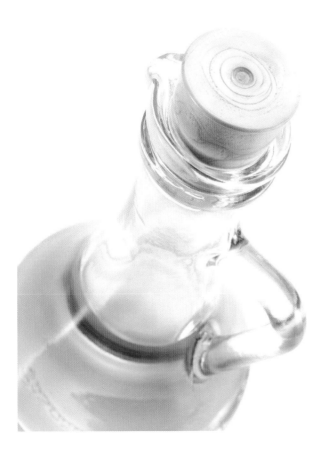

The Science of Fat

From a chemical standpoint, fat, oil, cholesterol, lecithin and other compounds fall into a group called **lipids**. For chefs, the most important lipids are fats, which are generally solid at room temperature; oils, which are generally liquid at room temperature; cholesterol, a wax-like substance found in the body and in food, and lecithin, a lipid-compound that acts as an emulsifier.

Types of Fat

Dietary fats are found in both plant and animal sources. The basic chemical units of fat are **fatty acids**. There are three types of fatty acids — saturated, monounsaturated and polyunsaturated. The type depends on how many hydrogen atoms are in the chemical structure. Basically, fats are chains of carbon molecules with hydrogen molecules attached. At some places, there can be a double bond in the chain, which means that a hydrogen molecule is missing. Fatty acids may have anywhere from 4 to 30 carbons, with double bonds at different places on the carbon chain.

If there is one double bond, the fatty acid is mono-unsaturated; if there is more than one, it is poly-unsaturated; if there are no double bonds and all carbons have hydrogen attached, the fat is saturated.

The more unsaturated fatty acids present in a fat, the more likely it is to be liquid at room temperature; the more saturated fatty acids present, the more likely the fat is to be solid. When fats that are predominantly monounsaturated and polyunsaturated replace saturated fats in the diet, they generally reduce blood cholesterol levels. Fats that are predominantly saturated tend to increase blood cholesterol levels.

Saturated fat is usually solid at room temperature and of animal origin, but there are some exceptions. Tropical oils such as coconut oil and palm oil are predominantly saturated and stay liquid at room temperature. Animal sources of saturated fat include dairy products, beef, veal, lard, tallow, pork, eggs and lamb.

(Saturated Fatty Acid)

Saturated fats in the diet tend to cause an increase in cholesterol, particularly LDL (bad) cholesterol, and are generally linked to increasing the risk of heart disease. High levels of fat in the blood (triglycerides) are also predictors of heart disease.

Most fats in food and in the bloodstream are in the form of triglycerides, three fatty acids linked together. Fats can have three of the same or three different fatty acids forming the triglyceride. When food fat comes from saturated fat, the body tends to make more triglycerides, thus elevating fats in the bloodstream.

Realistically, if you are eating a mixed diet including baked goods, meat, and dairy products, you can't avoid eating some saturated fats. The *Dietary Guidelines* advise replacing saturated fat in the diet with mono-unsaturated and polyunsaturated ones as much as possible. Government advice is to consume less than 10% of total calories from saturated fats, and lowering levels to 7% of calories reduces cardiovascular risk even more. Major sources of saturated fat include regular full-fat cheeses, pizza, grain-based desserts, dairy-based desserts, chicken dishes, franks, sausages, bacon and ribs, burgers, tortillas, burritos and tacos. Several saturated fat sources, particularly processed meats, sausages and bacon, have been linked to increased risk of colorectal cancer as well as cardiovascular disease.

Research in the last decade suggests that stearic acid, one of the shorter-chain saturated fatty acids, which is found in butter, meat and chocolate, does not have a cholesterol-raising effect in the body. Stearic acid can be converted in the body to oleic acid, a monounsaturated fatty acid with heart-healthy benefits.

Monounsaturated fat contains a carbon chain with one point of unsaturation. The structure contains one ("mono") double bond where the carbon molecule is not saturated with hydrogen. Food sources include olives, peanuts, avocados, almonds and their corresponding oils as well as canola, grapeseed and hazelnut oils. Monounsaturated fats are typically flavorful, with the exception of canola and grapeseed oils, which are bland.

(Monounsaturated Fatty Acid)

Monounsaturates are generally considered the healthiest form of fat because they do not elevate LDL cholesterol levels and do not lower protective HDL cholesterol. When possible, substituting monounsaturated fats for saturated ones is a heart-healthy choice. Because all fats have lots of calories, substituting with monounsaturated fat is better than adding it.

Polyunsaturated fat refers to a carbon chain with two or more ("poly") double bonds or two or more points of unsaturation. These fats tend to be of plant origin and are generally flavorless. Food sources include soybean, corn, sunflower, sesame, safflower and walnut oils. Sesame oil is often toasted to create a unique flavor. Mustard oil also contains polyunsaturates but is always used sparingly because of its intense flavor.

(Polyunsaturated Fatty Acid)

All food fats are really a mixture of the three types of fatty acids, but different fats vary in the amount of each type of fatty acid they contain (see table, Comparison of Dietary Fats). Although all food fats contain some of each type of fatty acid, foods are categorized by the type that is present in the greatest amount. Olive oil is called a monounsaturated fat (73% monounsaturated, 14% saturated, 11% polyunsaturated), while butter is called saturated (actually 63% unsaturated, 26% monounsaturated, 4% polyunsaturated). Sesame oil is sometimes categorized as a polyunsaturated fat and sometimes as a mono-unsaturated fat. It has 42% polyunsaturated, 40% monounsaturated fat and 14% saturated fat. The type of fatty acids consumed is now thought to be very important in influencing the risk of cardiovascular disease.

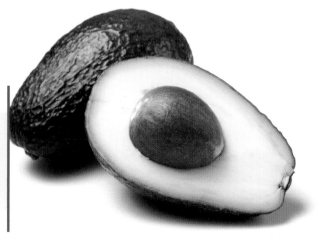

Comparison of Dietary Fats

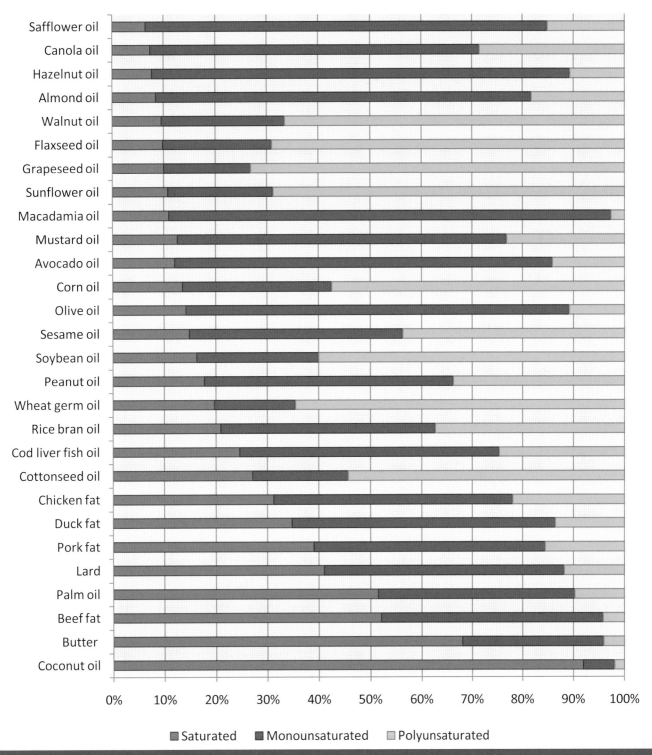

Adapted from: U.S. Department of Agriculture, Agricultural Research Service. 2015. USDA National Nutrient Database for Standard Reference, Release 28. Nutrient Data Laboratory, https://ndb.nal.usda.gov/ndb/

Trans Fatty Acids

When liquid oil is turned into a solid through the process of hydrogenation, some of its fatty acids, particularly those that are monounsaturated, are transformed and trans fatty acids are created. ***Trans fatty acids*** contribute to the stability of hydrogenated fats, helping them stay fresh, prolonging the shelf life of processed foods and baked goods, and keeping snacks, cookies and crackers crisp.

Although trans fats make up a very small portion of total dietary fat intake in the United States (approximately 2% to 6%), they are far more harmful to heart health than saturated fat. Medical research has indicated that trans fats should be reduced or eliminated because they can raise the level of LDL (bad) cholesterol while simultaneously lowering the levels of HDL (good) cholesterol.

Most trans fats are added during food manufacturing. In January 2006, the Food and Drug Administration began requiring that the Nutrition Facts panel on food labels list trans fat content. Mandatory disclosure has prompted food manufacturers to reduce sources of trans fat. Some cities have public health laws that ban the use of trans fat by restaurants. According to the law, food products can list zero grams of trans fat if the food contains less than 0.5 grams per serving. If you typically consume several servings of a food that has .49 grams of trans fat per serving then you could be consuming several grams of trans fats daily. Check the ingredient list for partially hydrogenated oils. This is a clue to the presence of trans fat.

Very small amounts of trans fats are produced naturally by grazing animals, so tiny amounts can be found in meat, milk and dairy products. Because these foods contain such small amounts of trans fat and since they contribute greatly to meeting total nutrient needs, elimination of these foods is not recommended by *Dietary Guidelines for Americans*.

Essential Fatty Acids

Omega-6 and omega-3 fatty acids are polyunsaturated fatty acids. Linoleic acid (LA), an omega-6 fatty acid, and alpha-linolenic acid (ALA), an omega-3 fatty acid, are considered ***essential fatty acids*** because they cannot be made by humans. Other fatty acids can be made by the body from the essential fatty acids. These essential fatty acids—linoleic and alpha-linolenic—help keep cell walls flexible and protect against hardening of the arteries and high blood pressure.

Research has shown that certain types of essential fatty acids are particularly important to health.

- ***Alpha-linolenic acid*** is the important member of the ***omega-3 fatty acids*** family. This fatty acid has been researched the most and has been found to reduce the risk of cardiovascular disease, reduce blood clotting, promote eye health and reduce the severity of autoimmune diseases such as arthritis. The best sources of omega-3 fatty acids are fatty fish such as herring, salmon, mackerel, trout, sardines, anchovies and oil-packed tuna. Grass-fed meats are also a good source. The American Heart Association recommends at least 2 weekly servings of fish, preferably omega-3-rich choices.

What Is Hydrogenation?

To transform liquid vegetable oil into a solid or spreadable form – for example, margarine or solid shortening – the oil must be hydrogenated. Hydrogenation is a commercial process by which hydrogen molecules are forced under pressure through the oil. In addition to hardening the fat, hydrogenation increases its stability and prolongs its shelf life and the shelf life of products made with it. During this process, the molecular structure of the oil is changed and the result is a partially saturated fat. The more an oil is hydrogenated, the greater the change and the more solid the final product. Sometimes the structure of the fat is changed and trans fats are formed. Squeeze bottle or soft tub margarines are less hydrogenated than hard stick margarines.

Food Sources of Essential Fatty Acids	
Fatty Acid	**Food Source**
Linoleic acid	Green leafy vegetables, seeds, nuts, grains, vegetable oils (corn, safflower, sesame, soybean, sunflower)
Alpha-linolenic acid	Oils (canola, flaxseed, soybean, walnut, wheat germ), nuts and seeds (flaxseeds, walnuts, soybeans), fish, grass-fed beef and lamb, soybeans, tofu

Plant sources include walnuts, ground flaxseed, flaxseed oil, canola oil, soybean oil, pine nuts, wheat germ, purslane and other leafy green vegetables. Some foods, such as eggs, milk, soft or liquid margarine, salad dressings and some cereals, have been modified to have more omega-3s. Read labels to identify these foods. The body does not use omega-3s from plant sources as well as omega-3s from fish.

- *Linoleic acid* is the important member of the *omega-6 fatty acids*. This fat is necessary to maintain healthy cell membranes, particularly to avoid skin disorders. In excess, some omega-6 fatty acids can stimulate inflammation and raise blood pressure. Food sources are safflower, sunflower, grapeseed, walnut, corn and soybean oils and green leafy vegetables. Most Americas get plenty of omega-6s from oils used in cooking, particularly fried foods.

Fun Fact

Oil packed tuna has more healthful fats than water-packed tuna. Some of the health promoting fats from the tuna go into water that is usually discarded. It is best to drain oil-packed tuna to avoid excess calories. Save the oil from oil-packed fish to use as the oil in salad dressings or cooking when "tuna" will add to flavor.

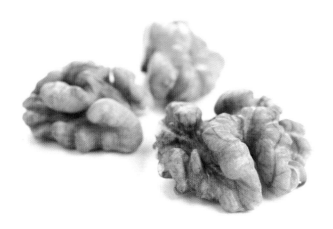

What's That Smell?

Free fatty acids, by-products of fat digestion or breakdown, are single fatty acids unbound to other substances. They are formed when a fat or oil spoils and turns rancid. They are easily noticed because they smell bad. Discard old or improperly stored butter and nut and vegetable oils that have an off odor. They should not be eaten.

Ratio of Omega-3 to Omega-6 Fatty Acids

Optimum balance between omega-3 and omega-6 fatty acids is important. Current thinking is that there is too much omega-6 and not enough omega-3 in most American diets. The popularity of French fries and processed foods has made overconsumption of omega-6 fatty acid a concern.

Cholesterol and Lipoproteins

Cholesterol is a wax-like substance produced by animals and humans and is essential to life. It is part of the outer membranes of cells, provides a fatty protective jacket around nerve fibers in the body and brain cells, and serves as a building block for certain hormones. The cholesterol molecule is also part of the structure of *bile acids*, which are produced in the liver, stored in the gallbladder and later necessary for the digestion and absorption of fat in the digestive tract. In the skin, cholesterol is transformed into vitamin D with the aid of sunlight.

Most cholesterol is made in the body (endogenous). Cholesterol is also in many common foods (exogenous). Endogenous cholesterol is made by the liver and in other body cells. The amount of cholesterol a person makes is largely determined by genetics but also is influenced by the type of fat eaten. Research has found that the most influential dietary components affecting blood cholesterol levels are total dietary fat, saturated fat and trans fatty acids. Dietary cholesterol is found only in animal products, never in plant products, even if plant products are high in fat.

Cholesterol in the human body is sometimes called **serum cholesterol** because it is found in the liquid part of blood, not in the red blood cells. Two main types of proteins in blood, **high-density lipoproteins (HDL)** and **low-density lipoproteins (LDL)**, carry cholesterol. In simple terms, LDL takes cholesterol into the bloodstream and HDL clears cholesterol out of the bloodstream. Thus they are sometimes called **good cholesterol** and **bad cholesterol**. Total cholesterol, when measured in the blood, is a combination of both types.

High levels of LDL are considered dangerous because LDL acts as the vehicle that helps deposit cholesterol on arterial walls, contributing to the buildup of plaque associated with cardiovascular disease, specifically **atherosclerosis**. LDL cholesterol levels in the blood are increased by saturated fat in the diet.

HDL carries less cholesterol and more protein. As it circulates through the bloodstream, HDL picks up cholesterol in the blood and returns it to the liver to be reprocessed or excreted. HDL cholesterol levels in the blood are decreased by the intake of polyunsaturated fats and remain unchanged with the intake of mono-unsaturated fats. For good health, it is beneficial to maintain a high level of HDL cholesterol in the blood.

Both endogenous and exogenous cholesterol create total cholesterol, which is measured by testing blood. When the total cholesterol or LDL cholesterol is too high, it becomes a health risk. A person with high cholesterol is usually advised to reduce dietary sources and may be prescribed medication to reduce the absorption or synthesis of cholesterol. Current medical thinking focuses on assessing the ratio of HDL to LDL cholesterol rather than total cholesterol, which combines both HDL and LDL. If the ratio is good, the risk of heart disease is of less concern so treatment may not be necessary.

Some people make excessive good or bad cholesterol independent of food intake because of genetics. Adults are typically advised to have their cholesterol and other blood fats checked every five years and make dietary modifications or take medications if total cholesterol, LDL cholesterol levels, or other blood fats are too high. Buildup of plaque, a forerunner of cardiovascular disease, often begins in childhood.

Current thinking is that the type of fat consumed is more important than the amount of dietary cholesterol eaten. Consuming less than 300 mg per day of cholesterol can help maintain normal blood cholesterol levels. Currently dietary cholesterol intake by men averages about 350 mg per day while average cholesterol intake by women is 240 mg per day.

The major sources of cholesterol in American diets include eggs, chicken, meat and burgers. All of the cholesterol is in the egg yolk; egg whites do not contain any cholesterol. Years ago, common dietary advice was to severely limit eggs. Much scientific evidence now suggests that one egg per day, including the yolk, does not result in increased blood cholesterol levels and does not increase the risk of cardiovascular disease in healthy people. Eggs are an excellent and economical source of protein and many other nutrients. Fat becomes a problem if eggs are served with bacon, sausage or with Hollandaise or other rich sauces. And while liver and organ meats have very high levels of cholesterol, as you will see on the chart, they are not eaten regularly or in large amounts by most Americans and they are the very best source of many vitamins and minerals.

Food High in Dietary Cholesterol

Food	Cholesterol (milligrams per 3.5 ounce portion)	
Organ meats		
Beef brains	3,010	mg
Goose or duck liver	515	mg
Lamb sweetbreads	400	mg
Chicken liver	345	mg
Turkey giblets	282	mg
Beef liver	275	mg
Egg yolks	185	mg per egg
Shrimp	195	mg
Red meats	60 - 80	mg
Poultry	60 - 70	mg
Seafood	90 - 120	mg
Fish	40 - 60	mg
Butter	33	mg/tablespoon

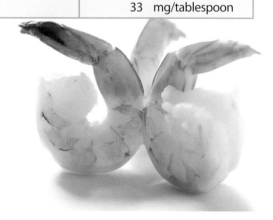

Dietary Fat and Heart Health

Heart disease is the number one killer of both men and women in America. Prevention of heart disease is a critical public health goal. Many Americans have elevated blood cholesterol levels, a key risk factor for heart disease and stroke. Both are caused by deposits of cholesterol-rich plaque in blood vessel linings. Over time, the vessels become hardened and narrow (atherosclerosis), and blood flow to the heart or brain is slowed down or blocked, causing a heart attack or stroke. Heart disease can begin in childhood, so heart health should be a consideration in planning and preparing food for children as well as adults.

Many factors, such as smoking, excess body weight, genetics and stress, are involved in elevating blood cholesterol levels. All fats, including the most heart-healthy varieties, have lots of calories; too many calories cause weight gain, which leads to a variety of health risks. As rates of overweight and obesity soar in both adults and children, every chef should be knowledgeable about fats for personal health and for the health of customers.

The American Heart Association makes the following recommendations for controlling fat and boosting heart health:

- Eat a variety of fresh, frozen and canned vegetables and fruits without high-calorie sauces or added salt and sugars. Replace high-calorie foods with fruits and vegetables.
- Choose fiber-rich whole grains for most grain servings.
- Choose poultry and fish without skin and prepare them in healthy ways without added saturated and transfat. If you choose to eat meat, look for the leanest cuts available and prepare them in healthy and delicious ways.
- Eat a variety of fish at least twice a week, especially fish containing omega-3 fatty acids (for example, salmon, trout and herring).
- Select fat-free (skim) and low-fat (1%) dairy products.
- Avoid foods containing partially hydrogenated vegetable oils to reduce trans fat in your diet.
- Limit saturated fat and trans fat and replace them with the better fats, monounsaturated and polyunsaturated. If you need to lower your blood cholesterol, reduce saturated fat to no more than 5 to 6 percent of total calories. For someone eating 2,000 calories a day, that's about 13 grams of saturated fat.
- Cut back on beverages and foods with added sugars.
- Choose foods with less sodium and prepare foods with little or no salt. To lower blood pressure, aim to eat no more than 2,300 milligrams of sodium per day. Reducing daily intake to 1,500 mg is desirable because it can lower blood pressure even further, but this level of intake severely restricts food choices and is hard to maintain. If you can't meet these goals right now, even reducing sodium intake by 1,000 mg per day can benefit blood pressure.

These recommendations have been incorporated into the current *Dietary Guidelines*. For chefs this means replacing butter, lard and shortening with vegetable oils, particularly canola and olive oils, replacing some meat with seafood, reducing the availability and portions of fried foods, trimming fat from meat, choosing cheeses with less fat, and using fat-free milk and lower-fat dairy products.

Dietary Fat and Cancer

Cancer is the second leading cause of death in America, right after heart disease. Research suggests that dietary fat may be involved in the development of some forms of cancer, particularly prostate cancer. In breast, colon and many other cancers, increased risk is associated with obesity. Since fat contributes many of the additional calories that lead to overweight, fat calories should be controlled to avoid obesity. The American Cancer Society's recommendations for cancer prevention include tracking body mass index (BMI), a statistical measurement indicating body fat through a ratio of weight and height. The ideal BMI is below 25. A BMI chart is found in Appendix E.

Shellfish and Cholesterol

Shellfish, like shrimp, lobster and crayfish, are moderately high in cholesterol. The form of cholesterol in shellfish, however, does not seem to elevate serum cholesterol levels. The American Heart Association says that shellfish do not need to be limited on heart-healthy diets, assuming they are not deep-fried or eaten with lots of butter. Shellfish are an excellent source of protein, low in fat and saturated fat, a good source of omega-3 fatty acids, and high in the minerals selenium, copper, zinc and iodine.

Fats Used in Cooking

Vegetable Oils

All liquid oils have almost the same caloric content, about 125 calories and 14 grams of fat per tablespoon. Oils contain primarily unsaturated fats and are predominantly of vegetable origin (although fish oil is also unsaturated). Vegetable oils contain different amounts of mono- and polyunsaturated fatty acids. Oils high in polyunsaturates include safflower, sunflower, corn, soybean and cottonseed. Oils high in monounsaturates include canola oil, peanut and other nut oils, and olive oil. The most highly praised member of this family is olive oil, which is 77% monounsaturated fat. In taste test comparisons, with few exceptions, monounsaturated fats are more flavorful than polyunsaturated fats. This factor is important for the cook who needs to create the greatest flavor from a minimum of fat.

Some manufacturers are now making blends of oils that are thought to be heart healthy, often with added vitamins, antioxidants and other protective substances.

Olive Oil

Widely promoted as a heart-healthy monounsaturated fat, olive oil is always cholesterol free and is the primary fat used in Mediterranean cuisine. Italian law defines types of olive oil based on pressing, flavor and acidity; olive oils from other countries generally use the same terminology. Olive oils differ in intensity of color, flavor and fruitiness. Some have a strong olive flavor while others are very mild (light in color and flavor). From a nutritional perspective, however, calories per tablespoon remain the same. When an olive oil is labeled "refined," it means the oil has been filtered; it does not mean the olives are top quality or first pressed. When an olive oil is described as "light" that refers to flavor and not calorie content.

Olive oil is an excellent choice for salad dressings, drizzles and marinades. Pure olive oil is fine for sautéing and cooking; extra virgin olive oil is more flavorful and better for other uses. The smoke point of olive oil is fairly low, so it is not very good for frying. Very mild olive oil can be used in baking or when you want an oil without much flavor.

Seed and Nut Oils

Peanut, canola, almond, avocado, mustard seed and hazelnut oils are like olive oil in that they are primarily monounsaturated. Safflower, sesame, sunflower and walnut oils are rich in polyunsaturated fats. Chinese peanut oil, dark sesame oil, macadamia nut oil and walnut oils have very distinct nutty flavors, so just a little has a full-flavor impact. Most light-colored oils are much milder in flavor.

Flax oil and wheat germ oil have robust flavors but are heat sensitive and fragile in chemical structure. They are usually used as food supplements rather than cooking ingredients, but can be added to finished dishes in small amounts, particularly in spa cooking.

Tropical Oils

Tropical oils were once the favored fats for processed foods. Palm and coconut oil had good shelf stability, creamy texture, and other features desired by food manufacturers. However, in the late 1980s these oils fell out of favor because of their saturated fats, which were linked to elevated blood cholesterol. We now know that replacing them with partially hydrogenated vegetable oils, which are high in trans fats, is even worse for the heart than tropical oils.

Some research suggests that coconut oil may not be as unhealthy as once thought. Coconut oil is composed of mostly medium-chain fatty acids, which are metabolized differently from long-chain fatty acids. They tend to be used for energy rather than stored as fat, and they have antimicrobial and antiviral properties. While coconut oil shouldn't be considered off-limits, it doesn't quite live up to the hype. Clearly more research needs to be done on coconut oil.

Chefs should not be particularly concerned about using small amounts of shredded coconut in cooking or as a garnish; it's not the same as deep-frying in coconut oil. A tablespoon of dried, shredded coconut has 33 calories, 3.2 grams of fat and 2.9 grams of saturated fat.

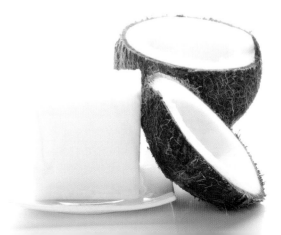

Vegetable Oil Spray

Non-stick vegetable oil cooking sprays are an excellent way to grease pans for cooking while using a minimum amount of fat. Choose brands that leave no unpleasant aftertaste on delicate cakes and other foods. Non-stick spray oils contain lecithin (a fat-related substance), which is added as a release agent so that cakes and muffins can be easily removed from their pans. Parchment paper or foil pan liners are not required when these sprays are used. Coating a pan with cooking spray (or brushing it with oil) and then dusting the pan with flour helps with removing certain types of cakes. A light vegetable oil (canola, safflower or corn, for example) brushed onto the pan with a pastry brush or sprayed from a pump-spray bottle also works. Commercial oil can be purchased in either aerosol-spray or pump-spray forms.

For those with ecological concerns, the Aerosol Education Bureau confirms that since 1978, nearly all United States aerosol manufacturers have stopped using chlorofluorocarbon propellants (CFCs), which are thought to injure the ozone layer. This move is in compliance with bans by the Environmental Protection Agency, Food and Drug Administration, and Consumer Product Safety Commission. Most commercial oil spray products use a hydrocarbon propellant blending propane, isobutane and ebutane, all gases that are environmentally safe.

casebycase | Designing a Restaurant Nutrition Strategy

Maria Caranfa, RDN, LDN, ACSM, EP, developed a multi-faceted nutrition strategy for one of the world's largest casual-restaurant companies, Bloomin' Brands Inc., which includes Outback Steakhouse, Carrabba's Italian Grill, Bonefish Grill, and Fleming's Prime Steakhouse and Wine Bar.

Maria knows her way around a menu. She developed Bloomin' Brands' product-to-plate nutrition strategy and has been instrumental in national menu labeling compliance, nutrition communications, and menu re-engineering. Under her direction, the company removed more than 20,000 calories from its menus by maximizing flavor and minimizing fat. And, she did all of this without sacrificing the experience guests come to expect.

Here are Maria's tips for designing a nutrition strategy:

Environment. Start by understanding the restaurant's customers and the regulatory nutrition environment. Ask your customers what is important to them in terms of health and nutrition when dining out, and develop relationships with national and state restaurant associations to better understand laws affecting the menu.

Business Plan. Embed nutrition into the business plan. Nutrition needs change and grow, new regulations are enacted, and nutrition analysis will change as the menu develops over time.

Resources. Employ registered dietitian nutritionists (RDNs) to lead your nutrition program. RDNs will work collaboratively across all business functions to develop a viable business strategy and a meaningful program for customers.

Platforms. Plan for multiple menu platforms – including paper and digital, menu boards, online ordering, delivery, third-party delivery, corporately owned stores and franchises.

Time. Give yourself more time than you think you will need. Determining and implementing menus, suppliers and products, recipes, operations, resources and organizational culture will be more time consuming than you imagine.

Database. A nutrition database is essential for recipe analysis, including nutrition values, allergens and ingredients. Look for a database designed for nutrition compliance with a strong technology platform and reputation.

Standardization and Methodology. Build standardized processes and strong, defendable methodologies for collecting supplier nutrition information, developing and writing recipes, and applying nutrition analysis techniques.

Communication. Internally, establish how the organization will embed nutrition into the business and foster organizational buy-in. Determine the frequency, audience and subject of nutrition updates. Ensure messaging is truthful and does not violate any FDA content or structure-function claims.

Re-analysis. A nutrition program is a part of the business. Review your strategy regularly to confirm that it is meeting current and addressing future needs.

Connection. Connect with industry professionals to ensure your organization is following best practices; is in-tune with consumer needs; and in compliance with all laws.

Nuts

While nuts are high in fat, most of the fat is the heart-healthy monounsaturated type. Eating some unsalted peanuts and tree nuts, specifically walnuts, almonds and pistachios, can reduce cardiovascular disease risk and lower LDL cholesterol levels. The Food and Drug Administration has also recognized the potential heart-health benefit of nuts and allows a qualified health claim that states that most nuts may reduce the risk of heart disease.

In modest amounts, nuts may also aid weight loss and weight control. The fat, protein and fiber in nuts help people feel full longer, so they may eat less during the day. But nuts should be consumed in small portions. They are high in calories and also can contribute to weight gain.

Nut butters, like almond butter, have become increasingly popular in recent years, showing up next to peanut butter on grocery store shelves. As far as nutritional value is concerned, there is very little

Avocado

Avocados are high in healthy, monounsaturated fats. One cup of avocado has 21 grams of fat, of which 14 grams is monounsaturated. Avocados provide fiber and potassium and are low in sodium. Of course, because it is a plant product an avocado doesn't contain cholesterol.

Avocado can be used to replace foods high in saturated fats, such as sour cream or mayonnaise. Slice avocados on sandwiches, puree and use in a dip or salad dressing.

difference between the two. Almond butter is slightly higher in fiber and calcium and lower in saturated fat; however, peanut butter has higher concentrations of plant sterols and stanols, which may decrease levels of LDL (bad) cholesterol. When choosing a nut butter, make sure to select those with no added sugars or hydrogenated oils and be aware that peanuts are a common allergen.

Nutrient Content of Various Nuts (per ounce)

Nuts (number per 1 ounce)	Calories	Protein (g)	Carbs (g)	Total Fat (g)	Saturated Fat (g)	Monounsaturated Fat (g)	Polyunsaturated Fat (g)
Almonds, 24	160	6	6	14	1	9	3.5
Brazil, 6	190	4	3	19	4.5	7	6
Cashews, 16	160	5	9	12	2	7	2
Chestnuts, 3	60	1	14	0	0	0	0
Hazelnuts or filberts, 21	180	4	5	17	1.5	13	2
Macadamia, 11	200	2	4	21	3.5	17	0
Peanuts, 32	160	7	5	14	2	7	4.5
Pecans, 20 halves	200	3	4	20	2	12	6
Pine nuts, pignoli, 167	190	4	4	19	1.5	5	10
Pistachio, 49	160	6	8	13	1.5	7	4
Walnuts, English, 14 halves	190	4	4	18	2	2.5	13
Walnuts, black, 14 halves	180	7	3	17	1	4.5	10

Source: U.S. Department of Agriculture, Agricultural Research Service. 2015. USDA National Nutrient Database for Standard Reference, Release 28. Nutrient Data Laboratory, https://ndb.nal.usda.gov/ndb/

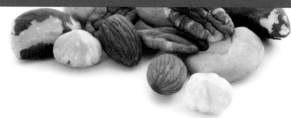

Butter

More than 120 different flavors contribute to butter's unique taste. In many cuisines, butter is considered the best-tasting fat for both cooking and baking. Most chefs prefer unsalted butter. Salt can be added to butter for flavor and to prolong shelf life; it often masks "off" flavors in older butter. **Butter** is made from pasteurized sweet cream. It is an animal fat that contains cholesterol (33 milligrams per tablespoon) and a solid fat that contains saturated fat (7.1 grams per tablespoon). By law, the minimum fat content of butter is 80%; premium and European-style butters have 82% to 88% fat. Water content varies from 10% to 18%, plus 2% milk solids. Whipped butter can be used as a spread to reduce fat and calories per table-spoon, but can't be used reliably in cooking or baking. The culinarian might consider butter a luxury to be used moderately and enjoyed wholly. Use it sparingly but smartly.

Margarine

A French chemist invented margarine during the late 19th century as an inexpensive butter substitute for the army of Napoleon III. **Margarine** is a blend of oils and solid fats that is heated and combined with water, milk or milk solids, emulsifying agents, flavorings, preservatives, coloring and vitamins. Margarine is partially hydrogenated to make it firm and spreadable. Solid (stick) margarine looks like butter.

Although margarine was once considered the perfect alternative to butter because it has no cholesterol, it is now under scrutiny along with other hydrogenated products because of the presence of trans fatty acids. The Nutrition Facts label on margarine lists the amount of total fat, saturated fat and trans fat per tablespoon.

Soft (tub) margarine spreads contain water and air and about 60% fat. Diet imitation margarine and reduced-fat spreads can contain about 40% fat and at least 50% water. These products, as well as soft-tub margarine, are unreliable for baking and cooking. When heated, their chemistry changes and water is released.

While it lacks the unique taste of butter, solid, **stick margarine** has roughly the same fat content – approximately 80% – but it is much lower in cholesterol. In fact, most brands contain no cholesterol. To satisfy kosher dietary laws (separating meat from dairy products), select margarine made without milk solids

or animal fats for cooking or serving with meat meals. Check the label for ingredients. Such margarines are labeled Kosher or Pareve. Select a margarine whose first ingredient is liquid oil high in polyunsaturates (such as liquid safflower oil); avoid products that have hydrogenated or partially hydrogenated oil as the first ingredient.

Several currently available margarines have added plant stanols. These margarines are called functional foods or **nutraceuticals** – that is, foods with ingredients specifically added for health effects. In this case, the plant **stanols** in the margarine can lower blood cholesterol levels if eaten regularly and in quite large quantities. It still is high in calories, so large quantities are a questionable choice.

Solid Shortening

Most **shortening** is made of highly polyunsaturated vegetable oil and contains about half the saturated fat of butter. Solid shortening is designed to go in, not on, food. Because it does not have to taste good or feel good in the mouth, it can contain a generous quantity of emulsifiers to preserve the suspension of the fat in liquid, to hold more air and to stabilize the moisture content of batter. One popular shortening contains 80% liquid soybean oil suspended in a honey-comb matrix of 20% hardened (hydrogenated) oil. It is 100% fat, contains no water and has high levels of emulsifiers added to stabilize the structure of baked goods and increase their absorption of moisture. Recently, many shortenings and cooking fats have been reformulated to remove trans fats.

Lard and Bacon Fat

Lard is rendered pork fat, plus a very small amount of water. It is 100% animal fat and has 14 milligrams of cholesterol per tablespoon. It is 39.2% saturated fat – not as much as one might think. Lard seems to be less harmful to the diet than previously believed; nevertheless, it is not really an option in low-fat cooking because of calories and amounts usually used. Lard is often used in piecrusts and baked goods to impart flakiness and tenderness. It is also a primary cooking fat in cuisines where pork is widely used. Bacon grease (fat released when bacon is cooked) can be used in small amounts to add a distinct flavor. Often with cooking greens or spinach, a small amount of cooked, chopped bacon can add a lot of flavor and pizzazz to a salad or vegetable dish, making it special. **Bacon fat** is nutritionally similar to lard but contains more sodium. Bacon fat, like lard, has slightly more unsaturated fat than saturated fat but does contain almost 40% saturated fatty acids and is not a great choice. One tablespoon of bacon fat has about 115 calories, 13 grams of fat, 12 milligrams of cholesterol and 20 milligrams of sodium.

Schmaltz

Schmaltz is rendered chicken, goose or duck fat. In kosher cooking, chicken fat is commonly used in cooking meals with meat when dairy products such as butter cannot be used. Goose fat is traditional in cassoulet; duck fat is often used, especially in French cuisine, for frying potatoes. Duck fat has a particularly high smoke point and crisps fried foods especially well.

Each of these poultry fats imparts a unique flavor. While traditional dietary guidance suggests removing the skin from chicken because of its fat, chicken fat is primarily monounsaturated. There is little point in removing chicken skin if one must add more fat or oil to cook skinless chicken. As with many fats, the issue is not so much type of fat but rather the amount used.

Cream and Sour Cream

Types of **cream** are grouped by fat content. By law, heavy cream, also called whipping cream, must have at least 36% milk fat; light whipping cream, 30% to 36% milk fat; light cream (coffee cream), 18% to 30% milk fat; half-and-half, 10.5% to 18%. Two exceptions to the regulations are fat-free half-and-half and whipped cream in a squirt can. Fat-free half-and-half is usually a blend of nonfat milk, sweeteners, thickeners, artificial colors and flavors, preservatives, and added vitamins. Typically, it is used to lighten coffee, but it can be substituted for half-and-half in recipes to reduce fat content and calories. Squirt-can "whipped creams" and whipped toppings have widely varying amounts of fat; some have no fat at all.

Sour cream is generally light cream soured with lactic acid bacteria and then homogenized until smooth and pasteurized. Light sour cream with reduced fat is also available. Nonfat sour cream is an emulsion of nonfat milk solids, thickeners and stabilizers. While this version does cut calories and fats, it does not usually impart the flavor, mouth feel and richness of sour cream. Sometimes a better substitution is Greek-style yogurt, another yogurt product or silken tofu.

Should You Use Butter, Margarine, Solid Shortening or Oil?

Butter tastes great and enhances many foods, but contains cholesterol and saturated fat. Margarine lacks butter's flavor and contains some saturated fat – slightly less than one-third that of butter. Margarines may have some trans fat but no cholesterol. You can bake with margarine. Solid shortening has a neutral (or an artificial butter) taste, is reliable for achieving certain qualities in baked goods and has about half the saturated fat of butter. Solid shortening has no cholesterol, but some brands contain trans fats. Because both margarine and shortening are hydrogenated, vegetable oil plus a small amount of butter is sometimes a good alternative. For many uses and in many cuisines, olive and other vegetable oils – with varying flavors and levels of mono- and polyunsaturated fats, but little saturated fat and no cholesterol – are the best choice for healthful cooking.

When using butter as a spread, allow it to come to room temperature. When the butter is soft and spreadable, less is often used.

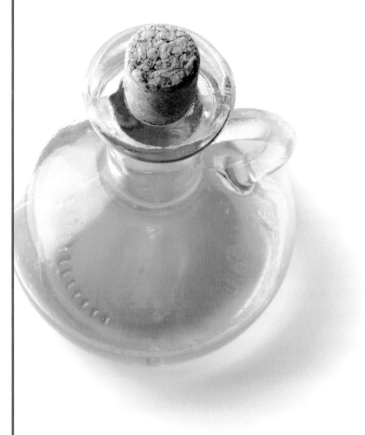

Nutrient Content of Dairy Products and Dairy Substitutes

All values are for 1 cup.

Item name	Calories	Protein (g)	Fat (g)	Saturated Fat (g)	Cholesterol (mg)	Calcium (mg)
Milk, nonfat (skim)	80	8	0	0	5	299
Milk, evaporated skim	200	19	1	0	10	740
Buttermilk, low-fat	100	8	2	2	10	284
Milk, low-fat, 1% fat	100	8	3	2	10	305
Milk, 2% fat	120	8	5	3	20	293
Milk, whole, 3.25% fat	150	8	8	5	25	276
Milk, evaporated	340	17	19	12	75	658
Half-and-half	310	7	28	17	90	252
Light cream	700	5	74	46	265	166
Heavy cream	830	5	89	55	330	156
Yogurt, plain, 0% fat	140	14	0	0	5	488
Yogurt, plain, low-fat	150	13	4	3	15	448
Yogurt, plain, whole milk	150	9	8	5	30	296
Yogurt, Greek, 0% fat	120	20	0	0	0	150
Yogurt, Greek, 2% fat	150	19	5	3	15	150
Kefir	150	8	8	6	35	250
Sour cream, light	320	8	24	15	80	340
Sour cream	440	5	45	26	120	253
Cottage cheese, nonfat	100	15	0	0	10	125
Cottage cheese, 1% fat	160	28	3	2	10	138
Cottage cheese, 2% fat	190	27	6	2	25	206
Cottage cheese, 4% fat	240	24	10	6	50	160
Cheese, ricotta, part-skim	340	28	20	12	76	670
Cheese, ricotta, whole milk	430	28	32	21	125	510
Goat milk	170	9	10	7	25	327
Buffalo milk	240	9	17	11	45	412
Sheep milk	260	15	17	11	65	473
Rice milk	110	1	3	0	0	283
Soy milk	130	8	5	0	0	61

Source: Adapted from: U.S. Department of Agriculture, Agricultural Research Service. 2015. USDA National Nutrient Database for Standard Reference, Release 28. Nutrient Data Laboratory, https://ndb.nal.usda.gov/ndb/

Nutrient Content of Various Cheeses

All values are for 1 ounce. The cheeses listed are among the most commonly used cheeses. Check food labels of other cheeses used in cooking or served.

Item name	Calories	Protein (g)	Fat (g)	Saturated Fat (g)	Cholesterol (mg)	Calcium (mg)
Cream cheese, fat-free	30	4	0	0	5	100
Cream cheese, low-fat	60	2	5	3	15	42
Cream cheese	100	2	10	5	30	28
Mexican queso fresco	40	3	3	2	10	81
Mozzarella, part-skim	70	7	5	3	20	222
Mozzarella, whole-milk	90	6	6	4	20	143
Feta	70	4	6	4	25	140
Goat cheese, soft	80	5	6	4	15	40
Brie	90	6	8	5	30	52
Camembert	90	6	7	5	20	110
Asiago	100	7	8	5	25	202
Provolone	100	7	8	5	20	214
Blue	100	6	8	5	20	150
Gouda	100	7	8	5	30	198
Gorgonzola	100	6	9	6	25	150
Muenster	100	7	9	5	25	203
Edam	100	7	8	5	25	207
American	110	6	9	6	25	175
Cheddar cheese	110	7	9	6	30	204
Cheddar cheese, reduced-fat	80	8	5	4	15	257
Swiss	110	8	8	5	25	224
Monterey jack	110	7	9	5	25	211
Fontina	110	7	9	5	35	156
Colby	110	7	9	6	25	194
Mascarpone	120	2	13	7	35	40
Havarti	120	5	10	7	25	202
Parmesan	120	11	8	5	25	314
Gruyere	120	8	9	5	30	287

Source: Adapted from: U.S. Department of Agriculture, Agricultural Research Service. 2015. USDA National Nutrient Database for Standard Reference, Release 28. Nutrient Data Laboratory, https://ndb.nal.usda.gov/ndb/

Storing Fats

Fats have a tendency to absorb strong odors, so they should be stored covered or well wrapped and away from strong-scented ingredients. Take special care to prevent rancidity, which alters taste and is potentially toxic as well. Rancidity can result when fats are exposed to air and combined with oxygen and water. Research shows that by-products of rancid fats can cause damage to the lining of blood vessels, which may lead to cardiovascular disease.

In general, unsaturated fats (oils) have a less stable molecular structure than saturated (solid) fats. They are more vulnerable to changes from exposure to heat, light and moisture. Oils should be stored in opaque containers in a cool, dark location or should be refrigerated. Cold temperatures sometimes turn oil cloudy. This cloudiness is not harmful; clarity returns as the oil reaches room temperature. Dark-colored specialty oils, such as walnut and hazelnut, are the least stable. Once opened, they should be refrigerated. Their shelf life is from 4 to 6 months. Refined vegetable oils (such as canola, safflower and corn) should be stored in a cool, dry location away from air, heat and light. They generally stay fresh for 6 to 10 months. Many vegetable oils naturally contain vitamin E or similar antioxidants that will help prevent rancidity. Safflower oil is an exception and must always be refrigerated.

Saturated fats such as butter and cream contain enzymes that can affect and accelerate rancidity. It is best to use unsalted butter because salt may mask the smell of rancidity. Butter and margarine should be refrigerated or frozen for short-term use; for long-term storage, they should be frozen.

Tips for Reducing the Fat in Recipes

When cooking with fat, chefs need to choose the right fats and oils and use the correct temperature and cooking techniques. The special qualities of fat are hard to replicate. Successful substitutions, especially in low-fat and low-calorie baked goods, are tricky. Generally, when you cut back or cut out fat, you also must adjust a whole range of carefully balanced components in the recipe. Enhance flavors by increasing or adding agents such as citrus zests, various extracts and, sometimes, sugar. To maintain the desired texture in baked goods, you will need a suitably viscous aerating and moisture-holding fat substitute such as fruit purees (prune, apple or banana), corn syrup, various vegetable oils, whole eggs or stiffly whipped egg whites. Sometimes, adding a little butter will help achieve the proper taste.

To restore the tenderness when fat is removed, try cake flour instead of higher-protein all-purpose flour. Since cake flour absorbs a different quantity of moisture, you must adjust liquids as well. Try acidic dairy products such as yogurt or buttermilk; they inhibit gluten development so that the item remains tender. Sometimes when acids are added, they can be balanced with some neutralizing baking soda.

Fat not only carries flavor but also helps to blend flavors and soften or mute strong or harsh flavors and sweetness. When fat is reduced, other flavors might have to be toned down to prevent them from becoming overpowering. High-fat recipes are more forgiving of mediocre ingredients because of the softening and blending properties of the fat. Thus, when fat is at a minimum, ingredients of the highest quality become even more important. Fat also stabilizes flavors. A lean sauce may taste fine one day but not so good the next.

When reducing the fat in a recipe, think of fat as a limited resource. The more you use in some menu items, the less available for others. Identify which fat or fats will contribute the most to the recipe and get the most flavor and function from the fat used.

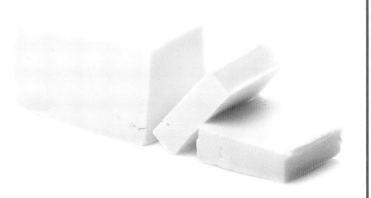

More Healthful Cooking Tips

- Choose low-fat dairy products, such as non-fat yogurt, part-skim ricotta cheese, part-skim mozzarella cheese, buttermilk and evaporated skim milk. For example, using canned evaporated skim milk as an alternative to cream can help create a low-fat sauce that still feels "rich."

- For sauces, concentrate flavors through reductions of stocks and vegetable or fruit juices.

- Rather than a roux, use fruit and vegetable puree or pure starch (arrowroot or cornstarch), gelatin, potato flakes or tapioca as a thickening agent for a sauce or soup.

- Bread and butter on the table can be made more interesting by supplying a variety of tasty whole-grain breads with alternative spreads such as olive oil, fruit butters and chutneys, vegetable pâtés or bean purees. Consider adding red pepper, fresh herbs or a variety of spices to the bread itself (either before or after baking).

- Replace some or all of the saturated fat (butter, cream, etc.) in a recipe with healthier fats such as olive, nut, canola or avocado oil.

- Certain foods require a lot of fat to create the flavor and texture people expect and want. For these foods, consider reducing the portion size or change plate presentation to provide a smaller amount of the "real thing."

- Test fat-free half-and-half, evaporated skim milk, Greek yogurt or reduced-fat sour cream as a replacement for some of the cream or sour cream in a recipe. Adjust seasonings and add thickeners if necessary.

Reading the Label

The Food and Drug Administration and the Department of Agriculture have set specific regulations on allowable product descriptions. The following claims apply to 1 serving.

Fat Free	less than 0.5 grams of fat per serving
Low Fat	3 grams or less of fat per serving
Reduced or Less Fat	at least 25% less fat than the usual product
Light	one-third fewer calories or 50% less fat than the usual product

- Add some brewed tea, vegetable stock or fruit juice to salad dressings to increase volume and decrease calories per tablespoon.

- Use small amounts of toasted nuts or some nut oil in salads to increase monounsaturated fat and create interesting flavors and textures.

- Shift the balance of entrée plates by increasing low-fat vegetables and whole grains and serving smaller portions of high-fat meats or cheeses.

- Use a small amount of strong-flavored cheeses that pack a punch rather than milder high-fat cheeses that melt well. Use cheese on top rather than mixed in dishes to create more visual and taste impact with less cheese (and fat).

- Use buttermilk in some soups and salad dressings to provide creamy texture and interesting flavor without fat.

- A little sesame oil mixed with rice vinegar makes a fine Chinese-style slaw or chicken salad dressing.

- Experiment with pureed potato or potato flakes as a thickener to replace some or all of the cream in some soups.

- Check out eggs that have more omega-3 fat and less cholesterol. Specific branded eggs are from chickens fed special feeds to change the fat and cholesterol content of their eggs.

- Try some of the butter and fat replacers available to the food service industry. Some oils are useful for frying and are altered to provide fewer calories per gram. A variety of fat replacers, including some fruit purees, can be used in place of some of the fat in baked goods that are supposed to be soft and chewy.

- Commonly used food substitution charts often create culinary failures. Real fat provides flavors and textures that are not easily replicated. The same recipe with fat-free yogurt substituted for sour cream will be different. Test, taste and adjust as necessary to create healthful foods to meet your culinary standards and goals. Healthful food must be delicious as well as nutritious.

- Sliced avocados can be used as a substitute of mayonnaise on sandwiches. Mashed avocado can be used in some dips and spreads replacing mayonnaise and sour cream.

Spinach Salad with Green Goddess Dressing

Serves: 10

Brent Ruggles,
CEC, Regional Executive Chef, Las Colinas Country Club, Irving, Texas

Selecting a healthful fat or oil and moderating the amount of fat used are two goals in healthful cooking. This recipe does both! The salad dressing combines the healthful fat of a creamy avocado for texture with a low-fat sour cream and mayonnaise and nonfat buttermilk. The smoked almonds in the spinach salad are reminiscent of a smoky bacon but substitute a healthier fat.

Green Goddess Dressing	Yield 5 cups	
Mayonnaise, low-fat	2	cups
Sour cream, low-fat	1	cup
Chives or scallions, fresh, minced	½	cup
Parsley, fresh, minced	½	cup
Lemon juice, fresh	1 ½	ounces
Vinegar, white wine	1 ½	ounces
Worcestershire sauce	1	ounce
Avocado, fresh, peeled and seeded	2	each
Buttermilk	2	ounces

1. Place all ingredients in bowl of food processor fitted with metal blade.
2. Pulse for 6-8 seconds, 4 or 6 times or until well blended.
3. Taste and adjust seasonings as necessary.
4. Use immediately or cover and refrigerate.
5. Use 2 tablespoons of dressing for each salad. Reserve remaining for additional use.

Per Serving

Calories	70		Cholesterol	5	mg
Fat	6	g	Sodium	95	mg
Saturated Fat	1.5	g	Carbohydrates	3	mg
Trans Fat	0	g	Dietary Fiber	1	mg
Sugar	1	g	Protein	1	g

Spinach Salad with Green Goddess Dressing and Smoked Almond Garnish	Serves 10	
Baby spinach, washed well	1 pound 4	ounces
Green Goddess salad dressing	10	ounces
Red onions, fresh, peeled and sliced into thin rings	5	ounces
Smoked almonds, whole	10	tablespoons
Tomatoes, currant or grape	10	ounces
Pepper, freshly cracked or coarsely ground	¼	teaspoon

1. Place spinach on a chilled plate. Drizzle with Green Goddess dressing (or serve dressing on side if guest prefers).
2. Garnish salad with 3 thin red onion rings, 1 tablespoon smoked almonds, tomatoes.
3. Sprinkle cracked black pepper over top of salad at service.

Per Serving

Calories	150		Cholesterol	5	mg
Fat	11	g	Sodium	230	mg
Saturated Fat	1.5	g	Carbohydrates	13	mg
Trans Fat	0	g	Dietary Fiber	5	mg
Sugar	2	g	Protein	4	g

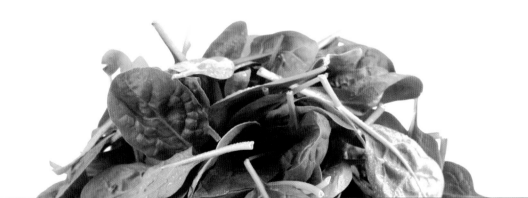

From the Kitchen
Jason Bruner, *Executive Chef*
1801 Grille
Columbia, South Carolina

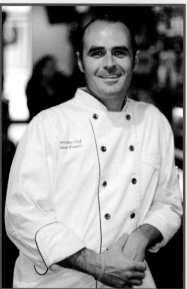

Nutrition plays a large role in both my professional and personal life, one influencing the other. I have worked at many establishments around the world, and all have allowed me to use healthy and fresh/local ingredients while learning how to source them. I love to use grains such as quinoa and farro, in addition to cooking techniques such as steaming and sous vide. I have always been a supporter of local agriculture, and at 1801 Grille we pride ourselves in using as many local, seasonal ingredients as possible.

As a chef, I feel I hold a certain level of responsibility to the community and serve flavorful yet healthy food options. My food is freshly prepared and often times locally sourced, and I'm able to take pride in the dishes I serve because I know I'm providing high quality meals. I want to leave this world a better place than I found it and fueling my community with healthy food is one way to achieve that.

Jason Bruner was born and raised on the bayou in South Louisiana, a region where the food culture is influenced by a melting pot of styles and traditions: Creole, French, Italian, and Mexican. His career began in New Orleans, where he worked as a line cook until Katrina hit and he moved north to Connecticut. There, he was accepted into the Culinary Institute of America, which opened doors for him and afforded him the opportunity to hone his craft in places as far-flung as Maui, Italy and China. Eventually, he returned to the south, planting his roots in Columbia, South Carolina, which is home now.

As the executive chef of 1801 Grille, Jason believes food is the great connector, bringing people together regardless of their background or politics. He also believes in cultivating the relationship between food and farmer, which ultimately translates to chef and farmer. He regularly travels to the source to see how things are being grown, how the food is handled. Whether it's strawberry shortcake featuring berries from the farm just up the street, or farm-raised boar and bison from just across the border in North Carolina, or grit fries made from grits milled right in Columbia, Jason knows that serving local, sustainable food is not only better for people's health, but ultimately for the community as well.

Trout Almondine with Mashed Potatoes and Green Beans   Serves: 10

Chef Jason Bruner
1801 Grille, Columbia SC

The crunchy almond coating on the trout with the creamy mashed potatoes and crisp green beans is a balanced meal in more ways than one.

Russet potatoes	10	each
Half & half	½	cup
Salt	½	teaspoon
White pepper	¼	teaspoon
Cut green beans, cut 2 ½ inch	2	pounds
Skinless rainbow trout filet	10	(6 ounces each)
Crushed almonds	¼	pound
Sunflower oil	¼	cup
Panko bread crumbs	1	cup

Per Serving

Calories	560	Cholesterol	95	mg
Fat	21 g	Sodium	400	mg
Saturated Fat	1.5 g	Carbohydrates	55	mg
Trans Fat	0 g	Dietary Fiber	8	mg
Sugar	6 g	Protein	40	g

1. Peel potatoes and cut into large dice.
2. Blanch potatoes until fork tender, drain, place on sheet tray in 350 °F oven and dry for 2 to 4 minutes. Once dry, place in a large mixing bowl.
3. Bring half & half to a simmer over medium heat. Add to mixing bowl with potatoes and whisk until smooth. Add salt and pepper.
4. Blanch green beans for 2 to 4 minutes and shock in cold ice water. Heat 1 tablespoon sunflower oil in sauté pan over medium heat. Add green beans to hot pan and sauté for 2 to 3 minutes.
5. Mix crushed almonds with panko bread crumbs and add 1 tablespoon sunflower oil to mixture. Press one side of each filet into the bread crumb mixture. Heat remaining sunflower oil over medium high heat. Place trout almond side down into the hot pan and cook for 2 to 3 minutes on each side. Place on a resting rack.
6. Using a piping bag, pipe the potatoes onto each plate. Place green beans alongside the potatoes and top with your trout filet, almond side up.

Fats at-a-glance

Type of Fats	Characteristics	Sources	Health Effect
Saturated Fats	Solid at room temperature (usually) Carbon chain is saturated with hydrogen	Mostly animal fats Tropical oils (coconut, palm)	Raise LDL cholesterol Raise total blood cholesterol
Trans Fats	Most formed during hydrogenation of oils and used in food processing	Partially hydrogenated oils	Raise LDL (bad) cholesterol May lower HDL (good) cholesterol
Monounsaturated Fats	Liquid One double bond on carbon chain	Olives, peanuts, avocados, almonds, canola oil, grapeseed oil, hazelnut, pecans, pumpkin seeds, sesame seeds	Improve blood cholesterol levels Reduces LDL (bad) cholesterol

Polyunsaturated Fats	Liquid
	Two or more double bond on carbon chain
	Types:
	  Linoleic acid
	  Omega-6 fatty acids
	  Linolenic acid
	  Omega-3 fatty acids
		Omega-6 Polyunsaturated Fats
		  Soybean, corn, safflower
		Omega-3 Polyunsaturated Fats
		  Soybean oil, canola oil, walnuts, flaxseed, Fatty fish (trout, herring, salmon, tuna, mackerel, sardines)
			Improve blood cholesterol levels
			Reduces LDL (bad) cholesterol

Opportunities for Chefs

Fats and oils are part of a healthful diet, but the type and total amount of fat used in food preparation are very important considerations in healthful menu planning. Dietary recommendations suggest that fat be limited to less than 35% of total calories. All fats are concentrated sources of calories, so total fat should be limited to avoid weight gain. Saturated fats, trans fats and dietary cholesterol should be reduced and/or replaced by healthier oils. Fats and oils come from a wide variety of sources. Animal fat is the primary source for saturated fat and cholesterol. Plant oils are generally more heart-healthy options. In general, healthful menus limit fried foods, and ingredients that are high in fat are used in moderate amounts.

Learning Activities

1. Determine the amount of fat and the equivalent in teaspoons of oil for the following foods:
   - 6-ounce filet mignon
   - half rack of pork spare ribs, barbecued
   - 2 pieces of fried chicken
   - 4-ounce grilled pork chop
   - 6 ounces of poached salmon
   - 1 ½ cups macaroni and cheese
   - 1 slice of pepperoni pizza

2. Determine the amount of fat in the following:
   - 12-ounce chocolate milkshake
   - 1 cup vanilla ice cream
   - 1 cup frozen yogurt
   - 1 cup Greek-style yogurt
   - 1 cup tapioca pudding

3. Select your five favorite cheeses and calculate the calories and amount of fat in 2 ounces of each using the chart on page 78 or food labels.

4. Using food labels, identify six foods that contain at least 5 grams of saturated fat, 5 grams of monounsaturated fat or 5 grams polyunsaturated fats.

5. Using the USDA database, figure out the amount of calories, total fat, saturated fat, monounsaturated fat, polyunsaturated fat and cholesterol in 1 ounce of chicken skin. Is using boneless, skinless chicken breast or thighs better? Why or why not?

6. Compare calories, fat and types of fat in one standard serving of potato chips, tortilla chips, baked potato chips, pita chips and popcorn using food labels.

7. Using the Fats at-a-glance chart on page 87, write a one-page report on the two best oils to have in each professional kitchen. Consider taste, practicality, nutrition and cost in justifying your choices.

For More Information

- American Heart Association, Heart-Check Meal Certification Program (Foodservice), **www.heart.org**
- *Dietary Guidelines for Americans, 2015-2020*, **www.dietaryguidlines.gov**
- *MyPlate*, **www.choosemyplate.gov**
- The International Tree Nut Council Nutrition Research & Education Foundation, **www.nuthealth.org**
- New York City No Trans Fat Help Center, **http://www1.nyc.gov/nyc-resources/service/2632/trans-fats**
- National Dairy Council, **www.nationaldairycouncil.org**
- National Livestock and Meat Board, **www.beefitswhatsfordinner.com**
- International Olive Oil Council, **www.internationaloliveoil.org**

Chapter Six

Water and Beverages

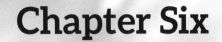

Learning Objectives | *After completing this chapter, you should be able to:*

- Identify functions of water in the human body
- Explain how much water the body needs
- List the signs and causes of dehydration
- Discuss the types of water available for foodservice operations
- List the pros, cons and sources of caffeine
- Compare the nutrient contributions of various non-alcoholic beverages
- Discuss the health benefits and potential harm of beverages containing alcohol

Humans can live for several weeks without food but only a few days without water. Liquids such as juice, milk, coffee, tea and carbonated beverages help meet the daily need for water as do foods, many of which contain more water than is readily apparent. A fluid is any liquid. **Water** is H_2O, two hydrogen molecules and one oxygen molecule. But all fluids, and many foods, are primarily water.

Water, Water Everywhere

About 60% of the adult body is water. In a 150-pound person, that adds up to about 90 pounds or the equivalent of more than 11 gallons of water. Fluid within cells (intracellular water) accounts for about 45% of body weight. Other fluids in the blood, including lymph, spinal fluid, secretions (extracellular water) and the fluid around and between cells, make up about 20% of body weight. The brain and muscles are mostly water (by weight); even bones contain about 20% water.

Water is a medium for the chemical reactions within cells. It transports nutrients to cells and waste and toxic substances away from cells. Water is a solvent for body compounds, lubricates the joints and plays a principal role in the regulation of body temperature through perspiration.

How Much Water Does the Body Need?

Actual water needs depend on many factors, such as food consumed, environmental temperature and humidity, age, activity level and state of health. Although there is no strong scientific basis to support actual quantities of water needed, Dietary Reference Intakes recommend 9 cups for women and 13 cups for men each day. [1] This estimate is based on national food surveys and does not include the additional water in solid foods. Keep in mind that the 9- to 13-cup recommendation includes all beverages, soups and other liquids.

Water...

- Is essential for life and is part of every living cell
- Represents about two-thirds of body weight
- Is the medium for all biochemical processes (digestion, absorption and excretion)
- Maintains blood volume and transports nutrients and oxygen throughout the body
- Helps maintain body temperature
- Acts as a lubricant for joints
- Cushions and protects organs and the fetus during pregnancy
- Is necessary for elimination and proper kidney functions
- Keeps skin and tissues in the eyes, lungs and air passages moist and supple

An Institute of Medicine report found that most healthy people get enough fluids and regulate body fluids well. There is little evidence that consuming more fluids is better or that drinking more water will increase moisture in skin for example. Thirst is a good indicator of the need for fluid. [2] Clearly, this finding excludes individuals with abnormally high needs due to illness, kidney disease, intense sweating or an inability to drink. Dark yellow urine can mean that the urine is too concentrated and that more liquids are necessary for good kidney functioning.

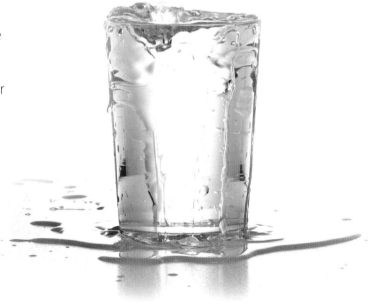

Fluid Balance

Getting water into the body is the first stage of hydration. But keeping water in the body in the amount cells need requires certain minerals. Fluid balance is maintained by **electrolytes**, which are minerals (sodium, potassium, chlorine, calcium, phosphate and magnesium) in the body that, when dissolved in water, have an electric charge (positively or negatively charged ions). Electrolytes regulate the electrical activity within cells, cellular acid base balance and proper fluid level. The human body can function only within a certain range of acid:base ratio. If the body becomes too acid or alkaline, nerve impulses are not properly transmitted, muscles can't function and fluid shifts disrupt normal cellular activity. The kidneys generally control electrolytes, which enter the body in food and are excreted primarily in urine and sweat.

Sodium and potassium levels require balance to maintain optimal hydration. Since most people eat too much sodium and too little potassium, eating less sodium and more good sources of potassium such as bananas, potatoes and other fruits and vegetables and yogurt improves fluid balance and helps maintain normal blood pressure. Foods rich in potassium provide other electrolytes as well. This is discussed in Chapter 7 in the section on minerals.

Water Intake and Output

Dietary sources of water include beverages and foods. Meat is 40% to 75% water, fruits and vegetables 70% to 95% water and bread approximately 35% water. Water also becomes available to the body when food is burned for calories. Fluid is lost through urine, feces, sweating and breathing.

Generally, consuming a varied diet and drinking beverages as thirst dictates meet the body's need for water to maintain adequate hydration. People who are physically active for prolonged periods of time and those exposed to hot temperatures or humid weather should consume extra liquids to compensate for losses from sweat. During times of profuse perspiration, the body can lose 2 to 4 gallons of fluid per day. (Keep this in mind in a hot kitchen.) Runners and distance cyclists need constant replenishment of fluids. Illnesses that include fever, vomiting or diarrhea cause fluid losses that require replenishing. Pregnant and breastfeeding women need additional water because of their increased blood volume and losses from milk production.

Thirst, the desire for water, which is controlled by the hypothalamus portion of the brain, serves as a regulator that keeps the body's water content within normal limits. Healthy people with well-functioning kidneys generally maintain fluid balance – that is, they take in about as much fluid as they excrete each day. If more water is consumed and retained, the result is swelling or edema, often in hands and arms or legs and feet. If too little water is consumed or secretion is excessive, **dehydration** results. In a state of dehydration, cells contain less liquid, and electrolytes become too concentrated. For many people, the first sign of dehydration is a headache. Severe dehydration causes aching muscles, disorientation, irregular heartbeat and even death. Children, seniors and people who are ill are more susceptible to dehydration than others.

Fluid Balance: Typical Intake and Output

Average Fluid Intake (in milliliters)*		Average Fluid Output (in milliliters)	
Beverages	1,300 ml	Urine	1,300 ml
Water from foods	900 ml	Feces	150 ml
Water from metabolism of food	300 ml	Skin (perspiration)	700 ml
		Lungs (expiration)	350 ml
Total average intake	2,500 ml	Total average output	2,500 ml

*237 ml – 1 cup of water

Dehydration: Signs and Effects

Causes	Signs
• Perspiration • Vomiting • Exercise • Burns • Diarrhea • High fevers • Kidney disease	• Dark yellow urine (the lighter the color, the higher the hydration) • Dry mouth (the last outward sign of dehydration) • Flushed skin • Fatigue • Impaired physical performance • Headache • Non-infectious recurring or chronic pain • Heartburn/stomach ache • Lower back pain • Mental irritation and depression

Safe Water

In the United States, fresh, pure water is taken for granted. The U.S. Environmental Protection Agency (EPA) regulates tap water (also referred to as municipal water or public drinking water). Most municipalities monitor water quality, filter water and add small amounts of chlorine and fluoride as a public health measure. Water sources generally meet standards set by the Safe Drinking Water Act (**https://www.epa.gov/sdwa**). The lead contamination of water in Flint, Michigan in 2015 focused public attention of the importance of monitoring water and water distribution systems.

Despite safeguards, however, each year there are thousands of cases of water-borne illness from contamination or improper water treatment techniques. Water contaminants include radon (which makes water radioactive), lead from old pipes, nitrates and pesticides from agricultural contamination of ground water, and chemicals from agricultural wastes. Severe storms can cause flooding that pollutes water systems. Municipal water is usually tested for these elements as well as for biological contaminants such as microscopic parasites that are not destroyed by routine chlorination. Areas that use well water, rather than municipal water, should be monitored carefully for water safety. The United States no longer has cholera or typhoid fever, but hurricanes, tornadoes and flooding are a constant reminder that maintaining a safe water supply is a worldwide concern.

How to Conduct a Water Tasting

Conducting a blind water tasting is useful in selecting bottled waters for a foodservice operation. Waters should be judged on the following characteristics:

- **Appearance**: Hold the glass up to the light. A good water will be clear, bright and show no floating particles. Watch out for lint in the glass.
- **Odor:** Sniff the water in the glass. Highest scores are given to those waters with no odor. Some waters will smell of minerals or sulfur.
- **Flavor**: Take a sip of the water and roll it around in your mouth, letting it flow over the tongue. Descriptors for flavor may include: alkaline, bitter, calciferous, cool, flat, fresh, lively, salty/saline, sour, stale or sweet.
- **Mouthfeel:** As you are swirling the water in your mouth, note how your mouth feels. You want a clean edge, a fresh and light texture – nothing flabby, cloying or musty. Carbonation, or its absence, together with the size, amount and distribution of bubbles, contributes significantly to the mouthfeel of water.
- **Aftertaste**: After you swallow the water, notice the sensation that remains. Tastelessness, thirst quenching and clean are the positive qualities.

Similar tastings can be done to determine which bottled, sparkling or mineral waters will be offered in your operation.

Chlorine and Fluoride

Chlorine is a chemical added in tiny amounts (chlorination) to water as a public health measure to reduce waterborne illness. Chlorine kills microorganisms such as typhoid and hepatitis.

Fluoride is a substance that contains the mineral fluorine, which is known to strengthen tooth enamel and makes bones stronger. *Fluoridation,* a public health policy for more than 40 years, adjusts the fluoride concentration in drinking water to 1 part fluoride per 1 million parts of water. According to the American Dental Association, tooth decay is reduced by 20% to 40% in fluoridated areas, even when fluoride from other sources – such as fluoride toothpaste, tea, canned salmon and sardines – is widely available. Excessively high fluoride levels, however, may cause spots on (or discolored) teeth.

Source: American Dental Association Fluoridation Facts, https://www.ada.org/~/media/ADA/Member%20Center/FIles/ fluoridation_facts.pdf?la=en

The Taste of Water

Minerals, trace elements and carbonation combine to create the taste of water. The most common tastes in tap water come from chlorine (from chemicals used in water treatment), iron (from pipes, storage tanks and nature) and sulfur (usually from natural hot springs). Some natural sources also contain algae, ranging from seaweed to pond scum, which imparts tastes and odors ranging from grassy and musty to spicy and septic.

The taste differences in water are very subtle, especially when compared to wine and other beverages, but they are discernible. A water's unique taste reflects its origin. Geological strata allow water to absorb minerals; each area's mix of minerals contributes to the unique characteristics of a single-source water (water drawn from one location).

Bottled water has varying degrees of minerals that create a range of flavor, mouthfeel and aftertaste, depending on one's sensitivity to taste. Some spring waters contain sodium, magnesium, sulfates, bicarbonates, chromium, copper, calcium and/or zinc. Some spring water also has a natural effervescence, often labeled as *sparkling water*.

Cucumber Lemon Refresher
Serves: 10

This refreshing beverage can be kept in the cooler both for staff working in the hot kitchen and for guests. It is especially nice served with fresh seafood salads.

Cucumber slices, 1/8 inch thick	20	each
Lemon slices, 1/8 inch thick	10	each
Water, hot	3	quarts

1. Put cucumber, lemon and hot water in a large pitcher or gallon container. Chill overnight or at least 8 hours.
2. Serve cold.

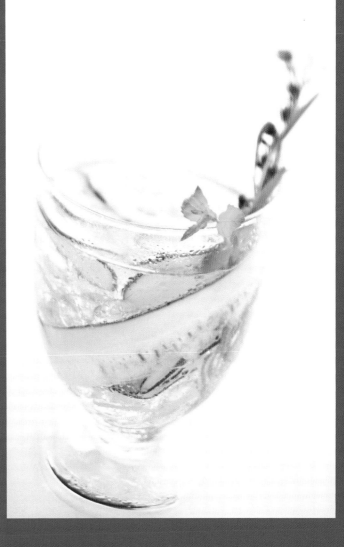

Bottled Water . . . and Water in Bottles

The Food and Drug Administration (FDA) regulates bottled water as a food. FDA established specific regulations for bottled water in Title 21 of the Code of Federal Regulations, including standard of identity, which are regulations that define different types of bottled water and have quality regulations that establish allowable levels for contaminants (chemical, physical, microbial and radiological). Some bottled water producers use municipal water as a source, filtering and removing minerals and chemicals. By FDA definition, **bottled waters** can contain no added ingredients except for antimicrobial agents or fluorides. Most popular brands of bottled water do not contain fluoride, a compound that is important to dental health.

Choose bottled waters from companies that belong to the International Bottled Water Association (**www. bottledwater.org**), an industry group that requires members to meet health and safety standards higher than federal government standards. NSF certification is also desirable. NSF International, a not-for-profit, non-governmental organization, is the world leader in standards development, product certification, education and risk-management for public health and safety (**www.nsf.org**).

Water with any added ingredients (other than anti-microbial agents or fluoride) is a multi-component beverage and must bear an ingredient list on the label. Waters with added carbonation (carbon dioxide), soda water (club soda), tonic water and seltzer water are regulated by FDA as soft drinks. Club soda has salt added for flavor. In the United States, carbonated water can be mineral water or processed water. The more carbon dioxide present, the more acidic the taste and the more active the bubbles.

Waters flavored and sweetened with sucrose or high-fructose corn syrup and/or sucralose are basically reduced-calorie fruit drinks. Children who drink them can be conditioned to think that all beverages, even water, should be sweet. Other bottled waters have some fruit juice added. Some are flavored with acai, pomegranate, blood orange, red grapefruit or other fruits with antioxidants or phytochemicals. The percentage of juice is always listed on the label. Some have sugar added, but many fruit-flavored sparkling waters have no calories or carbohydrates.

Flavored and/or nutrient-added water beverages are simply bottled water with flavoring. Some may also contain added nutrients such as vitamins, electrolytes (such as sodium and potassium) and amino acids. Ingredients in these flavored and nutrient-added water beverages must meet bottled water requirements if the term "water" is highlighted on the label. In addition, the flavorings and nutrients added to these beverages must comply with all applicable FDA safety requirements and must be identified in the ingredient list on the label.

Water is called "**hard**" when its mineral content is high, mostly as a result of calcium and magnesium. Because calcium firms the walls of plant cells, cooking with water containing more than 90 milligrams of minerals per liter can affect the texture of foods. For example, dried legumes and vegetables take longer to become tender when cooked in hard water. Coffee and tea made with hard water are weaker brews. "**Soft**" water, which is high in sodium, softens cell walls faster; vegetables cooked too long in soft water become mushy.

Flowing 'Green'

Bottled waters are not a "green" choice because of packaging and the energy and materials used to create bottles and cans and fuel used to transport them. Environmental awareness is causing some consumers and chefs to take another look at tap water. Some foodservice operations are serving water that has been filtered onsite using a reverse osmosis system. These waters can be offered still or sparkling, with or without ice. LEED (Leadership in Energy & Environmental Design) certification requires an examination of water use. Filtered tap water lessens impact on the environment.

Bottled water:

- Is more expensive than tap water
- Uses fossil fuels for manufacture and transport
- Creates a need for glass or plastic bottles or cans, caps and wrapping that produce additional waste, even if recycled

Types of Bottled Water

Type	Definition from Food and Drug Administration Labeling Rules
Artesian water	Water from a well that taps a confined aquifer in which the water level stands above the top of the aquifer
Purified water	Water produced by distillation, deionization, reverse osmosis or other suitable processes and meeting the definition of "purified water" in the *U.S. Pharmacopeia* (revision 23, January 1, 1995); also may be called "demineralized water," "deionized water," "distilled water" and "reverse osmosis water"; has virtually no flavor
Sparkling water	Water that, after treatment and possible replacement of carbon dioxide, contains the same amount of carbon dioxide that it had at emergence from the source
Spring water	Water from an underground formation from which water flows naturally to the surface of the earth at an identified location; may be collected at the spring or through a bore-hole tapping the underground formation feeding the spring; may or may not be carbonated or mineral water
Mineral water	Water containing at least 250 parts per million (ppm) total dissolved solids that come from a geologically and physically protected underground water source; minerals must be naturally present

Source: https://www.fda.gov/food/guidanceregulation/guidancedocumentsregulatoryinformation/bottledwatercarbonatedsoftdrinks/default.htm

Waters Not Defined by Government Standards

Type	Description
Flavored water	Bottled water with flavoring; must meet bottled water requirements if the term "water" is highlighted on the label; flavorings must comply with all applicable FDA safety requirements and must be identified in the ingredient list on the label
Nutrient-added water	Bottled water that contains added nutrients such as vitamins, electrolytes (sodium and potassium) and amino acids; may also contain flavor extracts and herbal supplements
Fitness water	Water that is lightly flavored to enhance taste; often contains small amounts of vitamins and added oxygen and/or antioxidants

Source: www.fda.gov/Food/ResourcesForYou/Consumers/ucm046894.htm

Coffee

Coffee is a socially acceptable and legal stimulant that helps many people get started and stay energized each day. It is the most popular hot drink in the United States. Contrary to popular belief, it is not made from a bean. Those so called "beans" are actually seeds of the coffee cherry. High heat used in roasting and processing coffee beans concentrates oils, tannins, tars and other chemicals that provide coffee's essential flavors and create its distinctive aroma. Coffee consumption is increasing annually, and the gourmet coffee trend remains strong. Coffee and its many variations are now sold everywhere. Iced coffee has gained popularity in the past decade, particularly among women and teenage girls. Although "a cup of coffee" is a common idiom, many people drink their coffee from mugs that hold far more than an 8-ounce cup.

Coffee is available in many forms including regular, decaffeinated, light (with half the caffeine), flavored and instant. Pure coffee has very few calories, but many people add milk, cream and/or sugar that alter nutrient value. Instant flavored coffee generally contains substantial amounts of non-fat dry milk, sugar and often also partially hydrogenated vegetable oil. Many "coffee drinks" contain a significant amount of fat and sugar, and some have 500 or more calories per serving. Lattes and cappuccinos (regular or decaf) contain milk and are an excellent way to boost calcium intake. Generally, lattes contain more milk than cappuccinos that have frothed milk. Both can be a very healthful choice if made with fat-free or low-fat milk.

Either chemical solvents or a water process is used to remove the caffeine from coffee. Swiss water-processed decaffeination is currently the safest method. *Chicory*, which has an aroma and flavor similar to coffee but no caffeine, is used as a coffee substitute or is blended with coffee to reduce caffeine content. Scientists at the University of Hawaii and elsewhere are working to create genetically engineered caffeine-free beans by isolating the protein that creates the caffeine gene and then growing plants without that gene.

In addition to caffeine, coffee contains two other stimulants – theophylline and theobromine – which are also present in chocolate, especially dark chocolate, and in tea. The effects of these stimulants is milder than caffeine.

Recent research suggests that those who drink coffee have a longer lifespan. One study found people who drank three to five cups of coffee per day had about a 15 percent lower risk of premature death compared to people who didn't drink coffee [3]. Coffee consumption has been linked to a decreased risk of stroke and may cut the risk of Type 2 diabetes. Coffee consumption is also related to lower risk of colorectal cancer. It is unclear which components of coffee cause this. While there is good news in growing evidence that moderate coffee consumption may play a role in optimizing health, moderation remains key.

Does Green Coffee Bean Extract Promote Weight Loss?

In January 2012, a very small 22-week study of 16 adults in India who took green coffee bean extract supplements was published and widely reported, raising hopes for a "magic bullet" for weight loss. The theory was that unroasted green coffee beans contain chlorogenic acid, an antioxidant substance that may boost metabolic rate. The extract must be taken as pills or capsules because it is so bitter. The small study was funded by the supplement manufacturer. The study found substantial weight loss among the subjects.

Chefs and others should be wary of publicized health benefits especially when:

- It is a single study
- The research is on only a small number of subjects
- The study is short in duration
- It is in a non-scientific publication or the popular press
- It is presented in a journal that is not peer-reviewed for validity of research methods
- The research is conducted or funded by companies or individuals that benefit from the sale of products tested
- It is aggressively marketed with testimonials (even by physicians) rather than science-based studies

Source: Vinson, JA, Burnham, BR, Negendran, MV. Randomized, double-blind, placebo-controlled, linear dose, crossover study to evaluate the efficacy and safety of green coffee bean extract in overweight subjects. Diabetes, Metabolic Syndrome and Obesity- Targets and therapy. 2012;2012(5):21-27

Tea

Tea is second only to water as the most consumed beverage in the world. In the United States, people drink much of their tea iced. Like coffee, tea contains no calories unless it is sweetened with sugar, honey or another sweetener with calories. All true tea comes from one plant, *Camellia sinensis*. Teas are made from various parts of the plant and with various processing methods. Varieties include many black, green and oolong teas.

Black tea is the most widely consumed tea in North America, Europe and India. It contains about half as much caffeine as coffee. Actual caffeine content depends on the length of time the tea is steeped and the amount of tea used. The leaves of black tea are oxidized (fermented) before drying, which gives this tea its dark color and full-bodied flavor.

Green tea leaves are processed using heat or steam, which preserves their beneficial phytochemicals. The pale green or yellow liquid is milder than black tea. Green and oolong teas are preferred in Asia.

Oolong tea is a compromise between black tea and green tea. The leaves are briefly oxidized before drying.

Several flavonoids (a type of phytochemical) are found in high amounts in tea. The most important and most studied is **quercetin**. Current thinking is that tea, particularly green tea, may help lower risk of heart disease and some cancers. For maximum health benefits, tea should be steeped about 5 minutes before drinking to allow maximum dispersion of flavonoids into the water. Flavonoids in tea interfere with the body's ability to absorb dietary non-heme (from plant sources) iron. Vegetarians and those who are dependent on iron from non-meat sources should avoid drinking tea with foods high in iron.

The concentration of caffeine and phytochemicals in tea depends on water temperature and length of brewing time. Americans tend to drink weaker tea than do people in many other countries.

Herbal teas and teas flavored with fruits, spices, flowers and nuts are not true tea. Herbal teas are infusions of dried flowers, roots and leaves from various plants. Many herbal teas have properties that relieve or treat health problems. For example, chamomile

Caffeine

Caffeine, a chemical with powerful physiologic effects, is present in many beverages, including coffees, teas, cola and other carbonated beverages. Caffeine is also found in herbs, guarana, yerba mate and cola nuts. Other common sources include chocolate, coffee-flavored yogurt and ice cream, and energy bars. Caffeine that is naturally present in food does not require labeling, but some manufacturers list caffeine content voluntarily. If caffeine is added to a food or beverage, it must appear on the list of ingredients.

Caffeine is absorbed rapidly, and its effects last from 3 to 12 hours. Caffeine has both positive and negative effects that vary from person to person. At one time, caffeine was prohibited for athletes because of its stimulant effects. In 2004, the World Anti-Doping Agency removed caffeine from its list of prohibited substances. [4] The National Collegiate Athletic Association allows minimal amounts of caffeine from food and beverages. [5]

In general, caffeine makes people feel better and more alert and potentially better able to exercise and think. Many find that eliminating caffeine in the late afternoon and evening allows them to fall asleep faster and sleep more soundly. But caffeine should be limited or avoided if there is any evidence of:

- Irregular heart beat or palpitations
- Severe PMS
- Sleep problems
- Bladder problems
- Anxiety or panic attacks

tea soothes an upset stomach, helps digestion and promotes sleep. Ginger tea relieves nausea. Peppermint tea may relieve bloating or indigestion after a heavy or spicy meal. Most herbal teas have no caffeine. Some contain antioxidant phytochemicals. Some herbal teas can trigger allergic reactions or other side effects; for example, comfrey tea may cause liver damage. In other words, "natural" does not necessarily mean safe.

Caffeine: Pros and Cons

The Good	The Bad	The Good and Bad
• Mental stimulant that improves alertness, sharpens thinking and lifts moods • Promotes the release of adrenaline starting at doses lower than 1 cup of coffee, black tea, cola and some soft drinks • Improves muscle coordination and strength if consumed before an athletic event; relaxes muscle tension; can enhance athletic performance of trained athletes • Relaxes the airways of the lungs and eases breathing • Acts as a laxative • 2 - 3 cups/day may lower the incidence of Parkinson's disease • Constricts blood vessels in the brain, easing headache pain for some people	• Increases risk of early miscarriage • May affect fertility in women who drink more than 2-1/2 cups/day • Can cause a brief rise in blood pressure • Can cause irregular or fast heartbeat • Speeds the kidneys' processing of fluid, thus increasing frequency of urination • Can irritate the bladder for those with incontinence • Affects brain chemicals, primarily melatonin, and can interfere with sleep • In high doses, can increase brain chemicals associated with anxiety • Increases production of stomach acid and can affect the valve between the esophagus and stomach that leads to acid reflux and heartburn • Exaggerates attention deficit disorder and hyperactivity • Can increase secretion of stress hormones and hamper the body's ability to regulate blood-sugar levels	• Prevents sleepiness • Does not cause cancer (unless people smoke when they drink coffee) • Does not increase breast cancer but may cause breast tenderness • Can cause drop in calcium if coffee is substituted for milk • Acts as a diuretic and can decrease bloating. Caffeine does not have a diuretic effect in most people unless more than 250 milligrams of caffeine (about 2 cups of coffee) are consumed. The liquid of the coffee adds to fluid intake

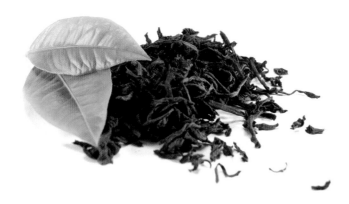

Dairy Drinks

Dairy beverages, which can include milk, kefir, shakes, lattes, lassis and smoothies, are a good way to supply shortfall nutrients such as vitamins A and D, calcium and phosphorus. Dairy beverages are also an important source of protein. *MyPlate* recommends 3 servings of milk and dairy products daily for children and 2 servings daily for adults, preferably from fat-free or low-fat sources. To achieve this, it is necessary to eat a dairy product at most meals or between meals as snacks. To help guests meet this guideline, foodservice operations should offer low-fat milk as a beverage at each meal plus other low-fat dairy options as alternative choices at each meal for those who do not choose milk as a beverage. Milk provides nine essential nutrients – calcium, phosphorus, potassium, protein, vitamins A, D and B12, riboflavin and niacin – and is one of the most nutrient-rich foods. Milk and milk alternatives are described in Chapter 5.

Federally funded programs such as school lunch and feeding programs for older Americans mandate that milk be served to help these vulnerable groups meet their needs for many key nutrients. Flavored milks, most often chocolate, strawberry, vanilla or banana, may be served in most of these settings. They provide key nutrients but also have added sugar. On average, low-fat chocolate milk contains the equivalent of 4 teaspoons of sugar and 56 calories more than plain low-fat milk. Some feeding programs offer flavored milk with the rationale that it will be more appealing and encourage milk drinking by those who do not like low-fat milk. Other programs do not allow flavored milks with the rationale that they encourage a preference for sweetened foods.

Other beverages such as buttermilk and kefir are generally equivalent in nutritional value to low-fat milk. Low-fat and skim milk can be used in cocoa, hot chocolate, lattes, iced coffee or other beverages to add milk to the diet. Milkshakes also contain dairy products, but the ice cream adds quite a lot of fat and sugar. Smoothies made with yogurt and fruit are a far better choice from a nutritional perspective.

Smoothies have become a popular drink, and small meal, as they have grown from a drink for dieters and athletes to a mainstream choice. Smoothies offer many creative opportunities, and the combinations and flavors are endless. Many smoothies are fruit drinks, but some contain yogurt or frozen yogurt, thus adding the nutrients that dairy products provide.

Beverages: Value-Added, High-Profit and Healthful

Italian-style sodas and fruit juices or syrups in carbonated water can be light and healthful. Some restaurants have added bottled artisanal teas, fruit and water beverages or have developed house-made infusions of herbal or citrus sodas, lemonades, root beers, fruit and vegetable juices, herbal beverages, and other drinks that are both popular and profitable. Customers are willing to pay for these types of beverages as long as ingredients are high in quality. Try these ideas or create your own:

- Apple ginger sparkler
- Aqua fresca
- Clementine soda
- Fresh kiwi grape juice
- Grapefruit sparkler
- Hibiscus-honey iced tea
- Iced ginger tea
- Jasmine spritzer
- Lavender spritzer
- Lemongrass soda
- Mint limeade
- Papaya melon citrusade
- Peach and rosemary spritzer
- Pomegranate-honey cooler
- Thai basil soda
- Watermelon ginger limeade

Lactose Intolerance

The enzyme lactase is required to break lactose, the sugar in milk, into its two component simple sugars. In some people this enzyme is present in insufficient quantities to digest milk products, so drinking milk can cause discomfort. Lactose intolerance is more common in non-Caucasian populations. The lactase enzyme is available commercially and can be added to dairy products to break down milk sugar. Offering milk with added lactase might be considered when serving populations who have a high incidence of lactose intolerance. Individuals who are lactose intolerant sometimes take lactase enzyme tablets before meals so they can consume small amounts of dairy products.

Juices and Fruit Drinks

One of the main recommendations made by *My-Plate* and the *Dietary Guidelines* is to increase intake of fruits and vegetables. Fruit and vegetable juices are nutrient-rich beverage choices that provide an array of essential vitamins, minerals and protective phytochemicals. Available as single juices, blended or exotic, some juices are also fortified with calcium, fiber and vitamins. Look for 100% pure juice or offer fresh juices and 100% juice combinations. Tomato, carrot, beet and vegetable juices are generally lower in calories and higher in nutrients than most fruit juices. Although 100% fruit juice is a good choice, it should be limited to 1 cup per day. Most fruit should be eaten whole or cut. Fiber and other protective substances are reduced when the fruit is juiced.

Citrus, berry, melon and tropical fruit juices are generally rich in vitamins and phytochemicals. Apple and white grape juices are not as high in many nutrients and are more likely to be fortified with added nutrients. Purple grape juice, cherry, pomegranate and cranberry juice are particularly rich in phytochemicals and have unique health benefits. Several fruit juices, including orange juice, can be fortified with calcium and are very useful ways for meeting the calcium and vitamin D needs of vegans and lactose-intolerant people. Some juices are fortified with fiber from fruit pulp to replace or exceed the dietary fiber removed when the fruit was juiced. Certainly, whole fruits are richer in fiber than most juices, but juices are a good way to boost fruit and vegetable intake.

Commercial fruit drinks are made with water and fruit juices and are often sweetened with high-fructose corn syrup. They can be lightly carbonated. Some fruit drinks are only 10% fruit juice and are high in calories from sugar but low in nutrients. Because of the added sugar, these juices should be limited in keeping with the *Dietary Guidelines* recommendation to reduce added sugars. Fruit drinks made with some fruit juice and carbonated or mineral water with little or no sugar added for flavor are healthier alternatives.

Fruit Smoothies

Smoothies can make a healthy snack or light meal and, when made with the right ingredients, can add valuable nutrients to the diet. Blended and chilled, smoothies can be made from fresh, frozen or canned fruit or vegetables. Smoothies often include ice, yogurt, frozen yogurt or milk. They have a milkshake-like consistency but unlike milkshakes, they usually don't contain ice cream. Many fruit smoothies are combinations of fruits with no dairy component.

Some popular smoothie flavors include:

- Avocado-mango
- Banana, coconut and mango
- Mixed berry
- Carrot-pineapple
- Cherry-almond
- Frosty pine-orange yogurt
- Grape and green tea
- Mango yogurt
- Blueberry-banana
- Sunshine lemon
- Sweet basil
- Vanilla-banana almond

Visit **www.3aday.org** for creative smoothie recipes.

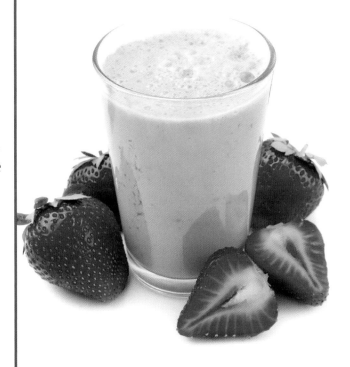

Coconut Water

Coconut water is one of the fastest-growing new beverages in the United States. Food manufacturers have added it to fruit juices, yogurt, sports drinks and sorbets. Not to be confused with **coconut milk**, which is derived from the meat of mature coconuts, coconut water is the clear liquid found in young coconuts. **Coconut cream** is similar to coconut milk but is made with a higher ratio of coconut to water.

Research on the health benefits of coconut water is limited, and recent claims have not been substantiated by scientific research. Compared to many other beverages, however, coconut water can be a healthier option. Like all plant-based foods or beverages, coconut water contains phytochemicals as well as minerals and vitamins. Because it contains electrolytes and minerals, coconut water is often marketed as a sports drink. One cup of coconut water has only 46 calories (less than many other popular beverages) and 9 grams of carbohydrate. It is a good source of fiber, potassium, magnesium and vitamin C. The drawback to coconut water, however, is that it is high in sodium: 252 milligrams per cup and it is often an expensive beverage option.

Soft Drinks

For many Americans, **soft drinks** – called soda pop in some parts of the United States – are a popular beverage. There are hundreds of flavors, sweetening ingredients and levels of sweetness. Soft drinks come in regular, diet, caffeinated and caffeine-free varieties. Some people drink these instead of morning coffee.

While diet soft drinks do not add pounds directly, drinking calorie-free, sweetened beverages alters brain chemistry to seek more sweets. In addition, diet drinks generally replace more nutrient-rich options.

Most regular soft drinks are low in nutrients and high in calories and sugar from high-fructose corn syrup or cane sugar. Regular soft drinks are like liquid candy, often with added chemicals, artificial colors and flavors. Few Americans need these extra calories. By some estimates, 37% of total daily liquid calories come from sugar-sweetened drinks, and consumers don't reduce their food intake when they drink

Functional Beverages

Functional beverages are drinks enhanced with added ingredients to provide specific health benefits beyond general nutrition. Popular ingredients include caffeine, green tea, guarana, yerba mate, vitamin C, ginger and ginkgo biloba.

- **Energy drinks** evolved from juice-bar drinks. They are intended to improve stamina and are usually high in carbohydrates and often have caffeine and nutrients added.
- **Sports drinks** are designed to replace fluids lost during physical activity. They are generally high in sodium and potassium.
- **Smart drinks** may contain amino acids and are often herb based. They provide energy with stimulants (often caffeine) without impairing motor functions. Despite aggressive promotion, little scientific evidence supports increased performance when consuming smart drinks.

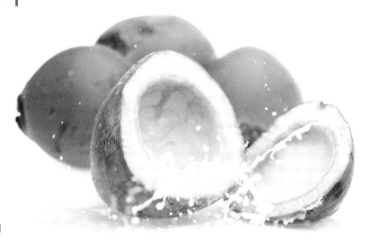

calories from soda and other beverages. [**6**] Children who consume soft drinks can become accustomed to very sweet flavors, which can cause them to cut back on nutrient-rich beverages such as milk, juice and water. While an occasional soft drink is okay, children should not drink soft drinks regularly. Providing healthful beverages on menus for children is an opportunity for menu development. Replacing a ginger ale-based kiddie cocktail with a fruit-based drink is a step in the right direction.

Alcoholic Beverages

Unlike other foods for which absorption begins in the small intestine, alcohol is absorbed quickly into the bloodstream through the lining of the stomach and the first part of the intestine. Foods that contain protein or fat slow the absorption and effects of alcohol. Sparkling wines and carbonated mixers stimulate the digestive tract and accelerate alcohol absorption. Once absorbed, 2% to 10% of alcohol is eliminated through the kidneys and lungs; the rest is broken down in the liver. It takes the body about an hour to eliminate 1 ounce of alcohol. Consequently, blood alcohol levels increase steadily when more than 1 drink per hour is consumed.

The health effects of alcohol can be beneficial or harmful, depending on the amount consumed and the age and other characteristics of the drinker. Children, adolescents, and pregnant and nursing women should not drink beverages or eat foods containing alcohol. For people who cannot limit their alcohol intake, no amount of alcohol is ever safe. People taking medications that interact with alcohol and those who have certain medical conditions should drink alcohol only with the advice of their doctor.

Diners also may choose to avoid alcohol for personal or religious reasons. Thus, any foods containing alcohol should be clearly identified, and beverages without alcohol should be readily available.

Current research suggests that **moderate drinking** – 1 drink for women per day or 2 drinks for men per day – does not endanger health and may actually promote health. These amounts are primarily based on two assumptions: size and weight (assuming men are larger and have more muscle mass) and the fact that men metabolize alcohol more quickly and efficiently than women. Women metabolize alcohol more slowly than men because they produce less alcohol dehydrogenase, which is an enzyme that breaks down alcohol and helps remove its toxic byproducts from the body. [7]

Beverages containing alcohol supply calories but few essential nutrients. Each gram of alcohol provides 7 calories, almost twice the number of calories in a gram of protein or carbohydrate. Although consuming 1 to 2 drinks per day is not associated with increased nutrient deficiency, heavy drinkers may be at risk for malnutrition if alcoholic beverages are substituted for nutrient-rich foods.

Hazards of excessive alcohol consumption include increased risk of liver cirrhosis, cancers of the upper

A Drink Is a Drink Is a Drink

One drink is considered 1.5 ounces of 80-proof liquor or 1 ounce of 100-proof, 12 ounces of beer (5% alcohol), or 5 ounces of wine (12% alcohol). Each of these beverages contains about 1 ounce of pure alcohol per serving. These are quite modest portions and many "single" orders, or drinks, are equivalent to 2 servings of alcohol, especially when drinks are served in oversized glasses.

gastrointestinal tract, injury, violence and death. Drinking too much alcohol can raise the levels of triglycerides in the blood and can lead to high blood pressure and heart failure. Consuming too many calories from alcohol can lead to obesity and a higher risk of developing diabetes. Excessive drinking and binge drinking can lead to stroke as well as increased risk of accidents and impaired decisions and performance. Other serious alcohol-related problems include fetal alcohol syndrome and increased risk of birth defects, cardiac arrhythmia and sudden cardiac death.

The National Cancer Institute reports an elevated risk of breast cancer for women who drink alcohol and theorizes that alcohol affects the hormonal levels of older women. Women who drink moderate amounts of alcohol, however, had fewer other cancers, heart disease, stroke, hip fractures and dementia than non-drinkers. [7]

While choosing to have an alcohol-containing beverage is a personal choice for restaurant patrons, and there is profit made from sales of alcohol, a wise restaurateur is careful not to "oversell" and never serves alcohol to minors. Many restaurants are creating interesting alcohol-free drinks as specials. Virgin cocktails, also called mocktails, continue to be a top trend.

Alcohol and Calories

In mixed drinks, wine and beer, most calories come from the alcohol, but some calories also come from carbohydrates in the grain or fruit used to make the alcohol and from mixers. When meal planning is done and certain percentages of carbohydrate, protein and fat are recommended, there is usually no provision for additional calories from alcohol because it is not an essential nutrient. When controlling calories, it is important to reduce calories from added sugars and fats in the diet. If a person eats the same amount and adds alcohol-containing beverages, the result will be weight gain. One or two drinks each day, adding hundreds of calories, may be why some people have trouble managing their weight.

What Is Moderation?

The *Dietary Guidelines* define moderate consumption as 1 drink per day for women and 2 drinks per day for men. Research suggests that this amount provides the most beneficial health effects; greater amounts may increase particular health risks.

Moderate consumption of beer, wine or spirits may have beneficial health effects in some individuals. The pattern of drinking is also important. One or two drinks a day maximizes the benefits and minimizes the adverse effects of alcohol. But "saving up" to have 7 or 14 drinks in one or two nights is not a viable option. Binge drinking maximizes the adverse effects and eliminates the positive effects of alcohol consumption.

Over the past several decades, many studies have been published in research journals about how drinking alcohol may be associated with reduced mortality from heart disease. Several studies have shown that moderate amounts of alcohol increase HDL (good) cholesterol. Other studies indicate that drinking moderately lowers risk of dementia and loss of cognitive function in aging adults.

Wine

The health benefits of wine, particularly red wine, have been extolled in the popular press. Evidence continues to mount that regular, moderate wine consumption (1 to 2 glasses daily) helps prevent or delay heart disease, type 2 diabetes, dementia, rheumatoid arthritis and osteoporosis. In the Mediterranean Diet, wine is regularly consumed with meals. Some senior care and nursing homes offer a glass of wine with dinner and report that this increases socialization, relaxation and better sleep patterns - all beneficial outcomes.

Wine contains the phytochemical ***resveratrol***, which became a household word in 1991 when a 60 Minutes segment about the French Paradox described it as not only healthful but also a powerful anti-aging agent. Resveratrol, first isolated in the 1960s by Japanese scientists, is the most studied of the phytochemicals known as polyphenols. The compound functions as a plant's defense against damage from bacteria and fungi. It is being studied in clinical trials as a medication, but findings are not yet available. Resveratrol may prevent platelets in the blood from sticking together, which may reduce clot formation and the risk of heart attack and stroke. It also may play a role in reducing LDL cholesterol and slowing the aging process.

Resveratrol is found in the skins of grapes and other fruits. Red wines and red/purple grape juice have more resveratrol than white wine because they are exposed to grape skins for a longer time during fermentation. Red wine and dark grape juices contain many other polyphenols. For example, some researchers believe that polyphenols in the coating of grape seeds are even more potent than resveratrol. Researchers are not sure which of the compounds in red wine provide health benefits but generally agree that a combination of substances in red wine provides health benefits. Concord or red grape, acai, pomegranate and cherry juice provide similar health benefits.

Calories in Alcoholic Beverages

Beverage	Portion		Calories	
Beer	12	ounces	150	calories
Light beer	12	ounces	100	calories
White wine	5	ounces	115	calories
Red wine	5	ounces	110	calories
Liquor	1.25	ounces	80	calories

Wine Headaches

Most people think it is the sulfites in wine that can cause headaches. An allergic reaction to sulfites, however, usually involves breathing trouble and rashes, not headaches.

Sulfites are found not only in wine but also in foods such as dried fruits, baked goods and pickled vegetables. A serving of dried apricots contains almost 10 times the amount of sulfites in a serving of wine.

Research indicates that tyramine is the active substance in wine that causes the dilation and contraction of blood vessels that can result in headaches. Tyramine is an amino acid by-product produced during fermentation. It is suspected for triggering migraines in up to about 40% of the migraine population. Wine contains several different tyramine compounds. Younger and unfiltered wines contain higher amounts.

Source: The National Headache Foundation, **www.headaches.org**

Red wine also contains the phytochemical *quercetin*, an anti-inflammatory found in fruit and vegetable skins. Quercetin has antiviral effects that help the body resist flu, infections and lung inflammation and inhibit growth of prostate cancer. [6] More information on phytochemicals is found in Chapter 7.

Beer

Some studies indicate that beer may have the same health benefits as wine. Ales, lagers and stouts in modest amounts (1 glass per day) may reduce the risk of heart attack and stroke, probably because of the presence of phytochemicals known as polyphenols (see Chapter 7). Low-alcohol and non-alcohol beers seem to offer the same heart-protective effects as regular beer. In modest amounts, beer has a relaxing effect on the body, improves blood circulation, reduces stress and promotes urination.

While most calories in beer come from alcohol, beer also contains carbohydrates – about 1 gram per ounce of beer. A 12-ounce glass of beer contains about 150 calories and 13 grams of carbohydrate. Beer also contains some folate, magnesium, niacin and potassium.

In cooking, beer can be used as a marinade to flavor and tenderize meat. It can be used in the batter for some fried foods and, like wine, can be added to gravies or sauces to boost flavor. Beer also can be used in the steaming liquid for sausages and shellfish. Malty beers add a sweet, slightly nutty taste, while lagers add a bitter or herbal flavor.

The microbrew industry has doubled from 2012 to 2016, with approximately 2500 craft breweries in the US in 2012 to more than 5300 in 2016 and more growth since then. And with that, comes flavorful artisan beers that present an expanded role in cooking. Rich thick porters can be used in desserts, Belgian ales lend themselves to soups, and hoppy IPA's braises, and chilis. [8]

Avoid cooking with beer if food is served to children, pregnant women, or people with alcoholism, liver disease or gout. In excess, beer contributes to all health problems associated with excessive alcohol and/or calorie consumption. Individuals with diabetes should follow their doctor's advice about drinking beer, wine or other alcohol-containing beverages.

Cooking with Alcohol

Like salt, alcohol brings out the flavor of foods and improves flavor perception. In very small amounts, alcohol molecules are volatile and evaporate rapidly. This is why a splash of brandy or liqueur on fruit brings the fruit's aroma to the nostrils and enhances enjoyment. Alcohol also has a unique ability to bond with both fat and water molecules; some alcohol in a marinade will help the marinade and its aromatics permeate the food. When deglazing a pan with wine after searing meat, the browned bits dissolve in the wine and add additional flavor and aroma to a sauce. Other liquids used to deglaze do not offer the same flavor intensity. With almost any use of alcohol in cooking, small amounts of alcohol will create the desired effect. Larger amounts overwhelm flavors and can create unpleasant aromas.

A common misconception is that when alcoholic beverages are used in cooking the alcohol disappears because of the heat. This is not true. Only some alcohol burns away. The amount remaining depends on the temperature and length of cooking. It is important that alcohol not be in foods of people who, for various reasons, should not drink alcohol. If a food contains alcohol, that fact should be in the menu description or mentioned by servers to inform guests who may not want to consume alcohol for religious, health or other reasons.

The amount of alcohol that remains after cooking is listed on the following table.

Preparation	Remaining Alcohol
Immediate consumption	100%
Overnight storage	70%
Stirred into a hot liquid	85%
Flamed	75%
After baking/simmering:	
15 minutes	40%
30 minutes	35%
1 hour	25%
1.5 hour	20%
2 hours	10%
2.5 hours	5%

Source: USDA Table of Nutrient Retention Factors, Release 6, www.ars.usda.gov/SP2UserFiles/Place/12354500/Data/retn/retn06.pdf

From the Kitchen
Jonathan B. Howard
Head Bartender
Henley Modern American Brasserie, Nashville, TN

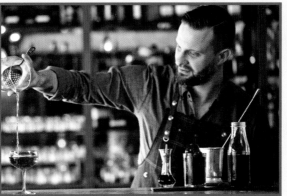

My personal food philosophy is less is more. I love eating small bites. I like being able to try different flavors and also being able to stop when I am getting too full. I love bright, fresh flavors which is why I feel I make drinks that way. But I can also get down on my grandmother's Southern cooking at any point.

Nasturtium is a plant I really love using. Its citrusy and peppery flavor always acts as a firecracker in cocktails, plus it imparts this really amazing color to a drink when shaken into it. I'm also a massive proponent of vinegar in drinks. The health benefits are amazing but it also packs a punch when used properly to balance a drink. Try ¼ ounce of vinegar in place of ¾ ounce citrus juice for a balanced yet nuanced cocktail option. We use everything from rose vinegar to chamomile to sorghum, and I keep finding vinegars I can't wait to use.

As simple as it sounds, serving healthful recipes allows you to show the amount of flavor held within a simple ingredient. Carrots and beets carry a really good amount of sweetness so the needed sugars to balance a drink are not as high, and those fresh healthy flavors can come through. Also, it is a good feeling when your guests can leave invigorated rather than weighed down and serving healthier food and drinks can achieve that idea, which they will thank you for.

Jonathan B. Howard brings his simple food philosophy to the art of bartending. He feels strongly that a drink should be delicious and easy to drink, first and foremost. After all, drinking is a social interaction, so why complicate things by serving a drink that takes too long to prepare or is too odd to understand? His style is bright, light and refreshing, incorporating all types of bubbles and rare herbs, and his drinks feature a range of fortified wines, eau di vie, sherries and vinegars.

At Henley, an American Brasserie and Bar located in the Kimpton Aertson hotel in Nashville, he and Executive Chef Daniel Gorman focus on locally grown produce and purveyors, executing food and drink that speaks to the Southern earth from which things are grown, while also tipping their hat to some of their favorite cuisines and drinks along the way.

They use only use fresh ingredients brought in by the kitchen team and look at the alcohol-to-nutrient ratio during conception. A drink might incorporate juiced carrot with scotch, parsley and ginger, for example. Or a drink with rum and Lillet might get a hit of fennel, snap pea and vinegar. The result is a healthful drink that excites the palate without losing sight of the basics.

Spanish Shoemaker
Serves: one

Jonathan Howard
Henley Modern American Brasserie, Nashville, TN

Grapefruit quarter	1	each
PX Sherry Steeped Figs	2	each
Simple syrup (1:1)	½	ounce
Palo Cortado Sherry	1	ounce
Fino Sherry	1	ounce
Rivulet Pecan Liqueur	½	ounce
Fresh mint		garnish
Dehydrated grapefruit slices		garnish
Freshly grated cinnamon		garnish

1. In a mixing tin, add grapefruit, 1 fig, and simple syrup. Lightly muddle.

2. Add remaining ingredients and 2 cubes of ice. Shake very briefly and fine strain into a deep cocktail glass.

3. Top with crushed ice and garnish with mint, a dehydrated grapefruit slice, and 1 fig cut in half. Finish with freshly grated cinnamon.

casebycase | Move Over 'Virgins' and 'Mocks'

Dry January started in 2013 in England as a public health campaign to reduce alcohol consumption after a holiday season of frequent imbibing. As the idea migrated to the U.S., some bars and restaurants added adult cocktails to their menus beyond the usual mocktails and Virgin Marys. These more sophisticated mixed drinks also appeal to patrons who, for whatever reason, have chosen never to drink alcohol, but want to socialize over "drinks" without experiencing the stigma that can come with abstaining. For operators, promoting no-alcohol drinks that look and taste like traditional cocktails but stand on their own merits can be good business. The patron who may order club soda or a soft drink now has the opportunity to choose something more fun – and better for the bottom line.

And the opportunities are endless, from fruit- and herb-infused seltzer to cider sangria, Moscow mules, negronis, and Mojitos – all with lots of flavor and cachet but no buzz. The Barn, a popular steakhouse in Evanston, Illinois, owned and operated by Amy Morton, created three "faux spirits," bourbon, gin and curacao, which can be used to make classic drinks like a "gin" and tonic, gimlet and cosmo.

And what about that old standby – water? According to Technomic's 2018 Beverage Consumer Trend Report, 65 percent of sparkling water consumers used to choose carbonated soft drinks. A majority of consumers say they are more likely to purchase beverages with an "all-natural" descriptor, with no artificial flavors or sweeteners.

In some quarters, water is assuming the stature of wine. The Fine Water Society was founded in 2008 to enhance the visibility of fine water and communicate that water is a natural product which, like wine, reflects the geology and environment of its origins. The society defines fine water as luxurious, high in quality, limited in distribution and expensive with a brand history and heritage. Proponents of fine water believe it is a healthy and stylish alternative to alcohol and that food, tea, coffee and artisanal crafted cocktails benefit greatly in taste and story from carefully chosen water.

If and until the fine water trend hits hard in U.S., however, operators, depending on their level of service would be wise to simply give patrons a few choices of still and sparkling H_2Os.

Opportunities for Chefs

Whether tap water or bottled sparkling water, fountain drinks or artisanal sodas, "mocktails" or sophisticated beer, wine and cocktails, there should be something for everyone on a comprehensive and creative beverage menu. Menus for both children and adults should include fat-free and low-fat dairy options and 100% fruit or vegetable juices should be available. Intakes of both low-fat dairy products and vegetables and fruits are too low in the diets of most Americans. Calorie-free beverages can help meet needs for water without adding sugar or calories.

Learning Activities

1. Conduct a water tasting with various still and sparkling waters. Compare appearance, aroma, taste and mouthfeel.

2. Develop a non-alcoholic beverage menu with selections appropriate for children and adults.

3. Compare labels of three products from each of the following two categories: artisanal sodas and traditional soft drinks.

4. Compare recommended beverage serving sizes with actual serving sizes in a local restaurant or bar.

For More Information

- Bottled Water Basics, Environmental Protection Agency, **www.epa.gov/safewater/faq/pdfs/ fs_healthseries_bottlewater.pdf**

- International Bottled Water Association, **www.bottledwater.org**

- National Coffee Association USA, **www.ncausa.org**

- Preston-Campbell B. *Cool Waters: 50 Refreshing, Healthy, Homemade Thirst Quenchers*. Harvard Common Press: Boston; 2009.

- Safe Drinking Water Hotline, Environmental Protection Agency, 800-426-4791

- The Tea Association of the USA, **www.TeaUSA.com**

- Water on Tap, What you need to know, Environmental Protection Agency, **www.epa.gov/ safewater/wot/pdfs/book_waterontap_full.pdf**

Chapter Seven

Vitamins, Minerals and Phytochemicals

Learning Objectives | *After completing this chapter, you should be able to:*

- Explain the roles vitamins play in growth and good health

- List and describe the general functions and food sources of fat-soluble vitamins and water-soluble vitamins

- List and describe the functions and food sources of major minerals

- List nutrients of concern that many Americans lack in their diets and foods that are the best sources of these vitamins and minerals

- Identify diseases caused by specific vitamin and mineral deficiencies

- Give tips to ensure that vitamin and mineral intake is sufficient

- Explain what phytochemicals are and give examples

- Identify cooking techniques that promote retention of nutrients and those that cause nutrient loss from foods

This chapter is primarily for reference and is essential information to provide in a nutrition text-book. While most chefs do not need to know specific roles, sources or values of the many vitamins and minerals, the information in this chapter will help chefs answer questions and meet challenges presented by customers with particular health concerns.

Unlike the macronutrients (protein, fat and carbohydrates), vitamins and minerals do not provide energy to fuel the body. Even though the body's need for vitamins and minerals is small enough to be measured in milligrams (1/1000th of a gram) or micrograms (1/1000th of a milligram), these nutrients are vital to maintaining good health.

Thirteen **vitamins** are essential nutrients because they have specific biological functions in the human body and must be obtained through food, either because they are not made in the body or because the body does not make a sufficient amount. All vitamins are organic compounds with carbon in their chemical structure. In some cases, foods provide substances, called precursors, that are converted in the body to the active form of the vitamin. Absence of a vitamin in the diet causes a specific deficiency disease.

Many minerals exist in nature; 15 of them are considered essential nutrients that must be obtained from food. Unlike vitamins, **minerals** are inorganic substances with no carbon molecules in their chemical structure. Different minerals have different biological functions – for example, as components of body cells, as regulators of metabolic reactions, for growth and development, to produce enzymes and hormones, and to protect cells from damage.

Phytochemicals, also called phytonutrients, are not essential nutrients. They are not vitamins or minerals. They are compounds with biological activity that aid cellular functioning and often protect cells from damage. Their presence in the diet is protective, but specific phytochemicals do not meet the criteria to be essential nutrients. They are discussed in this chapter because, like vitamins and minerals, many phytochemicals work at the cellular level to promote health and reduce risk of disease.

The body of knowledge concerning vitamins and minerals is fairly new, and the science behind phytochemicals is even newer. Our understanding of the delicate balance of vitamins, minerals and phytochemicals and the interaction of all nutrients is becoming clearer each year as research is conducted and reported in medical journals.

Americans consume significantly fewer vegetables, fruits, whole grains, milk and dairy products, and seafood than recommended. These foods provide key nutrients. Consequently, American diets are lacking in some nutrients and this is a public health concern. The *2015-2020 Dietary Guidelines for Americans* identifies potassium, dietary fiber, calcium and vitamin D as nutrients of concern. In addition, intake of iron, folate and vitamin B_{12} is of concern for specific population groups. It is recommended that everyone reduce intake of one mineral – sodium. [1]

While all nutrients have important functions, many are easily provided by diets most Americans eat. When a goal is providing healthful foods, increased focus on foods that provide the nutrients most likely to be lacking is a good strategy. This book provides information on many vitamins and minerals so that chefs will have an easy reference as to functions and food sources. Focus should be given to key nutrients, often those that have been identified as nutrients of concern.

Because this book is not intended as a comprehensive medical or nutrition text, it does not provide detailed information about biochemistry, physiology and medical nutrition therapy. That knowledge falls within the purview of the registered dietitian and/or nutrition scientist and is available in nutrition texts and on reputable Internet sites. Chefs and culinary professionals generally do not need to know the specific recommended milligrams or micrograms of particular vitamins or minerals but should know the general functions and best food sources for major vitamins, minerals and phytochemicals.

For vitamins and minerals the Daily Value (the amount designated for food labels) and the DRI (amount recommended for daily intake) for men and women are listed for a point of reference. The foods with the highest amounts of nutrients are on the top of the lists that follow. This knowledge will help guide ingredient selection. With few exceptions, a well-balanced and varied diet can provide all the vitamins and minerals a person needs, without adding supplements. Keep in mind that while providing a wide variety of foods makes vitamins, minerals and phytochemicals available, food storage and cooking techniques affect the final nutrient composition of any food served.

Nutrients of Concern

Because many Americans consume large amounts of **empty-calorie food** (food with calories but few nutrients), getting adequate amounts of essential vitamins and minerals can be a challenge. It is important to select nutrient-dense foods. **Nutrient-dense foods**, also called nutrient-rich foods, provide vitamins, minerals and other substances that have positive health effects, with relatively few calories. They are lean or low in solid fats, added sugars and sodium.

According to the *Dietary Guidelines for Americans*, intake levels of certain nutrients are of concern for specific groups. Four under-consumed nutrients of public health concern are vitamin D, calcium, potassium and dietary fiber. These four shortfall nutrients are clearly linked to nutrient inadequacy and increased likelihood of medical problems.

Additional shortfall nutrients include vitamins A, C, E, magnesium and phosphorus; iron and folate for women of childbearing age; and vitamin B12 for people over age 50. Foods high in saturated fats, sodium and added sugars should be replaced with nutrient dense vegetables, fruits, whole grains and fluid milk and milk products to increase intakes of shortfall nutrients and nutrients of concern.

Estimated Percentages of Americans with Adequate Nutrient Intakes

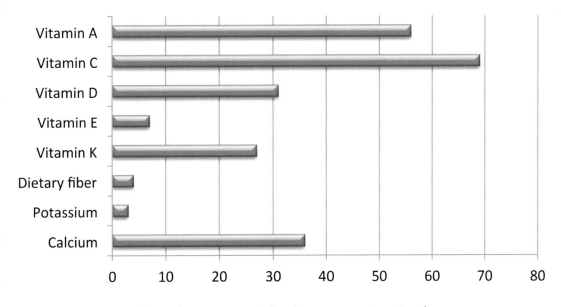

% of American with adequate nutrient intake

Sources: Moshfegh A, Goldman J, Cleveland L. *What We Eat in America, NHANES 2001-2002: Usual Nutrient Intakes from Food Compared to Dietary Reference Intakes.* U.S. Department of Agriculture, Agricultural Research Service. 2005, **www.ars.usda.gov/ba/bhnrc/fsrg**

Moshfegh A, Goldman J, Ahuja J, Rhodes D, LaComb R. *What We Eat in America, NHANES 2005-2006: Usual Nutrient Intakes from Food and Water compared to 1997 Dietary Reference Intakes for Vitamin D, Calcium, Phosphorus and Magnesium.* U.S. Department of Agriculture, Agricultural Research Service. 2009, **www.ars.usda.gov/SP2UserFiles/Place/12355000/pdf/0506/usual_nutrient_intake_vitD_ca_phos_mg_2005-06.pdf**

Interpreting Nutrient Source Lists

On lists of "excellent" or "good" food sources of specific nutrients, the foods that are considered best sources are found at the top. Some lists provide the grams, milligrams or micrograms for a standard measure of food as typically consumed – for example, 1 cup or 2 tablespoons. When a range is given, such as for the milligrams of a nutrient in ready-to-eat cereal, it is because different brands are fortified at different levels. Other formats list nutrients per 100 grams of food, regardless of the type of food. But some foods that seem to be excellent sources of a particular nutrient per 100 grams might have to be consumed in an unrealistic portion in order to truly qualify as an "excellent source."

For example, 100 grams (3 ½ ounces) of skim milk is less than ½ cup, but 100 grams of cinnamon equals 14 tablespoons. Based on a 100-gram portion, the cinnamon would rank as a terrific source of calcium, providing 1,002 milligrams. The 100 grams of milk provides only 125 milligrams of calcium. The reality is, however, that while one would be very likely to drink 1 cup of skim milk (providing 300 milligrams of calcium), one would eat only a pinch of cinnamon (containing about 5 milligrams of calcium) in a single portion of food. The lesson: Consider the realistic portion when comparing food sources of any nutrient.

You will notice that some foods, like salmon, greens and legumes are on many of the lists as best sources. Increasing these foods as menu choices ensures that your total menu will be more healthful.

Where to Find Nutrient Content Information

- USDA National Nutrient Database for Standard Reference, **https://ndb.nal.usda.gov** contains reports on foods by description or food sources by individual nutrients; free of charge
- Commercial nutrient databases
- Bowes & Church's *Food Values of Portions Commonly Used*, 19th edition, or a similar resource book
- The Nutrition Facts portion of the food label, including the percent Daily Value information
- Nutrient information from food manufacturers, distributors or trade organizations
- Smartphone applications that provide nutrient data

Vitamins

Vitamins are essential organic (carbon-containing) substances that the body needs in small amounts. Vitamins help the processes by which other nutrients are digested, absorbed, metabolized or built into body structures. Some vitamins function as **coenzymes**. This term means that they enhance and speed up actions of enzymes that are necessary in chemical reactions within cells of the body.

The absence of a vitamin may cause a nutrient deficiency. Symptoms of that deficiency go away when the vitamin is consumed. For example, inadequate vitamin C causes bleeding gums and easy bruising, which are the initial symptoms of scurvy. When a person with scurvy eats citrus fruits or other foods containing vitamin C, deficiency symptoms stop.

"Limey"
Originated in the late 19 century to describe British sailors who were forced to consume lime juice (high in vitamin C) to prevent scurvy. Before this, many sailors on very long voyages developed scurvy due to lack of fruits and vegetables that provide Vitamin C.

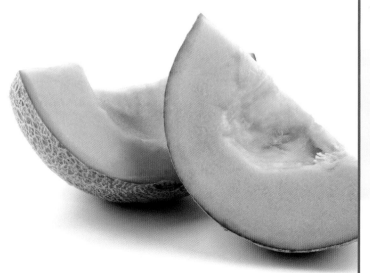

Vitamin Deficiency Diseases

One of the criteria to be a vitamin is that the absence of that substance causes a specific deficiency disease. What are those diseases?

Vitamin C	Scurvy
Vitamin A	Night blindness
Vitamin D	Rickets, osteomalacia
Vitamin E	Hemolytic anemia in infants
Vitamin K	Bleeding
Thiamin	Beriberi, Werneke-Korsakoff Syndrome
Riboflavin	Ariboflavinosis
Niacin	Pellegra
Pantothenic Acid	Parasthesia
Vitamin B$_6$	Anemia, neuropathy
Biotin	Dermatitis, enteritis

There are two categories of vitamins: fat-soluble (A, D, E and K) and water-soluble (thiamin, riboflavin, niacin, folate, vitamin B$_{12}$, vitamin B$_6$, biotin, pantothenic acid and vitamin C).

Fat-Soluble Vitamins

Fat-soluble vitamins are carried in lipids or food fats and are stored in fatty tissue and in the liver in the body. They can reach toxic levels if taken in excess over time.

Vitamin A

Vitamin A is an antioxidant and plays important roles in vision, bone and tooth growth, reproduction, cell functions, and the immune system. The active form of vitamin A, ***retinol***, is found in animal foods such as liver, egg yolks and dairy products. There are several precursors to retinol; the most active is beta-carotene (12 micrograms of beta-carotene equal 1 microgram or 1 RAE of retinol). ***Beta-carotene***, which is converted to vitamin A in the intestine, is a pigment found in fruits and vegetables that are bright orange, yellow and dark green. Beta-carotene's color makes it easy to identify foods high in vitamin A. Because beta-carotene and other vitamin A pre-cursors, known as carotenoids, do not have the same biologic activity as retinols, they must be mathematically converted to retinol activity equivalents (RAE) and international units (IU), an older measurement used in many food composition tables. Human need for vitamin A also is expressed in retinol equivalents (RE).

Inadequate vitamin A intake causes changes in eye tissues that can result in vision problems and blindness as well as changes in the cells that protect organs and skin and act as barriers to bacteria and viruses. Excessive vitamin A over a prolonged period of time can be toxic, causing hair loss, bone pain, fatigue, dry cracked skin, liver damage, high blood pressure, bleeding gums and birth defects. According to recent national consumption studies, more than half of Americans do not consume the recommended daily dietary requirement of vitamin A. Adding more fruits and vegetables to menus is a good way to provide vitamins and minerals while controlling calories and is a major recommendation of the *Dietary Guidelines for Americans*. [1]

Vitamin A		
Measure	**Population**	**Amount**
Daily Value		900 micrograms RAE
Dietary Reference Intakes (DRI)	Men, ages 14 and above Women, ages 14 and above	900 micrograms RAE 700 micrograms RAE

Best Sources of Vitamin A

Deep green and orange vegetables and liver are the best sources.

Food	Serving	Vitamin A (IU)	Vitamin A - RAE (micrograms)
Carrot juice	1 cup	45,133	2,256
Pumpkin, canned	1 cup	38,129	1,906
Sweet potato, cooked	1 potato	28,058	1,403
Carrots, cooked	1 cup	26,571	1,329
Beef liver, cooked	3 ounces	22,175	6,582
Squash, butternut, baked	1 cup	22,868	1,144
Spinach, cooked	1 cup	18,666	1,146
Carrots, raw	1 cup	18,377	919
Kale, cooked	1 cup	17,707	885
Turnip greens, cooked	1 cup	17,655	882
Collards, cooked	1 cup	15,417	771
Chicken liver, cooked	3 ounces	11,329	3,315
Mustard greens, cooked	1 cup	8,852	442
Braunschweiger	2 slices	7,967	2,393
Dandelion greens, cooked	1 cup	7,179	359
Melons, cantaloupe	1 cup	5,411	270
Lettuce, cos or romaine	1 cup	4,878	244
Peppers, sweet, red, raw	1 cup	4,665	234
Lettuce, green leaf, raw	1 cup	4,147	207
Vegetable juice cocktail	1 cup	3,770	189
Papayas	1	3,326	167
Lettuce, butterhead (Boston and bibb types)	1 cup	1,782	93
Cheese, ricotta, whole milk	1 cup	1,095	295
Eggs	2 each	658	178
Milk, nonfat, low-fat, whole, buttermilk	1 cup	500	149
Cereal, ready-to-eat	1 cup	500 - 990	90 - 297

Source: U.S. Department of Agriculture, Agricultural Research Service. 2015. USDA National Database for Standard Reference, Release 28. Nutrient Data Laboratory, **http://www.ars.usda.gov/services/docs.htm?docid=8964**

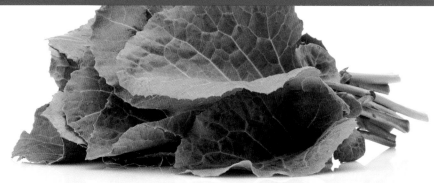

From the Kitchen

Deborah Madison, *Chef/Author*

Sante Fe, New Mexico

Ingredient No. 1: Seasonal, Fresh and Local

"Since the 1970s," notes Sante Fe, New Mexico-based chef, author and educator Deborah Madison, "every decade has had its token vegetarian menu item. In the '70s, it was fat-laden eggplant Parmesan, in the '80s, it was pasta primavera, which usually had little to do with spring vegetables, and in the '90s, it was the ubiquitous Portobello mushroom." Thanks in no small part to Deborah, the multi-award-winning author of 12 books about the glory of local produce, fruits and vegetables are no longer relegated to the side dish, the salad, and the single vegetarian menu choice. Her latest book, *In My Kitchen*, is a collection of 100 inspired vegetarian recipes, some old, some new, reflecting how Debrorah loves to cook now.

Seasonality and local sourcing are at the heart of Deborah's approach to food. "Whether you call it fresh or local or seasonal, the concept is the same – fruit and vegetables that have not traveled long distances and have not been stored for long periods of time," she explains. "It's only recently that we have had everything available all the time, but we take this variety for granted. The fact is," she continues, "you can eat seasonally and locally all year – even in the winter. It won't be what you are used to, but it can be done if you rely on local farmers."

Local farmers' traditional planting and growing practices also offer a solution to a problem Deborah refers to as the "elephant in the room" – tired soil. "Plants are only as good as the soil they are grown in," she says. "Plants developed for 'big agriculture' have been hybridized to be in the ground less time than usual in soil that has become little more than a planting medium. Fed with fertilizer and watered on demand, they don't develop good, deep roots to absorb nutrients, and with repeated plantings, the soil is not given time to replenish itself." Deborah notes that the pioneering farm-driven restaurant, Greens, in San Francisco, where she was founding chef in the 1970s, was successful from the start in part because they structured their dishes on a meat-as-center-of-the-plate idea – but without the meat. "Our customers never felt like something was missing," Deborah recalls, "because there was always something to focus on, something that assumed the role of meat on the plate."

Sweet Potato and Pineapple Salad

Yield: 8 cups **Serves: 10, 3/4 cup each**

William Reynolds,
Chef Owner, New Buffalo Bill's,
New Buffalo, Michigan

Originally developed for cooking classes at Washburne Culinary Institute, this colorful and flavorful salad is now a favorite at his restaurant. It is good with chicken or pulled pork and also an excellent buffet item and for box lunches.

Sweet potato, peeled, ½ inch dice	2	pounds
Celery, ¼ inch dice	4	ounces (¾ cup)
Red onion, ¼ inch dice	4	ounces (¾ cup)
Pineapple, ¼ inch dice	8	ounces (1 ½ cup)
Dates, chopped	3	ounces (½ cup)
Cashews or pecans, coarsely chopped	2	ounces (½ cup)

Dressing:

Canola oil	¼	cup
Lemon juice, fresh	2	tablespoons
Cider vinegar	¼	cup
Salt	½	teaspoon
Pepper	¼	teaspoon
Sugar	1	tablespoon

1. Combine all dressing ingredients and emulsify with a blender or stick blender.
2. Roast sweet potatoes at 350° F for about 30 minutes or until tender.
3. Combine warm potatoes, celery, red onion, pineapple, dates and cashews with dressing and mix gently. Cool before serving.

Per Serving

Calories	210		Cholesterol	0	mg
Fat	9	g	Sodium	190	mg
Saturated Fat	1	g	Carbohydrates	33	mg
Trans Fat	0	g	Dietary Fiber	4	mg
Sugar	14	g	Protein	3	g

Looking toward the future, Deborah is concerned about the impact of uneven weather patterns on food supply. "We have already seen the effect of drought on the price of grain and corn and thus livestock," she says. "People are used to buying the most expensive cuts of meat because they are the fastest and easiest to prepare, but those on the economic margins may not be able to afford this anymore. As chefs," Deborah continues, "it's our responsibility to teach people how to choose and prepare alternatives, not only the tougher cuts of meat, but also – and especially – plant foods."

Vitamin D

Vitamin D (calciferol) acts like a hormone to help the body absorb and regulate calcium and phosphorus for strong bones, teeth and muscle. Vitamin D, especially the most active form, ***D3 (cholecalciferol)***, may provide protection from osteoporosis, hypertension (high blood pressure), cancer and several autoimmune diseases. Vitamin D is also available as ***D2 (ergocalciferol)***.

Vitamin D is made in the body when a cholesterol-like compound in skin is activated by ultraviolet light and converted to a precursor of vitamin D, which is then converted to its active form by enzymes of the liver and kidneys. People who have little exposure to sunlight because they keep their skin covered or who are seldom outside need more vitamin D in their diet. People who are lactose intolerant and avoid milk should seek non-dairy sources.

Vitamin D deficiency can contribute to fragile bones (osteoporosis), which is a major problem among older Americans, and ***osteomalacia*** (soft painful bones).

Although uncommon in the United States, vitamin D deficiency in children causes soft bones resulting in ***rickets***. Low levels of vitamin D in the body may increase the risk of breast, colon and prostate cancers; depressed mood, poor brain functions and more severe dementia in older adults; bacterial infections and gum disease. There is a significant amount of current research related to vitamin D beyond the long-known functions of building bones and teeth. In great excess from high-dose supplements, vitamin D can be toxic, causing nausea, fatigue and calcium deposits in organs.

The mineral calcium needs vitamin D to form bone cells, which is why milk is fortified with vitamin D. In addition to fortified milk and cereals, food sources of vitamin D include fatty fish, egg yolks, butter, liver, shrimp and shiitake mushrooms. Cheese and yogurt are usually not fortified with vitamin D; be sure to check the label. One microgram of vitamin D3 is equal to 40 IU (international units) of vitamin D.

Vitamin D

Measure	Population	Amount
Daily Value		20 micrograms
Dietary Reference Intakes (DRI)	Men, ages 9 to 70 Women, ages 9 to 70	15 micrograms 15 micrograms

Best Sources of Vitamin D

Fatty fish and fortified milk are the best sources of vitamin D.

Food	Serving		Vitamin D (IU)
Herring, pickled	3	ounces	1,384
Cod liver oil	1	tablespoon	1,350
Halibut, cooked	3	ounces	510
Catfish, cooked	3	ounces	425
Salmon, canned	3	ounces	390
Mackerel, cooked	3	ounces	306
Sardines, canned	1.75	ounces	250
Tuna, canned	3	ounces	200
Milk, fat-free, low-fat, whole or buttermilk	1	cup	100
Egg yolk	1	yolk	20
Beef liver, cooked	3	ounces	15
Orange juice, vitamin D fortified	½	cup	68
Butter	1	tablespoon	9
Cheddar cheese	1	ounce	7
Cereal, ready-to-eat	1	cup	0.6 - 2.9

Source: U.S. Department of Agriculture, Agricultural Research Service. 2015. USDA National Database for Standard Reference, Release 28. Nutrient Data Laboratory, **http://www.ars.usda.gov/services/docs.htm?docid=8964**

Vitamin E

Vitamin E (tocopherol) acts as an antioxidant in cell membranes and is especially important for the stability of cells that are constantly exposed to high levels of oxygen – particularly lung, brain and blood cells. Vitamin E protects the polyunsaturated fats and other fat-soluble substances in cells from cellular changes thought to contribute to cardiovascular disease and cancer. Many Americans do not consume adequate vitamin E, which is found in plant foods. There is no evidence of toxicity from the consumption of vitamin E naturally occurring in foods. Toxicity is possible with supplements, causing bleeding problems. Vitamin E is destroyed by high heat.

Vitamin E

Measure	Population	Amount
Daily Value		15 milligrams
Dietary Reference Intakes (DRI)	Men, ages 14 and above Women, ages 14 and above	15 milligrams (mg) 15 milligrams (mg)

Best Sources of Vitamin E

Plant foods, especially seeds, nuts, dark green leafy vegetables, oil and salmon are the best sources of vitamin E.

Food	Serving	Vitamin E (IU)	Vitamin E alpha-tocopherol milligrams
Cereal, ready-to-eat	1 cup	2.33 - 28.17	1.26 - 13.5
Sunflower seeds	1 ounce	15.35	7.40
Almonds	1 ounce	11.08	7.43
Sunflower oil	1 tablespoon	8.32	5.59
Safflower oil	1 tablespoon	6.91	4.64
Hazelnuts	1 ounce	6.35	4.26
Spinach, steamed	1 cup	5.35	3.74
Wheat germ	2 tablespoons	4.50	2.28
Turnip greens	1 cup	4.03	2.71
Pumpkin, canned	1 cup	3.87	2.60
Canola oil	1 tablespoon	3.64	2.44
Peanuts	1 ounce	2.93	2.36
Olive oil	1 tablespoon	2.89	1.94
Mango	1 cup	2.75	1.85
Sweet red bell peppers	1 cup	2.17	2.35
Soybean oil	1 tablespoon	1.66	1.10
Sweet potatoes	1	1.21	1.47
Salmon, cooked	3 ounces	1.17	0.69
Avocado	1 ounce	0.89	0.56

Source: U.S. Department of Agriculture, Agricultural Research Service. 2015. USDA National Database for Standard Reference, Release 28. Nutrient Data Laboratory, **http://www.ars.usda.gov/services/docs.htm?docid=8964**

Vitamin K

Vitamin K (phylloquinone) is necessary to make the proteins involved in blood clotting and also works with vitamin D to help regulate blood calcium levels and form bone. Intestinal bacteria make about half the body's vitamin K; food provides the rest. Green leafy vegetables are a major source. Vitamin K deficiencies are rare. Antibiotics can reduce vitamin K synthesis, thus increasing dietary needs. Individuals on medication to reduce blood clotting may be instructed to avoid foods high in vitamin K.

Vitamin K

Measure	Population	Amount
Daily Value		120 micrograms (µg)
Dietary Reference Intakes (DRI)	Men, ages 19 and above Women, ages 19 and above	120 µg 90 µg

Best Sources of Vitamin K

Dark green leafy vegetables are the best sources.

Note: You will see that cooked greens have more vitamin K than raw greens. This is because it takes much more raw greens to make 1 cup of cooked greens. For example, it takes 10 to 12 cups of raw spinach to make 1 cup of cooked spinach.

Food	Serving	Vitamin K (µg)
Kale, cooked	1 cup	1062.1
Collards, cooked	1 cup	836.0
Spinach, cooked	1 cup	1027.3
Turnip greens, cooked	1 cup	530.0
Beet greens, cooked	1 cup	697.0
Dandelion greens, cooked	1 cup	579.0
Mustard greens, cooked	1 cup	419.3
Broccoli, cooked	1 cup	220.1
Brussels sprouts, cooked	1 cup	163.0
Cabbage, cooked	1 cup	163.1
Spinach, raw	1 cup	144.9
Asparagus, cooked	1 cup	91.0
Endive, raw	1 cup	115.5
Lettuce, green leaf, raw	1 cup	45.5
Broccoli, raw	1 cup	89.4
Lettuce, cos or romaine, raw	1 cup	48.2
Cabbage, raw	1 cup	67.6

Source: U.S. Department of Agriculture, Agricultural Research Service. 2015. USDA National Database for Standard Reference, Release 28. Nutrient Data Laboratory, **http://www.ars.usda.gov/services/docs.htm?docid=8964**

Water-Soluble Vitamins

Water-soluble vitamins – vitamin C and the B vitamins – need to be consumed daily because they are not stored (except for some vitamin B_6 and B_{12}) and are lost through body fluids. Water-soluble vitamins are found in basic foods such as meat, grains, fruits and vegetables. They can be leached out of foods or easily destroyed by incorrect storage or preparation. Excess water-soluble vitamins are generally excreted in the urine, so toxicity from foods is rare. Significant excesses from high-dose supplements can be toxic for some B vitamins.

B Vitamins

B vitamins assist the body in making energy from food and help form red blood cells to heal wounds. They are also important for growth and development, proper nerve function and healthy skin, proper digestion, and a healthy appetite. B vitamins are found in proteins such as fish, poultry, meat, eggs and dairy products. Leafy green vegetables, beans and peas also have B vitamins. Many cereals and

some breads have added B vitamins through enrichment or fortification. Not getting enough of certain B vitamins can cause deficiency diseases.

Thiamin, riboflavin and niacin are needed for energy metabolism to release energy from carbohydrates, proteins and fats at the cellular level. All three are needed for proper growth. Deficiencies of thiamin, riboflavin and niacin are rare in the United States because many breads and cereals are enriched with these vitamins along with iron and folacin. Alcoholism can create deficiencies, in part because of low food intake.

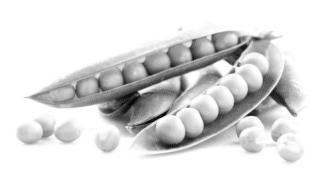

The B Vitamins

Common Names	Also known as
Thiamin	B_1
Riboflavin	B_2
Niacin	B_3
Pantothenic acid	B_5
B_6	Pyridoxine, pyridoxal and pyridoxamine
Biotin	B_7
B_{12}	Cobalamin
Folate	Folic acid and folacin

Thiamin

Thiamin, which is widely available in the diet, plays a critical role in the energy metabolism of all cells and in normal nerve and heart function. Thiamin is sensitive to heat and can be destroyed when food is cooked at temperatures higher than that of boiling water. Thiamin occurs in small amounts in many nutritious foods, especially lean pork and legumes, enriched, fortified or whole-grain products, bread and bread products, mixed foods whose main ingredient is grain, ready-to-eat cereals and nuts.

Thiamin

Measure	Population	Amount
Daily Value		1.2 milligrams (mg)
Dietary Reference Intakes (DRI)	Men, ages 14 and above Women, ages 19 and above	1.2 mg 1.1 mg

Best Sources of Thiamin

Lean pork is the best source, but thiamin is provided by many food groups.

Food	Serving	Thiamin milligrams
Cereal, ready-to-eat	¾ cup	0.4 - 1.5
Pork loin, cooked	3 ounces	0.53
Ham, cooked	3 ounces	0.58
Edamame	1 cup	0.47
Acorn squash, baked	1 cup	0.34
Long grain white rice, enriched, cooked	1 cup	0.33
Peas, cooked	½ cup	0.21
Long grain brown rice, cooked	1 cup	0.19
Pecans	1 ounce	0.19
Brazil nuts	1 ounce	0.18
Lentils, cooked	½ cup	0.17
White bread, enriched	1 slice	0.11
Whole-wheat bread	1 slice	0.10

Source: U.S. Department of Agriculture, Agricultural Research Service. 2015. USDA National Database for Standard Reference, Release 28. Nutrient Data Laboratory, **http://www.ars.usda.gov/services/docs.htm?docid=8964**

Riboflavin

Riboflavin is essential for the metabolism of carbohydrates to produce energy and amino acids. It also helps keep mucous membranes (such as those lining the mouth) healthy. Milk and dairy products are major sources of riboflavin and organ meats such as liver are rich in riboflavin. Ultraviolet rays of the sun and fluorescent light can destroy riboflavin, which is why milk should be stored in cardboard or plastic containers in a dark refrigerator.

Riboflavin

Measure	Population	Amount
Daily Value		1.3 milligrams (mg)
Dietary Reference Intakes (DRI)	Men, ages 14 and above Women, ages 19 and above	1.3 mg 1.1 mg

Best Sources of Riboflavin

Food	Serving	Riboflavin milligrams
Beef liver, cooked	3 ounces	2.4
Cereal, ready-to-eat	1 cup	0.4 - 1.7
Chicken livers, cooked	3 ounces	1.7
Yogurt	1 cup	0.35
Milk, nonfat, low-fat, whole, buttermilk	1 cup	0.45
Almonds	1 ounce	0.29
Mushrooms, raw	1 cup	0.28
Edamame	1 cup	0.28
Egg	1 large	0.23
Pork loin, cooked	3 ounces	0.22
Spinach, cooked	½ cup	0.21

Source: U.S. Department of Agriculture, Agricultural Research Service. 2015. USDA National Database for Standard Reference, Release 28. Nutrient Data Laboratory, **http://www.ars.usda.gov/services/docs.htm?docid=8964**

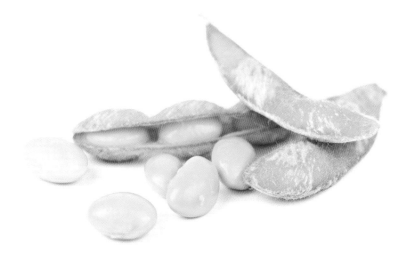

Niacin

Niacin is essential for the metabolism of carbohydrates, fats and many other substances in the body.

Protein foods rich in tryptophan (an amino acid), such as dairy products, can compensate for not consuming enough niacin in the diet. The body can convert tryptophan to niacin; 60 milligrams of tryptophan can be converted to 1 milligram of niacin. Dietary needs for niacin are stated as niacin equivalents (NE), a measure that takes available tryptophan into account. When large amounts of nicotinic acid, a form of niacin, are taken as a medicine or supplement, itching, flushing, nausea, liver damage and high blood sugar levels can result.

Niacin

Measure	Population	Amount
Daily Value		16 milligrams (mg)
Dietary Reference Intakes (DRI)	Men, ages 14 and above Women, ages 14 and above	16 mg 14 mg

Best Sources of Niacin

Most protein foods provide niacin.

Food	Serving	Niacin milligrams
Beef liver, cooked	3 ounces	14.7
Chicken, light meat, cooked	3 ounces	11.7
Tuna, in water	3 ounces	11.3
Swordfish, cooked	3 ounces	7.9
Salmon, Chinook, cooked	3 ounces	8.5
Turkey, light meat, cooked	3 ounces	5.8
Cereal, ready-to-eat	1 cup	5 - 20
Pork chop, cooked	3 ounces	3.9
Peanuts	1 ounce	3.4
Mushrooms, cooked	½ cup	3.5
Baked potato	1	3.3
Beef, lean, cooked	3 ounces	3.1 - 7.2
Pasta, enriched	1 cup	2.3
Lentils, cooked	1 cup	2.1
Peanut butter	1 tablespoon	2.1

Source: U.S. Department of Agriculture, Agricultural Research Service. 2015. USDA National Database for Standard Reference, Release 28. Nutrient Data Laboratory, **http://www.ars.usda.gov/services/docs.htm?docid=8964**

Vitamin B$_6$

Vitamin B$_6$ (pyridoxine, pyridoxal and pyridoxamine) is part of a coenzyme necessary for metabolism of carbohydrates, fat and especially protein. The nervous and immune systems need vitamin B$_6$ to function efficiently; it is also needed to convert tryptophan to niacin. The body needs vitamin B$_6$ to make hemoglobin, which carries oxygen to tissues, and to help regulate blood sugar levels. A vitamin B$_6$ deficiency can result in a form of anemia that is similar to iron deficiency anemia.

Vitamin B$_6$

Measure	Population	Amount
Daily Value		1.7 milligrams (mg)
Dietary Reference Intakes (DRI)	Men, ages 14 to 50	1.3 mg
	Women, ages 19 to 50	1.3 mg

Best Sources of Vitamin B$_6$

Food	Serving	Vitamin B$_6$ milligrams
Tuna, yellowfin, cooked	3 ounces	0.88
Beef liver, cooked	3 ounces	0.87
Potato, baked, with skin	3 ounces	0.70
Banana	1 large	0.5
Garbanzo beans, cooked	½ cup	0.53
Beef, sirloin, cooked	3 ounces	0.52
Chicken, light meat, cooked	3 ounces	0.51
Salmon, wild, cooked	3 ounces	0.48
Spinach, cooked	1 cup	0.44
Turkey, without skin	3 ounces	0.39
Beef, ground, broiled	3 ounces	0.33
Vegetable juice cocktail	6 ounces	0.26
Cereal, ready-to-eat	1 cup	0.5 - 2.5

Source: U.S. Department of Agriculture, Agricultural Research Service. 2015. USDA National Database for Standard Reference, Release 28. Nutrient Data Laboratory, **http://www.ars.usda.gov/services/docs.htm?docid=8964**

Vitamin B₁₂

Vitamin B₁₂ (cobalamin) is found only in foods of animal origin. B₁₂ assists in building all new cells including bone and red blood cells; is essential for breaking down carbohydrate, protein and fat for energy; and is needed to protect nerve fibers for normal functioning of the nervous system. Some B₁₂ is stored in the liver. Because vitamin B₁₂ is present only in animal foods, strict vegans may need B₁₂ supplements or injections. People who are unable to absorb vitamin B₁₂, due to a lack of a secretion in the digestive system, may develop a specific form of anemia with weakness, mental confusion, nervous system problems and paralysis. Vitamin B₁₂ is partly destroyed when foods are microwaved.

Vitamin B₁₂

Measure	Population	Amount
Daily Value		2.4 micrograms (µg)
Dietary Reference Intakes (DRI)	Men, ages 14 and above Women, ages 14 and above	2.4 µg 2.4 µg

Best Sources of Vitamin B₁₂

Food	Serving		Vitamin B₁₂ micrograms
Beef liver, cooked	3	ounces	70.7
Clams, raw	3	ounces	42.0
Mussels, steamed	3	ounces	20.4
Chicken liver, cooked	3	ounces	18.0
Oysters	3	ounces	16.4
Mackerel, king	3	ounces	13.2
Crab, steamed	3	ounces	9.8
Cereal, ready-to-eat, fortified	1	cup	1.8 - 6.0
Salmon, cooked	3	ounces	4.9
Beef, cooked	3	ounces	2.4
Cottage cheese	1	cup	1.4
Yogurt	1	cup	1.3
Milk, nonfat, low-fat, whole, buttermilk	1	cup	1.2

Source: U.S. Department of Agriculture, Agricultural Research Service. 2015. USDA National Database for Standard Reference, Release 28. Nutrient Data Laboratory, **http://www.ars.usda.gov/services/docs.htm?docid=8964**

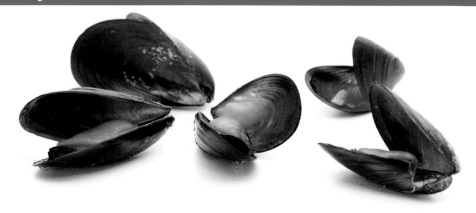

Folate

Folate is a component of the coenzymes necessary to form DNA; thus, all new cells require folate. It is important for red blood cell formation and helps the body use protein. Folate is critical early in pregnancy to prevent birth defects. Folate, folic acid and folacin are slightly different chemical forms with equivalent vitamin activity.

Folate is now added to enriched grain products as a public health measure to reduce birth defects. Because folate is lost during cooking, fresh and lightly prepared foods are good sources of folate and most legumes are excellent sources. The synthetic form of folate used for enrichment and fortification is quite stable and is well utilized by the body. To account for differing rates of absorption, folate is sometimes measured in dietary folate equivalents (DFE).

Folate

Measure	Population	Amount
Daily Value		400 micrograms (µg)
Dietary Reference Intakes (DRI)	Men, ages 14 and above Women, ages 14 and above	400 µg 400 µg

Best Sources of Folate

Food	Serving	Folate micrograms
Cereal, ready-to-eat, fortified	1 cup	200 - 700
Lentils, cooked	½ cup	179
Pinto beans, cooked	½ cup	142
Garbanzo beans, cooked	½ cup	141
Spinach, cooked	½ cup	132
Asparagus, cooked	½ cup (6 spears)	134
Rice, enriched, cooked	½ cup	119
Turnip greens, cooked	½ cup	85
Pasta, enriched, cooked	½ cup	84
Orange juice	6 ounces	54
Brussels sprouts, cooked	½ cup	47
Lima beans, cooked	½ cup	78
Romaine lettuce	1 cup	64
Beets, cooked	½ cup	68
Bread, enriched	1 slice	60
Potato, baked	1 each	57

Source: U.S. Department of Agriculture, Agricultural Research Service. 2015. USDA National Database for Standard Reference, Release 28. Nutrient Data Laboratory, **http://www.ars.usda.gov/services/docs.htm?docid=8964**

Pantothenic Acid, Biotin and Choline

The B vitamins pantothenic acid and biotin each act as coenzymes in metabolic processes. Both are available in a wide variety of commonly eaten foods. Deficiencies are uncommon, and toxicities have not been found. Bacteria within the intestine can make some biotin.

Choline was classified as an essential nutrient by the Food and Nutrition Board of the Institute of Medicine in 1998 and is usually grouped with the B vitamins. Despite the fact that humans can synthesize it in small amounts, choline should be consumed in the diet to ensure its availability to make neurotransmitters and lecithin, a substance in cell membranes necessary for fat transport in the blood stream and for cell structure and function. The *Dietary Guidelines* report lists choline as a shortfall nutrient. Food sources include eggs, beef, pork, lamb, salmon, chicken and fish.

Vitamin C

Vitamin C, also called ascorbic acid, helps make collagen, which is the structural foundation of cells. Vitamin C helps keep gums and other tissues healthy and aids in the healing of cuts and wounds. It also helps the body absorb iron. Vitamin C is necessary to form thyroxin, the hormone that regulates metabolic rate.

When vitamin C and iron are eaten at the same meal, the body absorbs up to three times more iron from non-meat (non-heme) sources. Iron from meat is well absorbed and does not require vitamin C for absorption.

Like vitamin E, vitamin C is a key antioxidant, protecting cells from damage that can increase risk of certain diseases, such as cancer. Vitamin C strengthens the immune system by supporting white blood cells; however, research has not shown that high doses of vitamin C will prevent or cure the common cold. It can, however, lessen symptoms.

Vitamin C has been identified as a shortfall nutrient because many Americans do not eat enough fruits and vegetables, the primary source of vitamin C. Some juices and cereals are fortified with vitamin C. Pregnant and nursing women, those who smoke, and people with injuries, infections or fevers require more vitamin C. Very high doses of vitamin C (more than 2 grams per day) through supplements can cause gastrointestinal symptoms. Deficiencies of vitamin C result in bleeding gums, easy bruising and poor resistance to infection. Severe deficiencies result in scurvy, which is seldom seen except in people who eat virtually no fruits and vegetables. Proper handling and storage of foods high in vitamin C is important because, as the least stable nutrient, vitamin C is easily destroyed by exposure to heat, leaches into water and is lost through evaporation. The amount of loss varies with time and temperature. Serving foods high in vitamin C in the raw state preserves this nutrient.

Vitamin C

Measure	Population	Amount
Daily Value		90 milligrams (mg)
Dietary Reference Intakes (DRI)	Men, ages 19 and above Women, ages 19 and above	90 mg 75 mg

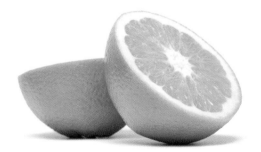

Best Sources of Vitamin C

Fruits and vegetables are the best sources.

Food	Serving		Vitamin C milligrams
Sweet red pepper	½	cup	115
Orange	1	medium	70
Orange juice	½	cup	62
Sweet green pepper	½	cup	60
Broccoli, cooked	½	cup	51
Strawberries	½	cup	49
Grapefruit juice	½	cup	47
Apple juice, with added vitamin C	½	cup	47
Papaya	½	cup	44
Grapefruit	½	medium	44
Brussels sprouts, cooked	½	cup	48
Tomato	1	medium	17
Cereals, ready-to-eat	1	cup	6 - 60

Source: U.S. Department of Agriculture, Agricultural Research Service. 2015. USDA National Database for Standard Reference, Release 28. Nutrient Data Laboratory, **http://www.ars.usda.gov/services/docs.htm?docid=8964**

Minerals

Minerals are inorganic substances that are essential for good health. They originate in the earth and cannot be produced by living organisms. Most minerals in the diet come directly from plants or indirectly from animal sources that have eaten plants. Minerals are also found in water.

Major minerals are those that the body needs in relatively large amounts (more than 100 milligrams/day). All the major minerals can be found in the body in amounts larger than 5 grams. *Trace minerals* have known biological functions in humans, but are necessary only in tiny amounts (less than 20 milligrams/day). Trace minerals are sometimes called microminerals.

Of the 92 known minerals, at least 21 are necessary for biochemical processes in humans. Minerals differ from other nutrients in that they remain intact during digestion and do not change in structure when performing biologic functions. Some minerals occur as part of the structure of organic compounds, such as hemoglobin and phospholipids in blood. Minerals are stable and not destroyed by heat, light or oxygen. In general, minerals maintain the body's fluid and acid–base balance; provide structural components

for building blood, bone and teeth; and sustain the immune system. Like vitamins, minerals act as cofactors in essential enzyme systems to repair cells and protect them from oxidative changes that cause aging, cardiovascular diseases and cancer. Minerals also participate in metabolic processes, energy production, muscle contraction and transmission of nerve impulses.

Minerals

Major Minerals	Trace Minerals
Calcium	Iodine
Chloride	Iron
Magnesium	Zinc
Phosphorus	Selenium
Potassium	Fluoride
Sodium	Chromium
Sulfur	Copper
	Manganese
	Molybdenum

Major Minerals

Calcium

Calcium, the most abundant mineral in the body, is essential for health in children and adults. Approximately 99% of the calcium in the body is used to form and maintain bones and teeth. The remaining 1% is found in other body tissues, aiding muscle and nerve functions and playing a role in blood clotting. Everyone knows that the body uses calcium to build and maintain strong bones and teeth, but calcium is also necessary for a regular heartbeat, muscle contraction and blood clotting. It also may help prevent high blood pressure and some forms of cancer.

Food sources of calcium typically come from the milk group and are needed throughout life. Calcium in bones needs to be replenished regularly to maintain structure and strength. Substituting other beverages for milk or calcium-fortified fruit drinks can compromise bone health. Children, teens and pregnant and lactating women need lots of calcium-rich foods to build and maintain bone mass.

Milk and dairy beverages, hard cheeses, yogurt, dark green leafy vegetables, dried legumes, tofu (soybean curd), fortified fruit juices, fortified cereals, canned sardines and salmon (due to soft, edible bones), and soft-shelled crab are the best sources of calcium. Blackstrap molasses is also very rich in calcium, but little is used per food serving. Dairy products that are high in fat such as cream cheese, ice cream and sour cream provide only modest amounts of calcium along with lots of fat and calories. The calcium in tofu comes from processing, not from the soy product itself. Small amounts of calcium are provided by calcium propionate, an additive used to keep bread fresh.

Milk, yogurt and other dairy products are the optimal sources of calcium because they come with protein, vitamin D and lactose, all of which maximize the absorption and utilization of calcium. Not all the calcium we eat is absorbed, however. Absorption rates are higher during pregnancy and childhood.

Those who are lactose intolerant, are allergic to milk or do not like milk can get calcium from fortified fruit juices. Generally, calcium citrate is the form of added calcium that is absorbed best. Calcium excesses are rare and only from over-supplementation. In great excess, calcium can lead to the development of calcium deposits in organs and tissues.

Broccoli as well as several greens such as collards, kale, and mustard and turnip greens provide significant amounts of calcium. Other greens, including spinach, Swiss chard, beet greens and parsley contain calcium but also contain **oxalic acid**, a substance that binds the calcium in the digestive tract and blocks some calcium from being absorbed. **Phytic acid** in whole grains and wheat bran inhibits both calcium and iron absorption.

Some people believe that because cow's milk allergies are common, children should drink rice milk or other beverages. In the presence of a true, diagnosed allergy or milk intolerance, milk and dairy products must be avoided and non-dairy sources of calcium must be provided. But for the vast majority of people, low-fat milk and other low-fat dairy products greatly enhance the nutrient quality of the total diet. All foodservice operations should have skim and low-fat milk available for health-conscious diners of all ages. To meet calcium requirements, it is also helpful to have a food rich in calcium available at each meal. Cooking with evaporated milk or yogurt and adding dried nonfat milk as a recipe ingredient also give a calcium boost.

Calcium and Bone Health

Bone cells die and are replaced throughout life. The majority of bone mass is built during childhood and adolescence and into early adulthood. Bone mass is lost in the normal process of aging but can be preserved with adequate calcium and vitamin D intake. Calcium deficiency is one of the factors associated with the onset of osteoporosis. It is more common in women than in men. One of every three people over the age of 65 suffers from osteoporosis, or adult bone loss, which can result in fractures and/or loss of height and pain from compressed vertebrae.

Children, teens and athletes are more likely to have fractures or break bones easily if they do not have strong bones from adequate calcium and vitamin D intake. Beverage choices should include milk when possible to promote healthy bones throughout life.

Calcium

Measure	Population	Amount
Daily Value		1,300 milligrams (mg)
Dietary Reference Intakes (DRI)	Men, ages 19 to 50 Women, ages 19 to 50	1,000 mg 1,000 mg

Best Sources of Calcium

Food	Serving		Calcium milligrams
Evaporated nonfat milk	1	cup	742
Nonfat dried milk	1/3	cup	498
Ricotta cheese, part-skim	½	cup	337
Parmesan cheese, grated	1	ounce	336
Milk, nonfat, low-fat, whole, buttermilk	1	cup	300
Yogurt	1	cup	300
Tofu, calcium set	3	ounces	294
Swiss cheese	1	ounce	220
Salmon, canned, with bones	3	ounces	212
Cheddar cheese	1	ounce	204
Mozzarella cheese, part skim	1	ounce	200
Rhubarb, cooked	½	cup	174
Collard greens, cooked	½	cup	133
Spinach, cooked	½	cup	122
Black-eyed peas, cooked	½	cup	105
Goat cheese, semisoft	1	ounce	84
White beans, cooked	½	cup	81
Bok choy, cooked	½	cup	79
Almonds	1	ounce	75
Turnip greens, cooked	½	cup	52

Source: U.S. Department of Agriculture, Agricultural Research Service. 2015. USDA National Database for Standard Reference, Release 28. Nutrient Data Laboratory, **http://www.ars.usda.gov/services/docs.htm?docid=8964**

Phosphorus

Phosphorus is the second most abundant mineral in the body. It helps build and renew bones and teeth. Phosphorus also assists metabolic reactions to produce energy from carbohydrates, protein and fat and helps maintain acid-base balance within body cells. Generally, calcium-rich foods also provide phosphorus.

Phosphorus is also found in meats, poultry, fish, eggs and legumes. Phosphorus from nuts, seeds and grains is about 50% less bioavailable than phosphorus from animal sources. Because it is provided by foods from several food groups, inadequate phosphorus intake is rare.

Phosphorus

Measure	Population	Amount
Daily Value		1,250 milligrams (mg)
Dietary Reference Intakes (DRI)	Men, ages 19 and above Women, ages 19 and above	700 mg 700 mg

Best Sources of Phosphorus

Phosphorus is found mostly in animal products and legumes.

Food	Serving	Phosphorus milligrams
Yogurt, plain nonfat	1 cup	356
Fish, salmon, cooked	3 ounces	252
Milk, nonfat, low-fat, whole, buttermilk	1 cup	247
Fish, halibut, cooked	3 ounces	231
Ricotta cheese, part skim	½ cup	225
Beef, sirloin, cooked	3 ounces	200
Cottage cheese	½ cup	179
Lentils, cooked	½ cup	178
Beef, cooked	3 ounces	173
Turkey, cooked	3 ounces	168
Swiss cheese	1 ounce	161
Chicken, cooked	3 ounces	155
Great Northern beans, cooked	½ cup	146
Navy beans, cooked	½ cup	143
Almonds	1 ounce	137
Peanuts	1 ounce	107
Egg	1 large	99

Source: U.S. Department of Agriculture, Agricultural Research Service. 2015. USDA National Database for Standard Reference, Release 28. Nutrient Data Laboratory, **http://www.ars.usda.gov/services/docs.htm?docid=8964**

Potassium

Potassium plays a major role in maintaining fluid, electrolyte and acid-base balance and cell integrity. It is also critical to the transmission of nerve impulses that maintain blood pressure, bone health and heartbeat. Deficiency, which occurs with dehydration, causes muscular weakness, paralysis and confusion.

Long-term low intakes have been linked to hypertension. Potassium has been identified as a nutrient of concern because so many Americans eat less than adequate amounts. In fact, less than 10% of Americans consume adequate potassium. Increasing fruits, vegetables and milk will help meet potassium needs.

Potassium

Measure	Population	Amount	
Daily Value		4,700	milligrams (mg)
Dietary Reference Intakes (DRI)	Men, ages 14 and above	4,700	mg
	Women, ages 14 and above	4,700	mg

Best Sources of Potassium

Mostly in fruits and vegetables and milk.

Food	Serving		Potassium milligrams
Potato, baked with skin	1	large	1,081
Prune juice	1	cup	707
Sweet potato, baked	1	each	542
Beet greens, cooked	½	cup	654
Plums, dried (prunes)	½	cup	637
Raisins	½	cup	618
White beans, cooked	½	cup	414
Tomato juice	1	cup	556
Yogurt	1	cup	531
Orange juice	1	cup	496
Halibut, cooked	3	ounces	421
Lima beans, cooked	½	cup	485
Acorn squash, cooked	½	cup	448
Banana	1	medium	422
Spinach, cooked	½	cup	420
Honeydew melon	1	cup	388
Milk, nonfat, low-fat, whole, buttermilk	1	cup	382
Avocado	½	cup	364
Artichoke, cooked	1	medium	343
Kidney beans, cooked	½	cup	327
Molasses	1	tablespoon	293

Source: U.S. Department of Agriculture, Agricultural Research Service. 2015. USDA National Database for Standard Reference, Release 28. Nutrient Data Laboratory, **http://www.ars.usda.gov/services/docs.htm?docid=8964**

Sodium

Sodium is an essential mineral that regulates body fluids, including blood volume. It also regulates acid-base balance, helps nerves and muscles function properly, and helps glucose and amino acids move across cell membranes to be metabolized. Surplus sodium is filtered out of the blood by the kidneys and is excreted in the urine. Sodium is also lost through the skin via sweating.

While dietary guidance recommends increasing or maintaining intakes of most minerals, sodium intake should be limited. In excess, sodium may contribute to hypertension (high blood pressure), which is very common in the United States and is a risk factor for heart attacks, strokes and kidney disease. For reasons that are not clear, some people seem to be "sodium sensitive." For them, there is a direct relationship between salt intake and blood pressure. Elderly individuals, people with diabetes or kidney disease, and African Americans are more sodium sensitive than young Caucasians. Too much sodium also can contribute to fluid retention, weight gain, stomach ulcers, stomach cancer and a form of osteoporosis.

The *Dietary Guidelines* recommend that sodium consumption be limited to less than 2,300 milligrams per day and to 1,500 milligrams per day (less than 1 teaspoon of table salt) for people over age 51, all African-Americans, and those with hypertension, diabetes or kidney disease. Americans typically consume two to three times this amount, about 3,400 milligrams daily. Processed foods – such as canned soups, prepared sauces, cured and deli meats, frozen or packaged meals, condiments (soy sauce, Worcestershire sauce and catsup), salted snacks, pickled foods, seaweed and salad dressings – account for more than 70% of the sodium Americans consume. Trying to reduce sodium in processed foods can be difficult. In many high-sodium foods – for example, breakfast cereals, gelatin desserts and instant puddings – the salty flavor is masked by high sugar content. For information on sodium-restricted diets, see Chapter 13.

Humans have a biological preference for sweet and salty flavors. This taste preference plus the wide-spread use of salt and sodium-rich ingredients, particularly in processed foods, creates a challenge for chefs who want to serve healthful foods. Choosing reduced or low sodium ingredients and reducing the use of salt over time seems to be a good strategy. Techniques for reducing salt and sodium are described in Chapter 9.

Sodium

Measure	Population	Amount
Daily Value		2,400 milligrams (mg)
Dietary Reference Intakes (DRI)	Men, ages 14 to 50 Women, ages 14 to 50	1,500 mg 1,500 mg

Sodium-Rich Ingredients

Sodium is in many compounds used as food ingredients. Sodium both preserves food and enhances flavor. Look for added sodium in ingredient lists. Check labels for sodium content.

Ingredient	Function
Monosodium glutamate (MSG)	Flavor enhancer
Sodium benzoate	Preservative
Sodium caseinate	Thickener and binder
Sodium citrate	Buffer used to control acidity in soft drinks
Sodium nitrite	Curing agent in meat
Sodium phosphate	Emulsifier and stabilizer
Sodium propionate	Mold inhibitor
Sodium saccharin	Artificial sweetener

Source: U.S. Department of Agriculture, Agricultural Research Service. 2015. USDA National Database for Standard Reference, Release 28. Nutrient Data Laboratory, **http://www.ars.usda.gov/services/docs.htm?docid=8964**

Sodium Content of Common Condiments and Recipe Ingredients

Food	Serving	Sodium milligrams
Table salt	1 tablespoon	6,900
Baking soda	1 tablespoon	3,775
Garlic salt	1 tablespoon	2,880
Baking powder, double-acting, sodium aluminum sulfate	1 tablespoon	1,464
Fish sauce	1 tablespoon	1,389
Tamari sauce	1 tablespoon	1,005
Soy sauce	1 tablespoon	901
Bacon, cooked	1 ounce	658
Soy sauce, reduced-sodium	1 tablespoon	533
Dijon mustard	1 tablespoon	360
Hoisin sauce	1 tablespoon	258
Capers	1 tablespoon	254
Catsup	1 tablespoon	167
Anchovies	1 each	146

Source: U.S. Department of Agriculture, Agricultural Research Service. 2015. USDA National Database for Standard Reference, Release 28. Nutrient Data Laboratory, **http://www.ars.usda.gov/services/docs.htm?docid=8964**

Top 10 Sources of Sodium

More than 40% of the sodium we eat each day comes from only 10 types of food. Many people are surprised to learn which foods are on the list because the foods do not always taste salty.

1. Breads and rolls
2. Pizza
3. Sandwiches
4. Cold cuts and cured meats
5. Soups
6. Burritos and tacos
7. Savory snacks (chips, popcorn, pretzels, snack mixes and crackers)
8. Chicken
9. Cheese
10. Eggs and Omelets

Source: U.S. Department of Health and Human Services, U.S. Department of Agriculture. *What We Eat in America* CDC. NHANES 2013-2014. Agricultural Research Service Website.

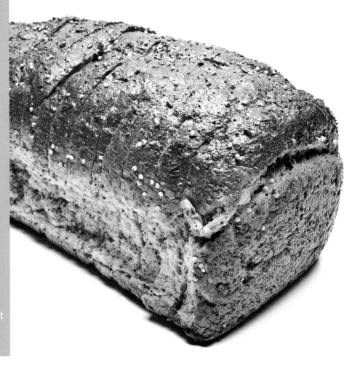

Food Category Sources of Sodium in the U.S. Population, ages 2 years and older

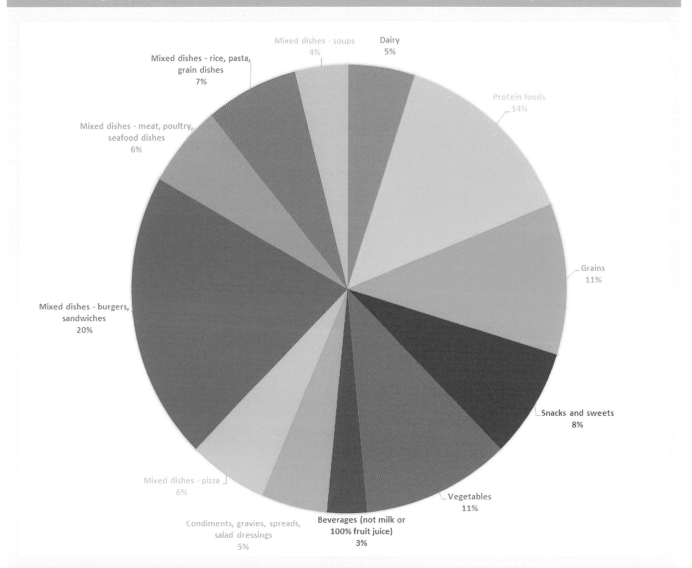

Mixed dishes - soups
4%

Dairy
5%

Mixed dishes - rice, pasta, grain dishes
7%

Protein foods
14%

Mixed dishes - meat, poultry, seafood dishes
6%

Mixed dishes - burgers, sandwiches
20%

Grains
11%

Snacks and sweets
8%

Mixed dishes - pizza
6%

Vegetables
11%

Condiments, gravies, spreads, salad dressings
5%

Beverages (not milk or 100% fruit juice)
3%

Source: U.S. Department of Health and Human Services and U.S. Department of Agriculture. 2015–2020 Dietary Guidelines for Americans. 8th Edition. December 2015. Available at **http://health.gov/dietaryguidelines/2015/guidelines/. Accessed November 20, 2018.**

How Much Sodium Is in Table Salt?

Table salt is fine-grained sodium chloride mixed with a trace amount of an anti-caking agent such as calcium silicate. Table salt is 40% sodium by weight and 60% chloride. One gram of salt provides 400 milligrams of sodium. One teaspoon (5.6 grams) of salt will add approximately 2,300 milligrams of sodium to a dish. By weight, all salt contains the same amount of sodium. Teaspoon for teaspoon, however, flaked kosher salt is lighter than table salt and will have somewhat less sodium per teaspoon.

Chloride

Chloride works with sodium to maintain fluid balance, helps transmit nerve impulses and helps regulate acid-base balance. It is also part of hydrochloric acid, a secretion of the stomach that is important to digestion. Americans get plenty of chloride because it is available in foods that contain salt (sodium chloride). It is also found in seaweed, rye, tomatoes, olives, meats and milk. The Daily Value for chloride is 3,400 milligrams.

Magnesium

Magnesium builds and renews bone and teeth and helps muscles and the nervous system work properly. It has a role in regulating blood pressure. It is necessary for carbohydrate, protein and fat metabolism and supports the immune system. According to the *Dietary Guidelines*, many adults do not meet the daily requirements for magnesium. Increasing magnesium and potassium in the diet lowers blood pressure and promotes the relaxation of muscles; thus, these nutrients are considered heart healthy. Magnesium is part of chlorophyll, which makes green leafy vegetables rich in magnesium. Eating plenty of vegetables and seafood regularly ensures adequate magnesium intake. There is a lot of current research to discover more about optimal magnesium intake.

Magnesium deficiency is sometimes seen but is usually associated with disease or medications. People with poorly controlled diabetes or who drink a lot of alcohol secrete magnesium. Signs of magnesium deficiency include muscle twitching or spasms, cramps, weakness and depression. Older adults are at risk of magnesium toxicity if they regularly take antacids or laxatives containing magnesium and do not have good kidney function.

Magnesium

Measure	Population	Amount
Daily Value		400 milligrams (mg)
Dietary Reference Intakes (DRI)	Men, ages 19 to 30 Women, ages 19 to 30	400 mg 310 mg

Best Sources of Magnesium

Food	Serving	Magnesium milligrams
100% Bran cereal	½ cup	121
Halibut, cooked	3 ounces	90
Oysters, steamed	3 ounces	81
Almonds	1 ounce	76
Spinach, cooked	½ cup	78
Swiss chard, cooked	½ cup	75
Lima beans, cooked	½ cup	63
Black beans, cooked	½ cup	60
Edamame	½ cup	54
Beet greens, cooked	½ cup	49
Peanuts	1 ounce	48
Molasses, blackstrap	1 tablespoon	48
Okra, cooked	½ cup	29
Hazelnuts	1 ounce	46
Yogurt	1 cup	29
Rice, brown, cooked	½ cup	42

Source: U.S. Department of Agriculture, Agricultural Research Service. 2015. USDA National Database for Standard Reference, Release 28. Nutrient Data Laboratory, **http://www.ars.usda.gov/services/docs.htm?docid=8964**

Sulfur

Sulfur is part of the structure of hair, nails and skin. It plays a role in collagen formation, acid-base balance and cellular function. Sulfur is part of two amino acids (methionine and cysteine) and two B vitamins (thiamin and biotin).

Manufacturers use sulfites, which are sulfur-based substances, to retard food spoilage and discoloration of foods such as dried fruits. Sulfites are formed naturally during wine fermentation and can be added to wine to prevent discoloration. Sulfites may cause headaches, sneezing, swelling of the throat or hives in some people. Foods containing added sulfites must provide that information on the label.

Food sources of sulfur include most protein foods, garlic, onions and Brussels sprouts. Some dietary supplements, such as glucosamine and chondroitin sulfate, also contain sulfate. Most people get adequate sulfur from protein foods in their diets.

Trace Minerals

Iron

Iron is present in the body in relatively small amounts but has vital functions. Iron combines with protein to form hemoglobin, the oxygen-carrying protein in red blood cells, and myoglobin, the oxygen-holding protein of muscles. Iron also helps body cells use oxygen.

Some iron is stored in the body in bone marrow, the spleen and liver. Only about 15% of dietary iron is absorbed, although more is absorbed when body stores are low. When iron stores are high, absorption decreases. The form of iron in animal foods (heme iron) is absorbed twice as readily as iron from plant foods (non-heme iron). Eating foods rich in vitamin C increases iron absorption from non-heme sources.

Similarly, the protein in meats, fish and poultry increases the absorption of iron from non-meat sources when eaten at the same meal. (A small amount of pork in beans increases iron availability of the beans.) Cooking acidic foods such as tomatoes in an iron skillet increases iron content of the food.

On the other hand, the tannins in tea and coffee, oxalic acid in dark leafy greens, and phytate in bran and whole grains decrease iron absorption. So while spinach looks like an excellent source of iron on food composition tables, not much of its iron is absorbable. More is absorbed when vitamin C is present – for example, when oranges are added to a spinach salad.

Iron deficiency anemia occurs when a person's diet lacks sufficient iron. As a result, less hemoglobin is produced and less oxygen is delivered to the cells, causing the person to become tired, irritable, indifferent and depressed; have difficulty maintaining body temperature; and experience decreased immunity. Women of all ages are at risk for iron deficiency due to menstruation, pregnancy and lactation. Frequent dieters, vegetarians and individuals who decrease their food intake as they grow older are also at risk. Iron deficiency anemia is the most common nutritional deficiency in Americans. Less common is a genetic disorder in which too much iron is absorbed and stored (hemochromitosis). Iron supplements can be toxic and should be kept in a well-sealed container and out of reach of children.

Odd Fact

Fresh fruit is fairly low in iron while dried fruits have more. This is because some dried fruits are dried on iron racks and some iron is absorbed. Check labels.

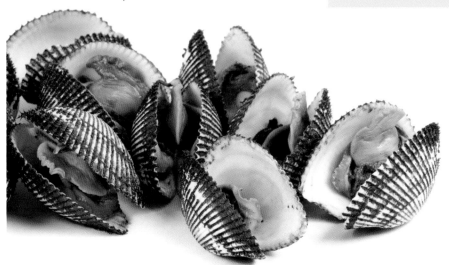

Iron

Measure	Population	Amount
Daily Value		18 milligrams (mg)
Dietary Reference Intakes (DRI)	Men, ages 19 and above Women, ages 19 to 50	8 mg 18 mg

Best Sources of Iron

Shellfish, liver, meats, legumes are the best sources. Vegetable sources of iron are not as well absorbed as iron from meat.

Food	Serving	Iron milligrams
Clams, cooked	3 ounces	23.77
Chicken livers, cooked	3 ounces	9.89
Beef liver, cooked	3 ounces	5.24
Oysters, raw	6 medium	5.04
White beans, cooked	½ cup	3.31
Lentils, cooked	½ cup	3.30
Spinach, cooked	½ cup	3.22
Jerusalem artichokes, raw	½ cup	2.55
Garbanzo beans, cooked	½ cup	2.37
Lamb, cooked	3 ounces	2.30
Beef, cooked	3 ounces	2.30
Pumpkin seeds	½ cup	2.29
Navy beans, cooked	½ cup	2.15
Tofu, firm	¼ cup	2.15
Kidney beans, cooked	½ cup	1.97
Cashew nuts	1 ounce	1.89
Potato, with skin	1 medium	1.87
Prune juice	4 ounces	1.52
Shrimp, cooked	8 large	1.36
Tuna, light	3 ounces	1.30
Chicken, dark meat, cooked	3 ounces	1.13
Chicken breast, cooked	3 ounces	0.89
Molasses, blackstrap	1 tablespoon	0.94
Raisins, seedless	1.5 ounces	0.81
Cereal, ready-to-eat, fortified	½ cup	5.79 - 18

Source: U.S. Department of Agriculture, Agricultural Research Service. 2015. USDA National Database for Standard Reference, Release 28. Nutrient Data Laboratory, **http://www.ars.usda.gov/services/docs.htm?docid=8964**

Iodine

The body needs **iodine** in very small amounts to synthesize thyroxin, a hormone responsible for regulating metabolic rate and body temperature. Too little thyroxin may cause fatigue and weight gain, while too much will cause weight loss and increased heart rate. Iodine is plentiful in the ocean, making many fish, shellfish and sea vegetables rich sources of this mineral. Other sources are dairy products and vegetables grown in iodine-rich soil. For many people, key sources of iodine are iodized salt and iodine residue from cleaning dairy and foodservice equipment. Average intake of iodine in the United States is higher than recommended.

Fluoride

Fluoride is important for the formation of bones and teeth. It helps make teeth resistant to decay and bones resistant to mineral loss. Sources of fluoride include fluoridated drinking water; seafood, particularly sardines and salmon canned with bones; and tea. Most communities have water fluoridated at 1 part per million parts water, the ideal ratio for dental health. If local water is not fluoridated, supplements may be prescribed. Excess fluoride can discolor teeth.

Molybdenum

Molybdenum is a necessary for the activity of several enzymes. It is found in peas, beans, grains and nuts. Too much or too little molybdenum is rare but an extreme excess can damage the kidneys.

Copper

Copper works with iron to build red blood cells; keeps the nervous system, bones and blood vessels healthy; is necessary to form collagen, an important protein in the body; and is a component of some enzymes. Beef liver is an excellent source of copper. Other copper sources include meat, organ meats, fish, shellfish, whole grains, seeds, legumes, textured vegetable protein, almonds and walnuts. Large doses of copper as a supplement can cause nausea, vomiting and other problems.

Selenium

Selenium helps maintain heart rhythm, is a component of essential enzymes and works with vitamin E as an antioxidant to protect cells against damage. The best selenium sources are shellfish, fish, tuna, turkey, whole wheat, barley, Brazil nuts and red meat. The amount of selenium in vegetables is determined by the soil where the vegetables were grown. Selenium needs are small and deficiencies are rare in the United States but common in China. Selenium deficiencies causes heart and thyroid problems. An excess of selenium from over-supplementation causes gastrointestinal upset, hair loss and nerve damage.

Manganese

Manganese is required for bone growth and development, reproduction, and cellular functions. Foods rich in manganese include whole grains, legumes, leafy vegetables, dried fruits, nuts and seeds, and pineapples. Excesses and deficiencies of manganese are very rare.

Chromium

Chromium works with insulin and is important in carbohydrate metabolism. Chromium deficiency causes abnormally high blood glucose levels. Rich sources of chromium include meat, cheese, whole grains, legumes, peanuts, broccoli and grape juice. Research on chromium is ongoing. It is claimed, but not proven, that chromium supplements promote muscle mass and weight loss.

Zinc

Zinc is in every cell and supports the activity of enzymes. Zinc is important for taste and smell perception, normal growth, sexual development, storage and release of insulin, and wound healing. Most animal protein foods provide zinc. Excellent zinc sources include oysters, clams, liver, beef, crabmeat, pork, the dark meat of poultry and fortified cereals. Only about 40% of zinc intake is absorbed. Phytates in grains and legumes can further decrease zinc absorption. Vegetarians and pregnant women are most likely to consume inadequate zinc. Symptoms of deficiency include poor appetite, diarrhea, skin rash, hair loss, growth problems and immunity problems. Long-term excesses of zinc can block copper absorption. Supplements should only be taken if prescribed by a doctor; an extreme excess of zinc can be fatal.

Phytochemicals

Phytochemicals, also called phytonutrients, are natural biologically active compounds found in plant foods. Although not nutrients themselves, phytochemicals work with nutrients and dietary fiber to protect against disease. Since phytochemicals are related to plant pigments, brightly colored fruits and vegetables – yellow, orange, red, green and purple – generally contain the most phytochemicals. Research suggests that phytochemicals help slow the aging process and reduce the risk of many diseases, including cancer, heart disease, stroke, high blood pressure, cataracts, osteoporosis and urinary tract infections. Although phytochemicals have biologic functions and health benefits, they are not vitamins or minerals. The absence of a specific phytochemical does not cause a dietary deficiency.

Each type of fruit and vegetable contains many different phytochemicals. And while their chemical structures differ, all phytochemicals – there may be as many as 8,000 – are protective, and their effectiveness increases when several are present. The concentration of phytochemicals in specific foods varies depending on how that food is grown, processed and stored, and what part of the plant is eaten. For example, broccoli crowns have more of some phytochemicals than broccoli stalks do.

Virtually all public health advice includes a recommendation to increase fruit and vegetable consumption. The American Institute for Cancer Research and the American Cancer Society say that some phytochemicals have the ability to stop a cell's conversion from healthy to cancerous at different stages. Recommendations for cancer prevention encourage high fruit and vegetable intake, including cruciferous vegetables. [2] The *MyPlate* eating plan includes 5 to 9 servings of fruits and vegetables daily. Americans of all ages consume too few vegetables and fruits. The *Dietary Guidelines* recommend shifting food intake patterns to a more plant-based diet that emphasizes fruits and vegetables thus increasing phytochemical intake. [1]

Media and consumer interest in phytochemicals is far ahead of established proof of the health benefits of these food components for humans. Although the Department of Agriculture website includes databases on carotenoids, flavonoids, isoflavonoids and other phytochemicals, much remains to be learned. [3] With data incomplete even for commonly eaten foods, it is impossible to calculate optimal phytochemical intakes for individuals.

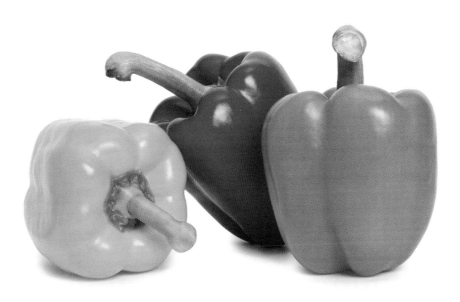

Phytochemicals: Potential Health Benefits and Sources

Carotenoids

Carotenoids are fat-soluble phytochemicals with a vitamin-A-like structure. They are the pigments responsible for the colors of many red, green, yellow and orange fruits and vegetables. Carotenoids have strong antioxidant and other potentially protective properties. Approximately 600 carotenoids have been identified. The table below lists some of the most common.

Carotenoid	Potential Health Benefits	Sources
Beta-carotene	• Slows aging process • Reduces risk of certain types of cancer • Improves lung function • Reduces complications associated with diabetes • Protects eyes	**Yellow-orange** fruits and vegetables such as mangoes, cantaloupe, dried or fresh apricots, papaya, carrots, pumpkins, sweet potatoes, butternut squash, nectarines, and green vegetables such as broccoli, spinach, collard greens and kale
Lutein	• Protects against cataracts and macular degeneration • Promotes eye health • Decreases risk of lung cancer	**Green** and **yellow** vegetables such as broccoli, collard greens, Brussels sprouts, Swiss chard, romaine lettuce, peas, corn, pumpkin and butternut squash
Zeaxanthin	• Protects against cataracts and macular degeneration	**Green** leafy and **orange** vegetables and fruit, especially spinach, green bell peppers, orange peppers, orange juice, oranges, honeydew, peaches, mango, winter squash, corn and egg yolks
Lycopene	• Reduces the risk of prostate cancer and heart disease	**Red** fruits and vegetables such as tomatoes, cooked tomato products, (catsup), red bell peppers, pink or red grapefruit, watermelon and guava

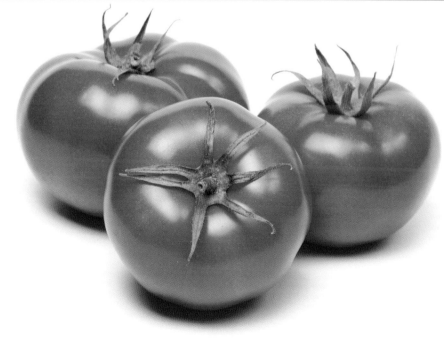

Flavonoids

Flavonoids are among the most potent and abundant antioxidants in the diet. More than 4,000 flavonoids have been identified. Flavonoids, particularly flavanols and proanthocyanidins, have been associated with reduction in the risk of cardiovascular disease.

Additionally, mounting evidence suggests flavonoids in black and green tea play significant roles in reducing the risk of cancer, stroke, insulin resistance, obesity, and declines in age-related brain functioning.

Potential Health Benefits and Sources of Flavonoids

Flavonoid	Potential Health Benefits	Sources
Anthocyanidins	• Delays diseases associated with aging • Helps prevent urinary tract infections • Aids circulation and nerve function	Purple and red fruits and vegetables, red wine, blueberries, cherries, raspberries, raisins, cranberries, strawberries, red grapes, kiwifruit, plums, red cabbage, kidney beans, beets, pomegranate, acai, tomatoes, eggplant peel, prunes, beets and some ripened olives
Flavonols Quercetin	• Antihistamine • Potent antioxidant • Inhibits the growth of head and neck cancers • Protects lungs from the harmful effects of pollutants and cigarette smoke	Apples, pears, cherries, cranberries, raspberries, grapes, red onions, kale, broccoli, leaf lettuce, garlic, green and black tea, red wine, cauliflower, capers and tomatoes (especially organically grown)
Flavanones Hesperidin	• Protects against heart disease and strengthens blood vessels • Prevents aches and night leg cramps	Citrus fruits and juices, such as oranges and orange juice with pulp, grapefruit and grapefruit juice, tangerines, lemons, limes, mandarins and tangelos
Naringenin	• May help prevent cancers • Potential cholesterol-lowering agent	Citrus peels, fruits and their juices
Flavanols Catechins	• May prevent heart disease and cancer	Green and oolong tea
Proanthocyanidins	• May contribute to maintenance of urinary tract health • May contribute to heart health	Cranberries, apples, red grapes, red wine, berries, chocolate, peanuts and cinnamon

Note: The health benefits of wine, especially red wine, have been highly publicized. Red or purple grape juice, pomegranate juice, cherry juice and acai juice have similar effects at varying prices and are non-alcohol alternatives.

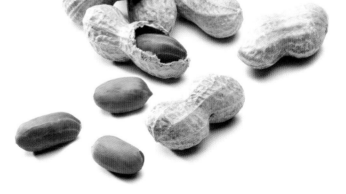

Phytoestrogens

Phytoestrogens are plant-derived compounds that are similar in effect to the hormone estrogen.

Potential Health Benefits and Sources of Phytoestrogens

Phytoestrogen	Potential Health Benefits	Sources
Isoflavones	• Lower blood cholesterol • Improve bone health • Help prevent hormone-related cancers and menopausal symptoms	Soybean, tofu, soymilk, soy-based foods, legumes, peanuts and chickpeas
Lignans	• Reduce risk of cardiovascular disease	Flaxseeds, sesame seeds, curly kale, broccoli, apricots, cabbage, Brussels sprouts, strawberries, tofu and dark rye bread

Glucosinolates

Cruciferous vegetables differ from other classes of vegetables in that they are rich sources of sulfur containing compounds known as **glucosinolates**. Because epidemiological studies provide some evidence that diets rich in cruciferous vegetables are associated with lower risk of several types of cancer, scientists are interested in the potential cancer preventive activities of compounds derived from glucosinolates. Guidelines for preventing cancer include eating cruciferous vegetables regularly.

Potential Health Benefits and Sources of Compounds Derived from Glucosinolates

Compounds Derived from Glucosinolates	Potential Health Benefits	Sources
Allium compounds (Allicin)	• May reduce the risk of certain types of cancer • May lower cholesterol and blood pressure • Contains anti-viral, anti-bacterial and anti-fungal agents	Mostly white vegetables – garlic, onions, chives, leeks, ramps and scallions
Sulphoraphane	• May reduce risk of colon cancer	Cruciferous vegetables such as broccoli, cauliflower, kale, Brussels sprouts, cabbage, bok choy, collard greens, turnips and turnip green sprouts
Indole-3 carbinol	• Blocks hormones that promote breast and prostate cancers	Garden cress, mustard greens, Brussels sprouts, horseradish, kale, watercress, turnip, Savoy cabbage, red cabbage, broccoli, kohlrabi, bok choy and cauliflower
Isothiocyanates	• Inhibit the development of chemically induced cancers of the lung, liver, esophagus, stomach, small intestine, colon and breast	Brussels sprouts, garden cress, mustard greens, turnips, Savoy cabbage, kale, watercress, horseradish, red cabbage, broccoli, kohlrabi and cauliflower

Other Phytochemicals

Potential Health Benefits and Sources of Other Phytochemicals

Phytochemical	Potential Health Benefits	Sources
Ellagic acid/Ellegotannins	• May reduce risk of certain types of cancer by inhibiting DNA binding of some carcinogens • May decrease blood cholesterol levels	Purple and red grapes, pomegranates and pomegranate juice, blueberries, raspberries, strawberries, blackberries, prunes, cranberries and currants
Capsaicin	• Improves digestion • Relieves inflammation • Can cause pain and/or euphoria effects from endorphin release	Hot chili peppers and cayenne
Curcumin	• Anti-inflammatory • Prevents colon cancer • Stimulates liver to break down toxins	Turmeric
Limonene (orange oil)	• May help to protect lungs and reduce risk of certain types of cancer • Blocks proteins that stimulate cell growth; possible cancer-fighting agent	Rinds and the edible white membranes of citrus fruits (zest), such as oranges, grapefruit, tangerines, lemons and limes
Resveratrol	• Keeps blood vessels flexible • Reduces risk of heart disease, cancer, blood clots and stroke	Red and purple grapes, red and purple grape juice, red wine and peanuts
Saponin	• Neutralizes enzymes in intestine that cause cancer • Boosts immune systems and promotes healing	Beans, soybeans, legumes, most vegetables and herbs
Phytosterols	• Lowers blood cholesterol	Wheat germ, sesame oil, corn oil, canola oil, peanuts, wheat bran, almonds, Brussels sprouts, rye bread, macadamia nuts and olive oil
Lentinan	• Immune booster • Has an anti-viral and anti-tumor effects	Shiitake mushrooms (fresh and dried)

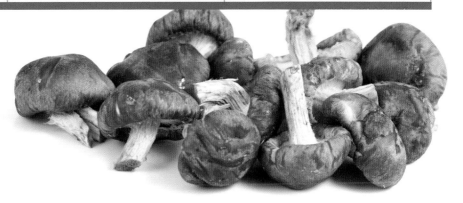

Antioxidant Protection

Although their structures differ, vitamins, minerals and phytochemicals can act as antioxidants, reducing cell damage caused by the oxidation that occurs naturally throughout the body. Antioxidants neutralize or inactivate highly unstable and extremely reactive molecules called **free radicals** that attack the body's cells every day. Free radicals are produced during food metabolism and by other triggers such as air pollution. Experts believe that antioxidants can help prevent free radical damage, which contributes to a variety of conditions, including cancer, heart disease and aging. Some vitamins and minerals and many phytochemicals provide this important biologic function. Examples include:

Vitamin A	Beta-carotene	Lycopene
Vitamin C	Selenium	Resveratrol
Vitamin E	Lutein	

How Much Is Enough? How Much Is Too Much?

The National Research Council sets estimated safe and adequate daily dietary intakes for key vitamins and upper limits above which toxic effects have been reported. More is not better. Vitamins and minerals in amounts found in food are generally safe. Fortified cereals are generally safe as are multivitamin-minerals that are age appropriate in moderate dosages. But sustained excessive intake of vitamins, particularly fat-soluble vitamins and some minerals (usually from supplements), can be harmful. Although water-soluble vitamins are not stored in the body, they can interfere with medications. And by taking large quantities of water soluble vitamins, one can develop a physiological reliance on the excessive quantity. For example, people who have taken vitamin C in excessively high doses may have bleeding gums, a symptom of deficiency, after they stop or reduce the dosage. Kidney stones have been reported among those who take mega-doses of vitamin C.

Taking vitamins and minerals in excess is costly, has no physiologic advantage and may create imbalances with other nutrients. Many vitamins and minerals are toxic at high levels. In supplement form, some can interfere with certain clinical laboratory tests and medications and can create stress on the liver and kidneys where they are metabolized.

Enrichment and Fortification

Enrichment restores vitamins and minerals lost during food processing. For example, when wheat is milled and refined into flour, thiamin, riboflavin, niacin and iron are among nutrients that are lost. Cornmeal also loses these nutrients in processing. The 1942 Enrichment Act restored the original levels of these four nutrients in flour. More recently, folacin was added at specified levels to enrichment nutrients to protect against birth defects from inadequate folacin.

Recently questions have been raised if the added folacin is food for brain function in the aged and thus is being studied. While enrichment has improved the healthfulness of refined flour, many nutrients in whole grains – including fiber, vitamin B6, magnesium, zinc and other trace minerals – are also removed during milling but are not replaced. Consequently, whole-grain breads and cereals are a better choice because of their more complete nutritional package.

In **fortification**, vitamins and minerals are added to food to boost nutrient levels beyond original values. Most milks and margarines are fortified with vitamins A and D. Some fruit drinks are fortified with vitamin C; soymilk and rice milk are fortified with calcium and vitamin B12; and salt has added iodine. Many breakfast cereals are fortified with a whole day's supply of vitamins and minerals, essentially making them a vitamin/mineral supplement encased in food. Many fortified foods are considered functional foods. See Chapter 8 for more on functional foods.

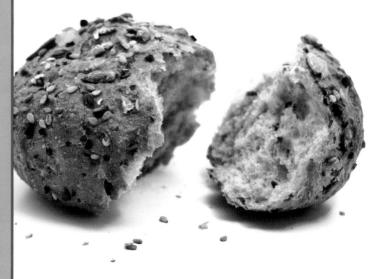

Bioavailability

Just because a food contains certain vitamins, minerals and phytochemcials does not mean the body can use those nutrients effectively. Many factors influence **bioavailability** – that is, the degree to which a nutrient is absorbed and utilized. The human body can adapt to varied levels of vitamin and mineral consumption. A well-functioning digestive tract generally regulates absorption and excretion to meet the body's needs. Ingesting extremely high amounts of specific nutrients overworks the body's ability to regulate. In addition, excessive intake of some minerals can lead to kidney failure and a host of other medical problems.

Nutrient bioavailability is enhanced by:

- Enzymes and bacteria within the digestive tract that can increase the amount of nutrients absorbed
- Vitamin C that boosts the absorption of iron present in plant foods
- Protein and vitamin D that boost calcium utilization
- A small amount of fat or oil that will increase the absorption of fat-soluble vitamins
- The form of a nutrient – for example, vitamin D_3 vs. vitamin D_2
- Fermentation processes, such as those used to make miso and tempeh, that may improve iron bioavailability
- Food preparation techniques, such as soaking and sprouting beans, grains and seeds as well as leavening bread that can reduce binding of zinc by phytic acid and increase zinc bioavailability
- Organic acids, such as citric acid, that can also enhance zinc absorption

Vitamins and minerals also may compete with each other for absorption through the gastrointestinal tract and bloodstream. For example, calcium, magnesium, iron, copper and zinc compete for the same protein carriers for absorption. Thus, too much of one can impede absorption of another.

Some substances bind minerals in the digestive tract, thus reducing the amount absorbed:

- Oxalates in vegetables such as spinach bind calcium so that most of it cannot be absorbed.
- Polyphenols in regular and herbal teas, coffee, and red wine bind iron.
- Phytates in whole grains, legumes and some vegetables bind calcium, iron, phosphorus and zinc.
- **Avidin**, a protein found in small amounts in raw eggs, will interfere with the absorption of biotin. Avidin is chemically altered by cooking so it is not present in cooked eggs.

On the positive side, cooking can also increase absorption of some vitamins and minerals either by softening cell walls so nutrients can be released or, in the case of legumes, by breaking down bonds between minerals and binders. For example, the vitamin A (beta-carotene) in cooked carrots is more available and absorbable than the vitamin A in raw carrots.

Oxalic and Phytic Acids

Oxalic acid binds some minerals, particularly calcium, so that they cannot be absorbed from the digestive tract. It is found in oranges, spinach, rhubarb, tea, coffee, bananas, ginger and almonds. Phytic acid binds some minerals, particularly iron and zinc, so that they cannot be absorbed from the digestive tract. It is found in cereals, nuts, sesame seeds, soybeans, wheat, pumpkin and beans. Thus, the full amount of minerals, as listed in food value tables, is not always available to the body.

The Raw Truth

Is raw food always healthier? Not really. Advocates of raw food diets claim that eating all foods raw (or heated no higher than 115 degrees) increases intake of natural enzymes and that a totally raw diet is healthful. While it is true that many raw foods contain active enzymes, it is unclear if this has much benefit to humans. Certainly, a raw food diet can cause weight loss because many foods are eliminated and total food intake decreases. Providing variety beyond raw fruits and vegetables involves extensive sprouting, soaking and specialized preparation methods.

Cooking destroys pathogens such as *salmonella* and *E. coli* found in some fresh fruits and vegetables. While most raw food diets are completely plant-based, some people also consume raw eggs and dairy. Less commonly, raw fish and meat may be included as well. Cooking these animal products will destroy pathogens and bacteria that may be in raw poultry, meat, fish and eggs making these protein rich sources safe to eat.

Cooked carrrots supply more beta-carotene than raw carrots. Boiling carrots, however, leads to a loss of polyphenols, an antioxidant. In addition, cooking can destroy some of the vitamin C in fruits and vegetables because vitamin C is highly unstable and easily destroyed when exposed to heat and water. Cooking softens food such as cellulose fiber in vegetables, allowing for easier digestion. Some foods such as whole grains and legumes are not palatable until cooked.

The bottom line is that eating more fruits and vegetables improves total diet – raw or cooked.

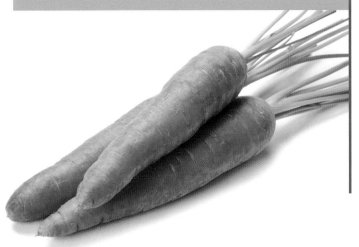

In general, vitamins and minerals are used more fully when they come from food rather than from supplements. When foods are fortified, usually a bioavailable form of a nutrient is added. For example, vitamin D in D3 form is added to milk; calcium citrate is added to orange juice. Some fortified breakfast cereals provide significant amounts of vitamins and minerals and can replace a multivitamin/mineral supplement in pill form. Supplements are generally safe in either pill, cereal or health bar form. Problems arise when nutrients taken in excessive amounts create imbalances with other nutrients or become toxic in large quantities. Individuals with allergies, intolerances or aversions to foods may need supplements to replace nutrients they may not get from food. A physician or registered dietitian should evaluate the person's diet and confirm with laboratory tests to ensure the appropriate type and amount of any supplement is taken. What advertisements, publicity and infomercials don't tell you is that overuse of self-selected supplements can be dangerous as well as an unnecessary expense.

Nutrient Retention

Nutrients in food are affected by many variables, including nutrients in the soil, degree of maturity at harvest, transportation time, storage, processing and cooking methods. The nutrients from animal foods are influenced by what the animal was fed or ate. Vitamins can be destroyed by exposure to heat, oxygen, light and extremes in pH and moisture. The extent of damage depends on the length of time food is exposed to each element. Careful storage and handling and close attention to proper cooking techniques will help minimize nutrient loss. Minerals are unaffected by high temperatures, but to preserve vitamins, avoid high heat and use the shortest appropriate cooking times. Water-soluble vitamins are particularly vulnerable.

Fresh, whole and minimally processed foods deliver high nutritive value and good appearance, taste and texture. Produce is often harvested unripe so it can withstand shipping. For optimal nutrient value, however, produce should ripen on the plant so the maximum nutrition is gained from the soil and plant.

casebycase | What's Smokin'?

One rarely sees the words "barbecue" and "healthy choice" in the same sentence, but at New Buffalo Bill's – in the heart of southwestern Michigan's Harbor Country – customers have been enjoying meaty wood-smoked barbecue, including brisket, award-winning ribs, pulled pork and chicken, along with an strong assortment of healthful side dishes since 2015.

William "Bill" Reynolds handles the barbecue side of the business and his 15-year partner in business and life, nationally known registered dietitian and a former president of the Academy of Nutrition and Dietetics, Mary Abbott Hess, makes sure the menu includes some choices with a healthier profile. New Buffalo Bill's offers various portion sizes, including a popular "taste of" serving and mini pulled pork or chicken sliders.

Bill, an honorary member of the Academy of Nutrition and Dietetics, spent 25 years at the Culinary Institute of America and 12 years at Chicago's Washburne Culinary Institute before "retiring" to his family's hunting ranch

in Del Rio, Texas, where the Lone Star State's unique barbecue flavor grabbed his attention. "A love for Texas barbecue and a commitment to preparing the best food we can – this is what fuels the passion behind New Buffalo Bill's," Bill explains. "Our 60-square-foot Ole Hickory Smokers allow us to mix old-world smoking techniques with modern technology."

To appeal more to children and for adults who are watching fat and calories, Mary urged Bill to add some lower-fat sides rich in micro- and phytonutrients, such as collard greens, sweet potato and pineapple salad, broccoli and cherry tomato salad with sunflower seeds, quinoa and whole-grain pilaf, several types of beans and strawberry applesauce. And for people seeking a non-meat alternative, there is smoked roasted salmon, smoked tofu, and portobello mushrooms and in 2019 we added a vegan sausage.

As Mary proudly notes, "Even vegans can get a healthy meal at New Buffalo Bill's."

Locally grown produce is more likely to be ripe when picked. To reduce nutrient loss, most produce should be chilled immediately and kept chilled until used.

Fruits and vegetables with cut skins should be covered so that vitamins are not exposed to air. Fruits and vegetables should also be removed from opened cans and covered before storage to avoid bacteria growth and altered flavors.

Frozen fruits and vegetables are equal, and sometimes even better, than fresh varieties because they are picked at flavor peak and quickly frozen after harvest to preserve nutrients. A "fresh" fruit may have spent considerable time in shipping or storage before it gets to your kitchen. Properly stored, frozen fruits and vegetables are not subject to nutrient losses from prolonged shipping or warehouse storage.

Whether or not organically grown produce has a higher vitamin and mineral content than traditionally grown produce depends on variables such as seed variety, soil condition and ripeness at picking.

Extensive validated research comparing organic and traditionally grown produce is not yet available. As explained in Chapter 8, there is much conflicting information.

A study from the University of California (UC) at Davis states that some canned foods actually provide higher levels of essential nutrients (in particular, the fat-soluble carotenoids) than similar fresh or frozen items. [4] The canning process locks in nutrients at their peak of freshness and shields them from oxygen. Look for fruits canned in natural juices, rather than heavy syrup, and for low-sodium or unsalted canned vegetables. Canned tomato products are more consistent in quality than their fresh counterparts and will have even more lycopene than fresh tomatoes. Canned fruits, vegetables and beans can be a nutritious and convenient alternative to fresh or frozen and more readily available for some foodservice operations. Canned legumes are convenient and save cooking time but can be higher in sodium. Draining and rinsing canned beans will reduce sodium by about 40%.

Additional conclusions drawn from the UC Davis study are:

- **Canned**: Canned foods are packed at their peak of freshness. Due to the absence of oxygen during their storage period, canned fruits and vegetables have a longer shelf life and remain relatively stable up until the time they are consumed.

- **Fresh**: Fresh is best if consumed within a short time after purchasing.

- **Frozen**: Frozen products are packed at their peak of freshness. Frozen fruits and vegetables may be more nutritious if stored for short periods of time under well-controlled temperatures.

- **All Forms**: Fresh, frozen and canned fruits and vegetables contribute to the nation's nutrition and make healthful choices available to everyone, everywhere.

Often, the same steps taken to preserve food quality also retain nutrients. For example, keeping vegetables fresh by washing them whole, covering and refrigerating them will help maintain freshness and nutrient content. Consider whether or not vegetables will be peeled before cooking. Removing the peel exposes more of the vegetable flesh and accelerates nutrient loss. Also, many nutrients are just beneath the peel and are removed during peeling. Edible peels and skins provide valuable fiber and phyto-chemicals; straining pulp from citrus discards fiber and many phytochemicals and vitamins. Juicing and straining fruits and vegetables extract liquids with many vitamins and minerals but discard the pulp and fiber. American diets need more, not less, fiber. Purees, coulis and smoothies that incorporate whole fruits and vegetables have broken cell walls that increase nutrient availability; fiber remains in the puree.

When possible, cook vegetables from the raw or frozen state and serve them immediately. To minimize nutrient loss, wash vegetables before cutting them. To cook most vegetables, steam them until just done. If not served immediately, stop the cooking process by plunging the vegetables into ice water, drain thoroughly, wrap and refrigerate until ready to serve. If steaming is not practical, blanch vegetables for a short period in rapidly boiling water. Then follow the necessary steps for maximum nutrient retention. Since water-soluble vitamins are released into cooking liquids, steaming and microwaving cause the least release and most vitamin retention. Reserve nutrient-rich cooking liquids for soups and marinades; to braise or poach meats, poultry and fish; and to cook starches. Note that adding baking soda (alkaline) to maintain a vegetable's color used to be popular trick, but doing so changes texture and destroys thiamin and vitamin C.

Avoid or limit frying vegetables and choose frying fats carefully. When serving fried foods, such as French fries, serve a small portion. The high heat used in frying, especially deep-frying, creates free radicals in the fat that are unhealthy. Free radicals that contribute to aging, heart disease and cancer risk are produced when oils are continuously oxidized by high temperatures.

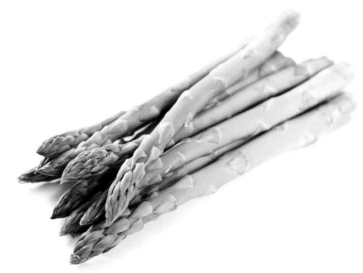

Opportunities for Chefs

Although needed only in small quantities, vitamins, minerals and phytochemicals perform very important functions in the body. Even the root word "vita" indicates the vital nature of these substances. The diets of many Americans are rich in calories, fats, sugars and sodium, but lacking in fiber, essential vitamins, minerals and phytochemicals. Planning, preparing and serving meals that are high in fruits, vegetables, whole grains, legumes, fish and seafood, lean meats and low-fat dairy products will help guests obtain these important nutrients. Using techniques to preserve nutrients and maximize their absorption adds to the nutrient density of the total menu.

Learning Activities

1. Collect 10 food labels. Highlight all ingredients that provide sodium. Identify the amount of sodium in a serving of each food.

2. Select one phytochemical and research its benefits and sources.

3. Review food composition tables or best source of nutrient lists. Identify 10 foods that provide at least 20% of the daily need for five or more vitamins or minerals.

4. Create three recipes that include ingredients rich in at least two nutrients of concern – potassium, dietary fiber, vitamin K, vitamin D, calcium or phosphorus.

For More Information

- Micronutrient Information Center, Linus Pauling Institute, Oregon State University, **https://lpi. oregonstate.edu/mic**

- Produce for Better Health Foundation, Phytochemical Information Center, **http://www.pbhfoundation.org/about/res/pic**

- USDA Database for the Flavonoid Content of Selected Foods, Release 3.1, Prepared by the Nutrient Data Laboratory, Food Composition Laboratory, Beltsville Human Nutrition Research Center, Agricultural Research Service, U.S. Department of Agriculture, May 2014, **https://www.ars.usda.gov/ARSUser-Files/80400525/Data/Flav/Flav_R03-1.pdf**

- US Department of Agriculture, Agricultural Research Service, Nutrient Data Laboratory. USDA National Nutrient Database for Standard Reference, Legacy. Version Current: April 2018. **https://ndb.nal.usda.gov/ndb/**

Chapter Eight

Planning Healthful Meals

Learning Objectives | *After completing this chapter, you should be able to:*

- Identify current major food trends related to nutrition and health
- Explain how to identify and purchase inherently healthful ingredients
- Describe the impact of the sustainable foods movement on planning healthful menus
- Discuss the benefits and disadvantages of using local and organic foods
- Find reliable sources of information on sustainable and organic foods
- List the benefits of functional foods and give examples
- Create healthful menu items
- Identify ingredients to use and limit when creating healthful foods
- Plan a healthful menu and specify appropriate portion size of each offering

The basic tenets of menu planning focus on balancing colors, textures and shapes, variety of ingredients, cooking methods, food cost, equipment availability, staff abilities, and guests' needs and preferences. Healthful menu planning adds careful consideration of total calorie count, type and amount of fat, nutrient density and retention, the amount of added sodium and sugar, and special dietary needs, such as gluten intolerance or food allergies. With so many factors to consider, planning excellent menus is a challenge.

The overall success of most menus, however, rests on flavor. No one can sell a healthy product (more than once) if it doesn't taste good. This dimension of menu planning is so important that Chapter 9 is devoted to creating flavorful healthful options.

Fruits, vegetables, whole grains, legumes, fish and seafood, lean meats, healthful oils, and low-fat dairy products are the key ingredients of a healthful menu. While Americans eat enough meat and total grains, studies show that most Americans do not eat enough fruit, vegetables (including legumes), whole grains and low-fat dairy products. Fruits, vegetables and whole grains are rich in vitamins, minerals, phyto-chemicals and fiber, and are relatively low in calories, fat and sodium. Dairy products provide calcium, an important mineral quite low in other food groups.

Focusing on fruits and vegetables makes seasonality an important aspect of menu planning. Generally, produce used in season is at its flavor peak, which allows for simpler preparation. Foods in season are also plentiful and available, which helps control food costs. Patrons look forward to seasonal foods – asparagus and morels in the spring, strawberries bursting with flavor in early summer, juicy tomatoes and peaches in late summer, crisp apples in autumn and hearty braised meats with root vegetables in the winter months. While many operations cannot revamp their core menu each season, most can run specials that focus on fresh foods and incorporate seasonal fruits and vegetables into salads, side dishes and desserts.

Menu Trends

Food fads come and go, but food trends have more staying power. The trend toward more healthful food preparations has been evolving for several decades. One of the most significant positive nutrition-related trends is serving traditional dishes from ethnic cuisines, such as Mediterranean and Asian, both of which rely less on meat and more on whole grains and vegetables. Other trends include lighter sauces, smaller meat portions, vegetarian options, small plates, greater emphasis on fruits and vegetables, more whole-grain offerings, and salads served as main courses.

With the increasing number of overweight and obese Americans, it may seem that the public doesn't care about nutrition. The fact is, however, that healthcare reform and public policies such as calories listed on menus and nutrient disclosure are focusing attention on making healthful foods and nutrition information more available to all. There is also an increased popularity of "getting back to nature" eating, with vegetarianism, organic and local foods on the rise.

Greater emphasis is being placed on menu items that are inherently healthy – that is, foods that are naturally "good for you." According to 2016 market research from Mintel, artificial is public enemy number one, with consumer demands for natural and less processed food and drink forcing companies to remove artificial ingredients. [1] Consumers are also looking for foods that include more whole and minimally processed ingredients. According to Mintel, "Eco is the new reality," with drought, worries about food waste and other natural phenomena affecting the worldwide food and drink supply, but influencing preparation and production." [1]

A National Restaurant Association publication, *Chef Survey: What's Hot in 2018*, showed restaurants can expect to see a growing demand for healthful kids' meals, sustainable seafood, housemade or artisan pickles and authentic ethnic cuisines. [2]

Many consumers are seeking foods that reflect their concerns about the environment, energy consumption, social justice, animal welfare and sustainable living. In fact, one of the principles from the Chefs Collaborative Statement of Principles states: Good food begins with unpolluted air, land, and water, environmentally sustainable farming and fishing, and humane animal husbandry. [3]

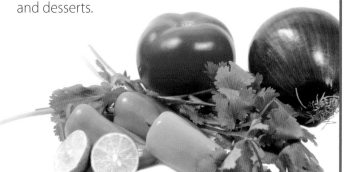

National Restaurant Association's Chef Survey: What's Hot in 2018

1. New cuts of meat
2. House-made condiments
3. Street food inspired dishes
4. Ethnic inspired breakfast items
5. Sustainable seafood
6. Healthful kids' meals
7. Vegetable carb substitutes
8. Uncommon herbs
9. Authentic ethnic cuisine
10. Ethnic spices
11. Peruvian cuisine
12. Housemade/artisan pickles
13. Heritage breed meats
14. Thai-rolled ice cream
15. African flavors
16. Ethnic inspired kids' dishes
17. Doughnuts with nontraditional filling
18. Gourmet items in kids' meals
19. Ethnic condiments
20. Ancient grains

Source: 2. National Restaurant Association. Chef Survey: What's Hot in 2018. Available at **http://www.restaurant.org/News-Research/Research/What-s-Hot.**

Flavor

Healthful flavors are explored fully in the next chapter, but flavor profiling is a significant food trend that must be mentioned here as well. Today's focus on flavor is reflected in customers' growing interest in ethnic cuisines. Many customers seek flavors they have enjoyed while traveling, have read or heard about, or have seen on the Internet or on television food programs. Chefs are cooking with condiments, herbs, spices and unique ingredients from all corners of the world. Various cuisines may fall in and out of favor, but continued public interest in authentic, ethnic flavors remains steady.

Food trucks have capitalized on our love of all things ethnic. More than 4,000 food trucks are feeding consumers each day, with annual sales exceeding $2.7

billion. Food-truck revenue jumped at an annual rate of 7.9 percent over the past five years. In fact, food truck growth is outpacing overall commercial food-service. [4, 5] Many food trucks offer an authentic food experience serving everything from Vietnamese street food to authentic Chinese steamed buns to Hawaiian shaved ice.

The *Dietary Guidelines* recommend significant reductions in sodium (salt), fats and added sugar. All of these components add to flavor. When salt, sugar and fat are limited, chefs have to work harder and are challenged to create alternative flavor enhancers. Salt reduction is discussed in Chapters 9 and 13, fat reduction in Chapters 4 and 13, and sugar reduction in Chapter 3.

Custom Food Preparation

Restaurant customers have always asked for custom food preparation such as degree of doneness for meats and "dressing on the side" with salads. Now there is even more interest in custom food preparation to accommodate individual nutritional needs, especially food intolerances (such as lactose and gluten) and allergies (such as peanuts). Menu items are also customized to meet specific dietary needs including weight loss. These special health considerations are addressed in Chapter 13.

The availability of half portions, fresh vegetables as sides, alternative sweeteners, low-fat salad dressing options, vegetarian entrées, sampler plates, skim milk as a beverage and hummus or olive oil with bread are easy ways to help customers meet their health needs without altering basic menu items or limiting selections.

Starters

Starters, or appetizers, are small portions of savory items served before the main course. Some patrons make a meal by ordering several starters – or "small plates" – rather than an entrée. Meze, tapas and dim sum are ethnic variations on the small-plate theme. If a starter must be fried, serve a small portion of the fried component as a part of a dish that includes other foods.

General guidelines for developing healthful starters include:

- Portions should be small to moderate, generally about 8 bites or ½ to ¾ cup.
- Incorporate vegetables, legumes and grains as primary ingredients whenever possible.
- Use endive leaves, mushrooms and cored vegetables to hold fillings for appetizers and hors d'oeuvres.
- Portion meat, fish or poultry at about 2 ounces.
- Include bread, fruit and pickled vegetables on charcuterie plates.
- Use whole grains and legumes creatively.
- Limit high-fat sauces to 1 or 2 ounces.
- Use healthful cooking techniques and heart healthy fats in preparing starters.
- Use yogurt or hummus as bases for dips and spreads.
- Place small amounts of smoked salmon, lean ham or prosciutto on canapes or with melon.

Starters: Guide to Appetizer Ingredient Choices

Recommended	Limit
• All vegetables • All fruits • Lean meats • Poultry • Seafood, any way except fried • Whole grains, such as barley, amaranth, quinoa, bulgur, wheat berries, wild rice, brown rice and farro • Moderate- or low-fat cheeses • Beans and other legumes • Whole-grain breads, crackers and pastas • Small amounts of sauces as garnish and for color, texture and flavor • Eggs • Vegetable and fruit sauces	• High-fat meats such as ribs, pate, foie gras and sausages • Fried seafood, poultry or vegetables • Cream • Patês, sausages and forcemeats • High-fat cheeses • Rich sauces • Fried garnishes • Fried potato or other chips

Soups

Soups can be hot or cold, hearty and filling, brothy and delicate, or creamy and smooth. They can be a start to a meal or a meal in themselves. Soups are inherently a great way to highlight seasonal vegetables and healthful ingredients such as beans and whole grains. When preparing house-made stocks, the chef can control sodium levels. These stocks are generally more flavorful than commercial varieties. Low-sodium stocks – some very high in quality – are available canned, frozen or as concentrates. Chilled soups made from cucumbers, asparagus, peas, melons or other fruits can be a healthful and interesting option.

Sodium in Chicken Base, Broth and Stock

	Amount	Sodium (milligrams)
Chicken base, standard	¾ teaspoon of base to make 1 cup of broth	704
Reduced-sodium chicken broth	1 cup	554
Low-sodium chicken base	¾ teaspoon of base to make 1 cup of broth	142
Low-sodium chicken broth, canned	1 cup	72
House-made chicken stock, no added salt	1 cup	70

Soup can also be low in calories and play an important role in creating satiety, according to Barbara Rolls, Ph.D., Guthrie Chair of Nutrition at Pennsylvania State University and author of *Volumetrics: Feel Full on Fewer Calories*. Participants in one of Rolls' studies consumed 20% fewer calories when they started their meals with a broth-based, vegetable soup. [6]

General guidelines for developing healthful soups include:

- Portion soups at about 8 ounces.
- Use evaporated skim milk or buttermilk for "creaming."
- Use vegetable purees or instant mashed potatoes as thickeners.
- Use defatted stocks for the foundation of soup.
- Emphasize vegetable-based soups.

- Include legumes and whole grains in soups, especially hearty soups used as a main course.
- Chill cooked soups and remove fat before reheating for serving.
- Use fresh herbs and spices to limit added salt. Turn up the heat with spice.
- Use lemon or flavored vinegars to add flavor and acidity.
- The liquid from canned beans can be drained and used in soups, sauces and salad dressings. It is a nutrient-rich thickener but does add sodium. Reduce salt if it is used as a soup thickener.
- Add a bit of butter, oil or cream just before service for gloss and mouthfeel.
- Top soups with chimichurri, pesto and other low fat flavorful condiments or sauces.

Soups: Guide to Ingredient Choices

Recommended	Limit
• Fresh stocks or low-sodium meat, poultry, fish or vegetable commercial stocks and broths	• Cream and sour cream
• Evaporated skim milk and buttermilk	• Commercial high-sodium bases
• Vegetables of all kinds	• Roux
• Cornstarch, arrowroot, tapioca or pureed starchy vegetables as thickeners	• Bacon, sausage
• Fruits	• Cheese
• Legumes	• Fried croutons
• Whole grains such as barley and wild rice	
• Yogurt	
• Lean proteins	
• Seafood	
• Tomato-based soups and chowders	
• Chopped chives, scallions, parsley or red pepper as garnishes.	
• Small amounts of chopped, crisp bacon, shredded cheese or tiny croutons may be used as garnish for added texture and flavor.	

Salads and Dressings

Salads can be the most healthful menu items, but add-ons such as cheese, olives, fried croutons and dressings greatly increase calories and fat. For example, a salad at a quick-service chain can sound like a healthful choice but in fact have more than 1,000 calories. A 2-ounce portion of vinaigrette (using a 3:1 ratio of oil to vinegar) can contain 42 grams of oil. At 9 calories per gram of fat, that vinaigrette will have 378 calories just from oil. A creamy (mayonnaise-based) salad dressing is comparable. On the other hand, for an Asian-style salad, cucumbers and other vegetables can be marinated in sweetened mirin or rice wine vinegar, yogurt and fresh herbs with no oil at all.

Calories, Fat and Sodium in 1 Ounce of Salad Dressings

	Calories	Fat (grams)	Sodium (milligrams)
French dressing	130	12.7	240
French dressing, reduced-calorie	55	3.7	285
Ranch dressing	140	14.5	230
Ranch dressing, reduced-fat	55	3.5	260
Blue cheese dressing	135	14.5	265
Blue cheese dressing, low-calorie	30	2.0	340
Italian salad dressing	80	8.0	470
Italian salad dressing, reduced-fat	20	1.8	390
House-made ranch dressing	35	2.5	50
House-made vinaigrette-style dressing	65	7.0	40

General guidelines for developing healthful salads and dressings include:

- Serve 1 to 2 cups of different leafy greens and a variety of fresh, raw, blanched, steamed, roasted or grilled vegetables.

- Choose dark greens most of the time – spinach, baby kale or arugula, romaine, watercress and leaf lettuces – rather than iceberg or pale-colored greens.

- Use plenty of red, orange and yellow fruits and vegetables in salads – sweet potatoes, mangos, pomegranate seeds, oranges, red and yellow peppers, and beets and carrots – for added vitamins and phytochemicals.

- Avocados and nuts provide flavor, texture and healthful fats but should be used in moderation because they are both nutrient dense and calorie dense.

- Use olives and dried fruits in moderation. They are healthful but high in calories.

- Try cut fresh fruits in salads – apples, pears, berries and citrus – or fruit and vegetable combination salads.

- Marinate vegetables, such as artichokes, cucumbers, sliced fennel and peppers, in flavored vinegars.

- Limit high-fat garnishes, such as bacon. Use them on top rather than mixed into the salad to control quantity and to have more visual impact.

- Use moderate-fat cheeses like goat, feta, part-skim mozzarella, or reduced-fat Cheddar or Swiss.

- If crisps or croutons are used, bake, rather than fry them.

- Limit salad dressing to 1 tablespoon for a salad course or 2 tablespoons for an entrée salad.

- Use less dressing by tossing greens with the dressing rather than serving it on top or on the side.

- Offer several low-fat dressing options – made from scratch or purchased.
- Have balsamic or wine vinegar and olive oil available for guests who want to mix their own ratio of dressing.
- Use reduced-fat mayonnaise or dressings in tuna, salmon, egg, chicken, pasta, bean, vegetable and potato salads.

- Use heart-healthy oils – olive, walnut, sesame, canola, safflower, soybean, corn and sunflower – but in moderate amounts. All oils are high in calories.
- Utilize super flavorful vinegars, such as pomegranate and tangerine, to boost flavor without fat.
- Use moderate amounts of egg, cheese, lean meat or seafood in main course salads.

Vegetable Salads and Dressings: Guide to Ingredient Choices

Recommended	Limit
• Fresh vegetables – raw, various cuts, blanched, steamed, grilled or roasted	• Mayonnaise, substitute reduced-fat
• Fresh fruits	• Nuts
• Dried fruits	• Cheeses
• Oils: olive, walnut, sesame, canola, corn, safflower, soybean and sunflower	• Meats, bacon
• Flavored vinegars	• Croutons, crisps, tortilla chips
• Lemon and citrus juices	• Dried fruits
• Herbs	• Oils, all
• Legumes	

Reduced-Calorie Vinaigrette Dressing Formula

Thicken low-calorie liquids if necessary with cornstarch, arrowroot or xanthan gum. Add appropriate seasonings. Examples are listed below.

Vinaigrette	Low-calorie liquid (2 parts)	Oil (1 part)	Acid (1 part)
Apple-Walnut	Apple juice	Walnut	Apple cider vinegar
Balsamic	Vegetable stock	Olive	Balsamic vinegar
Citrus	Orange juice	Canola	Lime and lemon juice
Asian	Vegetable stock or tea	Sesame	Rice wine vinegar
Vegetable	Tomato juice	Olive	Red wine vinegar
Raspberry	Apple juice	Canola	Raspberry vinegar

Creamy Dressing Formula

Blend 1 part non- or low-fat yogurt and 2 parts pureed part-skim ricotta cheese to form a creamy base for salad dressings. Other low-fat creamy ingredients such as buttermilk, nonfat mayonnaise and silken tofu can be used for the base. Blend 1 part acid to 3 parts creamy base and add seasonings to create the classic salad dressings. Roasted garlic or avocado may be added for flavor.

Dressing	Acid (1 part)	Seasonings (as needed)
Green Goddess	Lemon juice	Chervil, chives, tarragon and parsley
Ranch	Buttermilk	Chives, parsley, dill and garlic powder
Blue Cheese	White wine vinegar	Blue cheese, crumbled
Thousand Island	Catsup or chili sauce	Pickles, onions, scallions, finely chopped egg, pepper

Sandwiches

As simple as grilled Vermont Cheddar or as complex as the classic New Orleans Muffaletta, the sandwich is the ultimate portable meal – with a global passport. Sandwiches can be stuffed (falafel), grilled (panini), open-faced (tuna melt), wrapped (turkey wrap), folded (taco) or the traditional two slices of bread with filling. Bread – whole grain, rye, pumpernickel or raisin, to name a few – gives the sandwich size and shape and adds flavor, texture and nutrients. Whole-wheat bread, foccacia, naan, bagels, pita, tortillas, flatbreads, sandwich rolls or buns, English muffins and quick breads may be used for sandwiches. (When white bread is used, choose enriched varieties.) In general, a serving is a slice of bread (1 ounce) about 100 calories, small buns count as two servings. Many large rolls are equal to four bread servings. Unless weight gain is a goal, avoid using croissants and other high-fat bread or rolls for sandwiches.

Be aware that luncheon meats, cheeses, condiments and bread can be significant sources of sodium. These ingredients can easily exceed a day's allotment of sodium, even if the rest of the sandwich is made with healthful ingredients.

General guidelines for developing healthful sandwiches include:

- Select whole-grain breads for increased fiber and other nutrients. Choose breads that have 3 grams of fiber per slice.
- Do not refrigerate bread. It will become stale faster. The staling process occurs fastest just above freezing so is actually accelerated by refrigeration. Freezing is preferred if storage is necessary.

- Rich, high-fat breads, like croissants and brioche, easily double the caloric level of sandwiches. Check the label for fat, sugar and fiber content.
- Be aware of size and amount of bread. A 12-inch sub sandwich roll is equal to 4 to 6 servings of bread. Each ounce of bread counts as 1 serving.
- Flour tortillas or wraps can be high in calories. A 12-inch flour tortilla wrap can provide 355 calories, 60 grams of carbohydrate and 725 milligrams of sodium.
- Use reduced-fat cheeses such as part-skim mozzarella, reduced-fat Cheddar or feta.
- Use a variety of vegetables in sandwiches such as lettuce, peppers, tomatoes, spinach and shredded carrots.
- Use a seasoned bean puree, such as white bean and rosemary or hummus as a spread.
- Use lean meats and trim visible fat. Serve a moderate amount of the protein.
- Use grilled or roasted vegetables as fillings.
- Prepare tuna, salmon, chicken or egg salad for sandwiches with reduced-fat mayonnaise.
- Grill chicken, fish and other meats instead of deep-frying it for sandwiches.
- Use flavorful condiments.
- Use a minimum amount of fat when grilling sandwiches – vegetable spray or only 1 teaspoon of oil per sandwich.
- Limit or avoid fried ingredients or fried sandwiches.

Healthful, Flavorful Sandwich Fillings

Proteins	Vegetables	Spreads
• Low-fat or moderate-fat cheese • Turkey and chicken, nonprocessed preferred • Eggs • Bean spreads • Peanut butter or nut butters • Lean meats including lean ham, beef and roast pork • Salads (tuna, chicken, egg and seafood) with reduced-calorie dressing • Reduced-fat cold cuts and sausages • Grilled tofu • Sardines	• Bell peppers, raw or roasted • Cabbage • Grated carrot • Cucumber • Lettuce or other greens • Onion, raw or caramelized • Mushrooms, raw or grilled • Radishes • Salad mix and giardiniera (in water) • Tomato, fresh or grilled • Avocado • Roasted or grilled vegetables • Pickles, and pickled vegetables, in moderation	• Catsup • Mustard • Low-fat cream cheese or goat cheese • Miso spreads • Pesto • Almond butter • Cashew butter • Vegetable purees • Fruit or vegetable chutneys • Olive spreads • Roasted pepper spread • Hummus • Low-fat mayonnaise • Jam or jelly • Horseradish sauce • Chili sauce

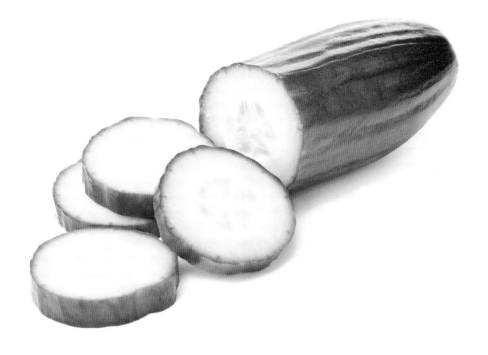

Sandwiches: Guide to Ingredient Choices

Recommended	Limit
• Turkey or chicken	• Large sandwich rolls or bagels
• Fish, shrimp, sardines, salmon or crab	• Large flour tortillas or wraps
• Lean meats or reduced-fat sausages	• Mayonnaise, regular
• Roasted red peppers	• High-fat breads such as croissants and brioche
• Grilled portabella mushrooms, zucchini or eggplant	• Fried taco shells
• Whole-wheat or other whole-grain bread (1- to 2-ounce portion)	• High-fat meats such as corned beef, bologna, bacon and sausages including hot dogs
• Mustards	• White bread
• Peanut or nut butters (2-tablespoon portion)	• Cream cheese
• Jams and jellies	• High-fat cheeses
• Pickled vegetables	• Anything fried
• Sliced apples and pears	• Butter
• Avocado	
• Eggs	
• Reduced-fat mayonnaise	
• Cheese with moderate fat	

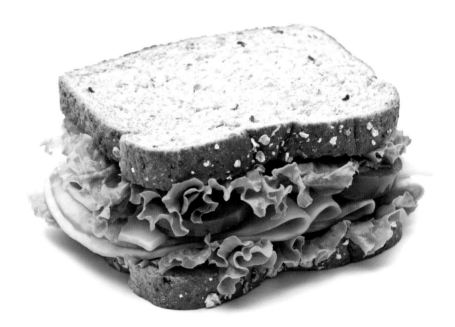

Main Courses

Traditionally, the main course showcases the chef's creativity and expertise. Healthful main courses can be vegetarian or meat-based. Current trends include locally sourced meats and seafood, sustainable seafood and newer cuts of meat such as pork flat iron, beef shoulder tender and other cuts.

General guidelines for developing healthful main courses include:

- Serve 3 to 5 ounces of cooked meat, fish, poultry, eggs or legumes. If this is not acceptable to your guests, provide protein in the lowest acceptable amount.
- Cook poultry with skin on to preserve flavor. Remove skin after cooking when practical. A 4-ounce, boneless, chicken breast with skin has 50 calories and 1.3 grams of saturated fat more than its skinless counterpart. Most of the fat in chicken skin is monounsaturated, which is the best kind of fat. Nevertheless, it does add calories. Remove excess fat, especially on duck, to moderate total fat and calories. Chicken wings have the highest skin to meat ratio.

- Do not limit poultry to breast meat. Dark meat has more iron and other minerals and although higher in fat, is considerably more tender and flavorful.
- Consider various poultry varieties like duck, quail, goose, pheasant, Cornish hen, guinea hen, squab, emu and ostrich.
- Include cooked whole grains or beans with entrées or as vegetarian entrées.
- Include low-fat dairy products.
- Use lots of vegetables and fruits as appropriate. Include a deep green, red or orange vegetable to add volume, color, flavor and nutrients to the plate.
- Use as little added fat as possible and choose healthful oils and fats.
- Trim visible fat from meats before serving.
- Skim fat from stews or liquids.
- Offer fish and seafood prepared any way but fried.
- Offer half portions for those who want a lighter main course or have a small appetite.

Main Course Salads and Dressings: Guide to Ingredient Choices

Recommended	Limit
Select or choice grades of beef, lean pork, veal, bison, buffalo, venison, lamb	High-fat meats such as ribs and brisket
Soy protein, tofu and tempeh	Prime meats
Poultry	Cured meats and sausages
Fish and seafood	Goose and duck (with skin and fat)
Lean sauces	Salted fish
Low-fat dairy products	Cheeses (melted or as sauces)
Vegetables	Fried meat, poultry, seafood
Grains, especially whole grains	Fried chips and croutons
Legumes	Butter, cream and sour cream
Fruits	Oils and items packed in oil
Herbs and aromatics	High-sodium marinades and sauces

Oven Roasted Cod* with Three Colored Peppers and Baby Potatoes

Yield: 10 servings each with 1 cup peppers, 1 fish fillet and 2 potatoes

Chef Nora Pouillon, Restaurant Nora
Washington, DC

It would be hard to find a better dish that helps diners meet the recommendation for plenty of fish and colorful vegetables. This beautiful and tasty entrée is filled with nutrient-rich ingredients.

Olive oil, divided	3	tablespoons
Onions, thinly sliced	2	medium
Garlic, minced	1	tablespoon
Green pepper, seeded and cut in julienne	2	each
Red peppers, seeded and cut in julienne	3	each
Yellow peppers, seeded and cut in julienne	3	each
Chicken stock or white wine	1 ½	cup
Mixed herbs such as thyme, oregano, rosemary, dill or parsley, chopped	1/3	cup
Sea salt	1	teaspoon
Black pepper, freshly ground	½	teaspoon
Cod fillets, cut into 10 portions	3	pounds,
	6	ounces
Small bouquet of assorted herbs for garnish		
Baby new potatoes, unpeeled	2	pounds

Rouille: Yield: ¾ cup

Red pepper, roasted, pureed	1	
Mayonnaise, light	½	cup
Garlic, minced	2	teaspoons
Saffron (optional)	1	pinch
Cayenne pepper	1	pinch

1. Preheat the oven to 450° F.

2. Heat 1 tablespoon of the olive oil in a large saute pan, add the onion, garlic and peppers and saute for about 5 minutes, stirring frequently. Add the stock or wine, herbs and season with salt and pepper and bring the mixture to a boil. Spoon the pepper mixture into a baking dish large enough to accommodate the fish fillets in one layer.

3. Clean the saute pan and heat until nearly smoking. Add the remaining 2 tablespoons of olive oil and immediately sear the seasoned cod fillets for 1-2 minutes on one side. Remove with spatula and place on top of pepper mixture, seared side up.

4. Bake 5-8 minutes or until desired doneness.

5. Steam the potatoes in a medium saucepan using a collapsible insert or boil them for 10-15 minutes, until a fork can be easily inserted in the potato.

6. Serve fish atop peppers with baby potatoes and a dollop of rouille (2 teaspoons per serving) or aioli (optional) and garnish with fresh herbs.

Rouille:

1. Mix ingredients together in a bowl.

* If Atlantic cod is not available, Alaskan black cod, halibut or any other firm fleshed fish is suitable for this dish.

Per Serving

Calories	300	Cholesterol	70	mg
Fat	10 g	Sodium	420	mg
Saturated Fat	1.5 g	Carbohydrates	23	mg
Trans Fat	0 g	Dietary Fiber	4	mg
Sugar	4 g	Protein	31	g

Sauces

Sauces add flavor, moisture and visual appeal to starters, main courses, vegetables, fruits and desserts. High-fat sauces such as white sauce (béchamel), cream sauce, mayonnaise and hollandaise sauce should be used in moderation. Salsa, tomato sauce, barbecue sauce and fruit sauces are naturally low in fat and can be used liberally to enhance the appeal and nutrient content of foods.

Most sauces contain a liquid, a thickening agent and other flavorings and seasonings. The liquid base for a sauce is typically:

- Stock
- Milk, yogurt or a dairy product
- Fruit or vegetable juice
- Wine, beer or spirits

The quality of the liquid base determines the quality of the sauce. Stock used for sauce can be made in-house where ingredients, particularly salt, can be controlled. Some high-quality bases and commercially available stocks that are low in sodium can also be used for sauces. Most sauces are thickened with a starchy product, such as flour, cornstarch, arrowroot, breadcrumbs, potato starch (or instant potatoes) or rice flour. Some commercial products use other starches for thickening. The thickening agent affects the appearance of the sauce. For example, a sauce thickened with flour has an opaque appearance, but when cornstarch is used, the sauce is clear. Servers should know if sauces are thickened with wheat flour or other ingredients containing gluten for those who may ask for gluten-free foods.

General guidelines for developing healthful sauces include:

- Use low-fat ingredients when possible.
- Use reductions for concentrated flavor.
- Reduce the fat in some sauces by replacing a roux thickener with a slurry.
- Use fruit- and vegetable-based sauces when possible. Examples include fruit or vegetable salsas, mango chutney, pureed corn, sweet potato puree, and black bean ragout. These are especially useful in banquet feeding, airline catering, hospitals or anywhere food is held before service. Vegetable and fruit sauces help retain moisture and heat in the main item.
- Whole-milk yogurt can sometimes be substituted for a higher-fat sour cream in a sauce. Greek yogurts are generally thicker and an excellent substitute. In hot sauces, blend 1 tablespoon of cornstarch into each 1 quart of yogurt and mix well with a wire whisk. This will prevent separation. Yogurt should be added at the end of the cooking process. Whole-milk yogurts are often preferable in texture and flavor to non-fat yogurts in cooking.

Sauces: Guide to Ingredient Choices

Recommended	Limit
• Fruit coulis	• Cheeses (full-fat)
• Cornstarch/arrowroot thickeners	• Cream
• Potato starch	• Butter or margarine
• Evaporated skim milk, buttermilk or fat-free half-and-half (for cream)	• Oil
• Fresh herbs, spices and aromatics	• High-sodium marinades and sauces
• Natural reductions	
• Low-fat or whole milk and yogurt	
• Fruit and vegetable juices and purees in sauces	
• Meat or poultry stock, reduced	

Side Dishes

Side dishes have evolved from an afterthought in menu planning to an integral component of the main course. Vegetarians and people wanting a light meal may order several side dishes as an entrée. Grains, legumes, pastas and vegetables can be prepared in both traditional and innovative ways to create variety and interest.

General guidelines for developing healthful side dishes include:

- Increase the amount and variety of vegetables offered. Serve vegetables that are red, orange, yellow, green, purple and white. Each color group provides different phytochemicals.
- Feature seasonal vegetables steamed, roasted or grilled.
- Limit salt and use herbs, spices, citrus fruits and aromatics to season foods.

- Use flavored salts sparingly.
- Rinse and drain precooked canned beans to reduce sodium content by about 40%, if desired. Packaged dry and fresh legumes are naturally low in sodium.
- Offer side vegetables prepared using different cooking methods, seasonings, and flavors – steamed, roasted, grilled, mashed and sautéed.
- Offer fruit such as grilled pineapple or peach halves and sautéed apples or pears as side dishes.
- Add interesting color and textures by using wild rice, red rice, black rice, quinoa, millet and nuts.
- Kale salad can be embellished with beans, tofu, fruit, nuts, wheat berries for a vegetable-based main dish.
- Dehydrated fruit or vegetable chips can be used as a garnish or side dish.

Side Dishes: Guide to Ingredient Choices

Recommended	Limit
• All vegetables	• Butter and margarine
• Fruits	• Cream
• Grains, especially whole grains	• Salt and seasoned salts
• Beans/legumes	• Oil
• Non-wheat noodles/pasta (quinoa, rice, buckwheat)	• Bacon and pork fat
• Whole wheat pasta	
• Nuts	
• Seeds	
• Herbs, fresh or dried	
• Vinegars	
• Spices	
• Stocks	
• Salsas	

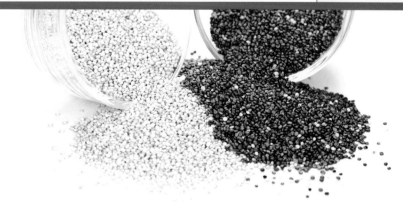

Breads

Both yeast breads and quick breads can be healthful additions to the menu—although many artisan breads (baguettes, boules, sourdough) contain little more than carbohydrates. The *Dietary Guidelines* recommend that at least half of the grains consumed be whole grains. [7] Breads make it easy to achieve that goal. Whole grains contain the entire grain kernel - the bran, germ and endosperm. Examples include whole-wheat flour, bulgur (cracked wheat), oatmeal, whole cornmeal and brown rice.

Look for the Whole Grain Council's product stamp, which indicates that a product contains 16 grams or more of whole grain per serving. The Council's website includes a list of restaurants that offer at least one whole-grain choice at each meal. Restaurants may also use a special symbol on menus to flag items that contain at least a half serving of whole grain. Likewise, a slice of whole-grain bread should contain at least 3 grams of fiber.

General guidelines for serving healthful breads include:

- Serve breads in 1- to 2-ounce portions. A 6-ounce muffin is 6 servings, not 1 serving.
- Offer whole-grain and multigrain options.
- White breads should be made with enriched flour.
- Serve small rolls and cut bread into modest portions.
- Use at least 50% whole grain in bread recipes where possible.
- Serve breads with lower-fat spreads such as rosemary white bean spread or hummus. Depending on the operation, olive oil may replace butter as an accompaniment for bread.
- Offer crisp crackers, flatbreads and thin breadsticks.
- Choose options with some seeds, dried fruits and/or nuts for added fiber and nutrients.

Courtesy Oldways and the Whole Grain Council,
www.wholegrainscouncil.org

Breads: Guide to Ingredient Choices

Recommended	Limit
• Whole-wheat bread	• Biscuits, scones
• Oatmeal, rye and other whole-grain or multigrain bread	• Croissants
• Italian and French bread, enriched	• Bagels, regular or large
• Crisp bread sticks, enriched	• Commercial muffins
• Whole-wheat pizza dough	• Cheese breads
• Flatbreads	• Sweet rolls and sweet breads
• Small rye bagels	• Quick breads such as banana bread and pumpkin bread
• Whole-wheat pita	• Corn bread
• Tortillas	• Large sandwich or sub buns
• Whole-wheat English muffins	• Garlic breads or breads with butter or oil toppings
• Seeded and nut breads	• Regular crackers
• Bran and fruit muffins	
• Reduced-fat crackers	

Desserts

Many people enjoy a sweet finish to their meal. Desserts, however, are typically high in sugar and fats. A philosophy of moderation – a small portion of something sweet and delicious – is wise.

General guidelines for adding healthful desserts to the menu include:

- Emphasize fruit – fresh, dried, pureed or frozen.
- Use lower-fat dairy products such as nonfat yogurt, part-skim ricotta cheese and reduced-fat cream cheese, when possible.
- Use sweet spices such as ginger, nutmeg or cinnamon.
- Serve a small but satisfying portion. A half-cup of vanilla ice cream has 140 calories; 1 ounce of angel food cake has 75 calories; 2 ounces of chocolate cake has about 200 calories; and ½ cup of rice pudding has about 185 calories.
- Use small (2 ½-inch) cupcake tins and other pans and utensils to make single-serving desserts.
- Use fruit rather than buttercream fillings and frost cakes lightly.
- Serve tarts, crepes and crumbles, and fruit desserts with one crust rather than two or with a nuts-and-oats topping.
- Reduce sugar and other high-calorie sweeteners where possible.
- Offer a small serving of a traditional dessert. Consider offering various portions of desserts from your dessert menu.
- Think small - a few small cookies rather than an oversized cookie.
- Serve gelato, with fewer calories and less fat, instead of ice cream.

- Serve cherries or berries in a meringue cup garnished with fresh mint.
- Serve a small amount of a "rich" dessert with fresh fruit or a fruit sauce to enhance and expand the portion.
- Use small, individual cups, molds or mini-soufflé dishes to control portions and enhance eye appeal.
- Drizzle small amounts of chocolate, fudge, caramel or fruit sauce atop a dessert or to dress the plate, or top desserts with a dusting of confectioner's sugar, only a few calories.
- Include a selection of small amounts of artisanal cheese with some dried fruit and/or nuts. While many of these cheeses are fairly high in fat, they are a nutrient-rich dessert option.
- Enhance desserts with nutrient-rich cherries, berries or other fruits as topping or garnish.
- Substitute finely ground whole-grain or legume flours for all or part of white flour in recipes.
- Eliminate trans fats from partially hydrogenated oils from your kitchen. Minimize saturated fats from butter and cream where possible and substitute with unsaturated plant oils.
- Use butter, where needed for flavor, in moderation.

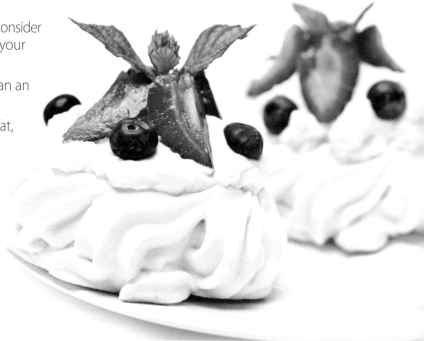

Desserts: Guide to Ingredient Choices

Recommended	Limit
• Fresh fruit	• Heavy cream and half-and-half
• Fruit coulis and purees	• Chocolate and white chocolate
• Fresh cooked fruits such as baked apples, poached pears, roasted apricots, and grilled peaches, figs or pineapple	• Butter
	• Canned fruits in heavy syrup
• Dried fruits	• Rich frostings, such as buttercream
• Cornstarch or arrowroot thickeners	• Caramel
• Fruit, berries or sliced melon on the dessert plate for added color, flavor and volume	• Nuts
	• Ice cream, frozen yogurt
• Grains such as brown rice, oatmeal and cornmeal	• Sherbet, sorbet, fruit ices
• Cocoa powder	• Poundcakes
• Dark chocolate	• Whipped cream, except as garnish
• Yogurt and Greek yogurt	
• Part-skim ricotta cheese	
• Phyllo (or filo) dough baked with little butter	
• Chocolate, caramel and other sauces as garnishes or in plate decor (squeeze-bottle technique)	
• Powdered sugar as garnish	
• Egg white souffles and meringues	
• Finely ground whole-grain flours including whole-grain white flour	
• Nuts, especially walnuts and almonds	
• Wheat germ, sesame, poppyseeds and other seeds	
• Sponge cake or angel food cake with fruit toppings or fillings	
• Pudding made with low-fat dairy products	
• Gelato made with milk and fruit	

Breakfast

It is true: Breakfast is a very important meal. For example, children who eat breakfast get more important nutrients such as calcium, dietary fiber, folate and protein. [8] In addition, children who consume breakfast show improved cognitive function, attention and memory, as well as improved performance on demanding mental tasks and in reaction to frustration. [9]

But children are not the only ones who benefit when they eat breakfast. Adults do, too. Many traditional breakfast items are healthful and, with minor modifications, those that are not so healthful can be given a makeover. General guidelines for developing healthful breakfast items include offering menu items such as:

- Hot and cold whole grains (steel-cut oats, brown rice, for example) and yogurt bars with various additions such as seeds, nuts and dried and fresh fruits.
- Eggs customizable, signature frittata and tofu scramble.
- Housemade chicken sausage patty, turkey bacon, grilled lean ham, Canadian bacon, poached salmon or salmon potato patty.
- Nutrient-rich waffles, pancakes or muffins made with whole-grain flour, pumpkin, banana, apple, flaxseed and/or nuts.
- Cereal buffet with muesli, assorted whole-grain cereals, fresh fruit and nut options.
- Skewers of melon and other cut fruits; baked apples, grilled pineapple, peaches or nectarines.
- Reduced-sugar or all-fruit jams.

- Breakfast items (omelets or sandwiches) with roasted or grilled vegetables, ratatouille, or vegetable stacks topped with a poached egg.
- Egg salad on multigrain toast.
- Yogurt, fruits, nuts, seeds, honey for build-your-own yogurt flavors or yogurt parfaits.
- Gluten-free menu alternatives such as cornmeal pancakes, buckwheat porridge, rice cereals, crustless quiche, waffles made with cornmeal, amaranth flour and brown rice flour.
- Daily specials that include healthful global breakfast small plates with tacos, flatbreads, corn griddle cakes, buckwheat pancakes, crepes, frittatas and panini sandwiches.
- Ready-to-eat cereals that are low in sugar (less than 5 grams per serving).
- Whole and cut fruits.
- Oatmeal with fresh or dried fruit and nuts.
- Cottage cheese or yogurt with fresh fruit.
- French toast made with low-fat milk and a minimum of fat, served with fresh berries.
- Grilled vegetable and cheese sandwich on whole-grain bread.
- Raw vegetable salads to complement breakfast sandwiches and egg dishes.
- Poached egg over sautéed spinach on whole-grain English muffin.
- Cinnamon toast made with multigrain bread.

Breakfast: Guide to Ingredient Choices

Recommended	Limit
• Whole-grain cereals	• Butter or margarine
• Whole-grain breads or rolls	• Bacon
• All fruits and fruit juices	• Sausage
• Cooked fruits, baked apples, stewed fruits, grilled grapefruit halves or sections	• Sugars and syrups
• Vegetables, such as broiled tomatoes, grilled asparagus, steamed spinach, grilled onions	• Fruit jams , highly sweetened
• Peanut or nut butter or spreads	• Cream cheese, sour cream
• Reduced-fat sausages, turkey bacon, Canadian bacon, lean ham	• Fruit drinks
• Cottage cheese	
• Reduced-fat cream cheese	
• Plain or fruited yogurt and yogurt parfaits	

- Rye bagel with smoked salmon, cucumbers, onions and reduced-fat cream cheese.
- Two-egg omelet with spinach and feta cheese or salsa and shredded cheese.
- Peanut butter and all-fruit jam on English muffin or whole-wheat toast.
- Fruit and yogurt smoothies.

Beverages

Beverages can be nutrient-rich and low in calories – think vegetable and fruit juices – or they can provide empty calories, such as soda laden with high-fructose corn syrup. Creating flavorful alternatives to alcoholic beverages is a way to showcase creativity and offer lower-calorie beverages to guests. (See Chapter 6 for more on beverages.)

Beverage Trends

Nonalcoholic Beverages
- House-made/artisan soft drinks
- Gourmet lemonade
- Specialty iced tea
- Mocktails
- Coconut water

Alcoholic beverages
- Craft/artisan spirits
- Locally produced beer/wine/spirits
- House-brewed beer
- Non-traditional liquors
- Craft beer
- Onsite barrel-aged drinks
- Culinary cocktails
- Regional signature cocktails
- Food-beer pairings
- Edible cocktails

Source: National Restaurant Association *What's Hot 2016 Culinary Forecast.* Available at: **http://www.restaurant.org/Downloads/PDFs/News-Research/WhatsHot2016**

Beverages: Guide to Ingredient Choices

Recommended	Limit
- 100% fruit juice - Fruit juice spritzers - Seltzer water, carbonated water or club soda - Mineral waters - Vegetable juices, low-sodium - Nonfat or low-fat milk - Buttermilk - Fruit smoothies - Kefir - Soy, nut or rice milk (for those with dairy intolerance) - Coffee, regular or decaffeinated - Black, herbal and green teas - Coconut water	- Sweetened soft drinks - Red and white wines - Spirits - Salted vegetable juices - Fruit drinks that often have only 5% to 10% fruit juice and added sugars - Flavored coffee mixes - Milkshakes and ice cream beverages - Beverages made with chocolate or fruit syrups

Presenting Food: Portioning and Plating

A goal to limit portions and types of foods may present an inherent conflict for restaurants and other places where food is sold. A restaurant wants to sell food, often in large quantities, and to provide a perception of value to the diner. The suggestion of restraint can impact the bottom line if the only change is reducing portion size. Strategies for success in offering healthier food are described in this chapter. In all types of food-service operations, from healthcare to college-dining to fine dining, there is value in caring enough about diners to offer foods to keep them healthy and coming back for more from your foodservice operation.

Often it is not the type of food served but rather the quantity served that compromises a healthful menu. Portion sizes have increased over the last 30 years; many items have more than doubled in size – and thus in calories, fat and sugar, too. For example, sodas have grown from a modest 8-ounce serving to 12- and 20-ounce cans to a 64-ounce Double Gulp. Research shows that commonly available portions almost always exceed U.S. Department of Agriculture and Food and Drug Administration standard portions, which are quite modest. For example, cookies, cooked pasta, muffins, steaks, sandwich rolls and bagels generally exceed standards by 200% to 700%. Eliminating larger-sized portions from the diet completely could reduce energy intake by up to 29% among US adults. [10] Chefs should know what standard servings are and should know the size of their portions by weighing or measuring them.

Since the 1980s, restaurants using oversized dinner plates, bakers using larger muffin tins and fast-food companies using larger drink, sandwich and French fry containers have supported this escalation in portion size. Even home recipes now suggest fewer servings for the same volume of ingredients.

Both larger portions and an increase in away-from-home food consumption have contributed to the weight management challenges so many Americans face. Larger portions provide more calories, encourage overeating and change consumer perception of what a normal, sensible portion looks like. Many experts agree that research on how to stop the obesity epidemic should focus on educating people to expect and eat smaller portions in general – fruits and vegetables being the exceptions to the rule. In a nation that has super-sized almost everything, many people simply don't understand the value of smaller portions. The goal is to right-size; it's healthier and less

expensive. Only recently have canned sodas become available in 8-ounce cans as a result of consumer demands.

The trick to making healthy indulgences is to provide them in small amounts. It may be time to recalibrate the restaurant kitchen by using scales to evaluate portions, switching to smaller scoops, using more single-serving dishes and bowls, and downsizing dishes, glasses and serving platters.

Consider portions carefully. Turn small into an advantage by offering bite-sized desserts, tasting portions, thin crackers and breadsticks. Focus on quality rather than quantity.

Moderating portion sizes and shifting focus from the center-of-the-plate protein require special attention to plating. Enhance the appeal of smaller portions by:

- Slicing meats and fanning (such as a chicken breast or sliced steak on salad greens).
- Using smaller plates to minimize white space.
- Using specialty plates that showcase smaller portions.
- Offering tasting menus.
- Garnishing with fresh fruits and vegetables that complement the dish.

Healthful garnishes are a good way to add fruit and vegetables to the plate without extra fat and sugar. Garnishes should bring color, texture, taste and interest to the dish without creating a distraction. Avoid using any item, edible or inedible, that does not contribute to the taste or texture of a dish. Ask yourself, "What purpose does this garnish serve?" Color is not enough. Colorful and healthful garnishes include shredded or finely diced vegetables, sliced or shredded sweet potatoes, carrots, daikon, parsnips, colorful peppers, fresh herbs, relishes, salsas, slaws, legumes, coulis, pomegranate arils, cooked grains, corn tortilla strips and baked wontons. Drizzle sauces, such as balsamic reduction or raspberry sauce, over food and on plates.

While much of this text has discouraged the use of high-fat ingredients like cheeses, deep-fried ingredients or whipped cream, these items can be effective garnishes to add texture or flavor to a dish. A dollop of whipped cream, a drizzle of fudge sauce, a sprinkling of crispy onion strips or fried sage leaves, or a few candied nuts add richness and visual appeal with just a modest amount of fat. Since the "topping" hits the palate first, it also boosts flavor from the first bite.

Healthful Plate Enhancers

Add color and textural contrasts that make plates beautiful as well as more nutrient rich:

Apple, fennel and walnut salad	Orange segments or rounds
Black beans and corn relish	Belgian endive
Carrot sauce	Pickled fruits or vegetables
Chimichurri sauce	Pomegranate seeds
Dried or fresh cranberry compote	Red pepper spread or vinaigrette
Eggplant caponata	Roasted red, yellow and orange peppers
Green tomato chutney	Salsas
Heirloom tomatoes	Sliced fresh or roasted pears in salad
Herb pestos	Sliced roasted beets
Jicama salad	Spicy peanut sauce
Mango, papaya, apricot or pineapple chutney	Winter fruit compote
Marinated bean salads	

Add Texture and Variety with Bread

- Pita triangles
- Thinly sliced olive bread
- Phyllo dough as cones or cups
- Lavosh, matzoh or flatbreads
- Seeded or herbed crisp, thin bread sticks
- Baked flour tortilla triangles
- Baked corn tortilla strips
- Baked croutons
- Mini-muffins
- Bruschetta
- Thinly sliced fruit and nut bread or toast
- Skinny, seeded bread sticks

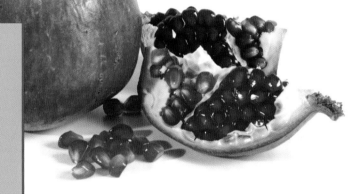

Children's Menus

Generation Z or the iGeneration is changing children's menus both in schools and across the food-service industry. Gen Z is the most culturally diverse group and they want ethnic and innovative cuisines on menus. Fresh, healthy and organic are norms for Gen Z as they pursue transparency in menus and food labels.

One in three of all children is overweight or obese. Childhood overweight and obesity rates have risen dramatically in the past 30 years. Seventeen percent of children ages 2 to 19 are obese and another 16 percent are overweight [12] Clearly major changes are urgently needed in the way we feed children, at home, at school and in the community.

The National Restaurant Association launched the Kids LiveWell program to help parents and children select healthful menu options when dining out. Restaurants that participate in the voluntary program commit to offering healthful meal items for children, with a particular focus on increasing consumption of fruit and vegetables, lean protein, whole grains and low-fat dairy, and limiting unhealthy fats, sugars and sodium. A study led by Harvard T.H. Chan School of Public Health found no meaningful improvements in the amount of calories, saturated fat, or sodium in kids' menu offerings during the first three years following the launch of the Kids LiveWell initiative in 2011. [13] This study also found that more than one in three children and adolescents consumed fast food every day. For kids, eating more restaurant food is associated with higher daily calorie intake from added sugar and saturated fats. Clearly, changing children's menus is an area of great opportunity.

According to the National Restaurant Association's 2018 survey of chefs, healthful kids' meals and ethnic-inspired kids' dishes are top trends. The survey also identified gourmet items, whole grain items and grilled items as trends in kids' meals. [2]

Must-Have Sides

- Fresh fruit – kid-sized pieces, single fruits or fruit medleys, such as orange wedges, apple wedges, melon balls, blueberries, whole strawberries, etc.
- Steamed or stir-fried vegetables – broccoli, asparagus or green beans with cheese sauce for dipping, corn on the cob
- Starches – brown rice, mashed sweet potatoes, baked vegetable strips, whole-wheat pasta in interesting shapes
- Carrot sticks or small carrots, red pepper strips, edamame, sugar snap peas or peapods

Perspectives on the Children's Menu: Food That Looks Good, Tastes Good and Is Good for You

What Appeals to Children	What Appeals to Adults for Children's Meals
• Small bites or hand-held food items	• Minimally processed whole foods such as fruits, vegetables, whole grains and lean proteins
• Identifiable foods or flavors	• Lean meats, preferably in an appropriate size for the child
• Foods that can be dipped in appealing sauces	• Accurate food descriptions revealing nuts, dairy, eggs or other common allergens
• Sweet flavors	• More grilling, baking and steaming; less frying
• Foods that can be customized to the child's preferences	• "Neat" foods with minimal sauce or sauce as a dip
• Menu descriptions that let the child know what's in the dish	• Low-fat milk, 100% fruit juice or water
• Interesting shapes	• Appropriate portions
• Crunchy textures	• Variety to accommodate different age groups and preferences
• Foods similar to the adult menu with minor modifications for the younger palate	• Appealing presentation of healthful choices
	• Menu items that make the chef's signature items available to children, too
	• Menu descriptions that let the parent know what's in the dish
	• Bendable straws, lids for beverage containers, small cups for small hands, non-breakable dishes

New Ideas and Twists on Old Favorites: Add Some Fun to the Children's Menu

- Quesadilla – whole-grain tortilla with Monterey Jack cheese and salsa
- Turkey mini-wrap – vegetables such as shredded carrots, lettuce and cucumber julienne along with lean turkey breast and cheese filling
- Vegetable mini-wrap – rice paper filled with hummus, julienne vegetables, lettuce and tomatoes; served with selected dipping sauces
- Peanut butter sandwich – on whole-grain bread with banana slices or apple wedges to add to the sandwich
- Veggie sticks and ranch dip – red peppers, carrots, celery, cucumbers, jicama, blanched green beans and sugar snap peas standing upright in a container to resemble French fries; served with dipping sauce
- Pot stickers – filled with lean meat and vegetables; served with Asian dipping sauce
- Kid's sushi rolls – filled with raw vegetables, with or without surimi (no raw fish), edamame
- Vietnamese salad rolls – served with dipping sauce
- Guacamole with corn chips – guacamole and salsa with baked chips
- Ham or turkey roll-up – tortilla rolled with turkey or ham, low-fat cheese, lettuce and mayonnaise or mustard
- Burger sliders – made with ground turkey, lean beef, fish or seafood, beans and added vegetables
- Penne pasta – with sautéed broccoli, carrots and peppers
- Macaroni and cheese – with steamed broccoli
- Pasta with tomato or meat sauce – served over whole-wheat or white pasta
- Chicken satay – served with peanut noodles
- Fish taco – served with guacamole
- Tuna melt – on whole-wheat English muffin with low-fat cheese
- Tuna salad cones – low-fat tuna salad scooped into flat-bottom ice cream cones; served with baby carrots
- Chicken fingers – grilled or baked and served with dipping sauces
- Asian treats – edamame, hoisin chicken strips and grilled shrimp
- Shrimp boat – steamed shrimp on romaine lettuce with chili sauce
- Mariner's special – 3 ounces of grilled fish with rice and green beans
- Vegetable stir-fry – with baby shrimp, chicken or beef strips
- Chicken, vegetable or tomato soup – served with whole-grain crackers
- Turkey meatballs and marinara sauce – with whole-grain pasta
- Mini caprese – grape tomatoes with tiny mozzarella balls or cubes; served with basil vinaigrette dressing
- Green eggs and ham – 1 egg scrambled with chopped spinach; served with 2 ounces of grilled ham and whole-wheat toast triangles
- Smashed vegetables – winter squash, sweet potatoes, peas and red skin potatoes
- Waffles with strawberries and blueberries – whole-grain waffles with fruit
- Patriotic oatmeal – small bowl of oatmeal topped with dried red cranberries and blueberries; served with 4 ounces of white, low-fat milk
- Ice cream sandwiches – graham crackers and frozen yogurt
- Fruit and cheese kabobs – cut fruit with cheese cubes
- Fruit smoothies – 6-ounce portion made with frozen fruit and low-fat milk
- Fruit fondue – pineapple, strawberries and banana served with chocolate or raspberry dipping sauce
- Banana split – half banana, sliced and topped with frozen low-fat vanilla and strawberry yogurt, a drizzle of chocolate sauce and a bit of crunchy granola
- Caramel apple slices – sliced apples with caramel dipping sauce
- Berry yogurt parfait – strawberry yogurt layered with sliced strawberries and blueberries; Teddy Grahams, chocolate covered raisins and sweetened dried cranberries as toppers
- Gelato made with milk and fresh fruit
- Serve it with a fun straw. Juices, smoothies, even soup is more adventurous when sipped through a colorful, even zany-shaped straw.

Selecting Healthful Ingredients

The trend toward using local, organic or sustainable ingredients is important to many guests and chefs. The number of farmers' markets has grown by almost five hundred percent in the last 25 years from about 1,700 in 1994 to almost 8,700 in 2017. [14] The number of community-supported agriculture organizations (CSAs) is difficult to accurately count because of the variety of CSA delivery models. Clearly there has been tremendous growth in this food delivery method. [15] Food hubs are another method of delivering local foods to consumers and foodservice operators. [14]

It is useful to remember, however, that including plenty of fruits, vegetables, grains and other inherently healthy products, in whatever form – frozen, canned, dried or fresh – is the single most important factor in planning healthful menus. The reality is that many Americans are not particularly interested in nor can they afford to eat "green." In addition, in many operations, the food budget does not allow for organic or other ingredients that are costlier than conventional produce, grain or protein sources. Thus, foodservice operations of all types – schools, community feeding programs, college and university, healthcare, nursing homes, quick service, family-style and fine dining – are seeking affordable "green" ingredients. Some restaurants have created their own gardens to provide some ingredients to use and feature.

Heritage and Heirloom Ingredients

Everything old is new again. Heritage meats and heirloom vegetables and fruits are finding a place on contemporary menus. "Heritage" is usually used to describe animals, while "heirloom" refers to plants. These terms describe varieties of animals and crops that have unique genetic traits, were raised many years ago and are typically grown in a sustainable manner.

According to Seed Savers Exchange (**www.seedsavers. org**), a nonprofit organization dedicated to preserving rare plant varieties, an **heirloom plant** is "any garden plant that has a history of being passed down within a family." While some argue that an heirloom variety must be at least 50 to 100 years old, all agree that heirloom fruits and vegetables are unique plant varieties that are genetically distinct from the commercial varieties popularized by industrial agriculture. Heirloom varieties are less consistent in size, shape and color than commercial varieties but often have more flavor and interesting textures and shapes. Heirloom varieties of beets, beans, carrots, cucumbers, lettuces, salad greens, spinach, radishes, peas, melons, pumpkins, squash, chard, corn, tomatoes, peppers and eggplant are available. For example, there are 60 varieties of heirloom beans to add interest and variety to the menu.

Seed Savers Exchange members have distributed an estimated 1 million samples of rare garden seeds since the organization was founded nearly 35 years ago. Those seeds now are widely used by small farmers supplying local and regional markets with unique alternatives to commercial produce.

Protecting the Past

Slow Foods (**www.slowfoodsusa.org**) is a global, grassroots movement with thousands of members around the world. The group links the pleasure of food with a commitment to community and the environment. The Slow Foods USA chapter has created a U.S. Ark of Taste, which catalogs more than 200 foods in danger of extinction. By promoting Ark products, Slow Foods helps ensure they remain in production and available.

The American Livestock Breeds Conservancy (**www. albc-usa.org**) is a nonprofit membership organization working to protect more than 150 breeds of livestock and poultry from extinction. Founded in 1977, the conservancy is the pioneer organization in the U.S. working to protect historic breeds and genetic diversity in livestock. Heritage varieties include breeds of cattle, sheep, pigs, chickens and turkeys.

Ancient Grains and Pseudograins

As nutrition policymakers and consumers continue to focus on increasing whole-grain consumption, ancient grains have found a place in stuffings, pilafs, crepes, salads, risottos, stir-fries, fritters, bread puddings, garnishes, breading for meats, grits, soups, crusts, pastries and cakes. These grains and grain alternatives can be good options for customers who are sensitive to gluten in wheat, oats, rye and barley.

Pseudograins

Sometimes called grain alternatives, pseudograins are foods that are prepared like grains but are actually seeds. Pseudograins are sometimes cooked but also can be ground into flour or used in cereals. Amaranth, millet and quinoa are pseudograins.

Amaranth

Amaranth's tiny beige granules have a nutty flavor and creamy-soft texture. These seeds (not grains) can be used as a breakfast cereal or side dish and make a healthful thickener for soups and stews. Amaranth's broad, leafy greens with red markings can be cooked as a vegetable and taste somewhat like spinach.

Millet

Millet is small and round. It can be white, gray, yellow or red and has a mildly nutty flavor and a soft texture. Millet is popular in Asian and African cooking but has not been fully appreciated in this country. The most widely available form of millet is the pearled, hulled variety. Many multigrain breads contain millet.

Quinoa

Quinoa, pronounced "KEEN-wa," is a seed that has been growing in the rugged highlands of South America for centuries. The small oval granules have a nutty flavor, soft texture and beige hue. Quinoa is particularly high in protein and can be combined with or substituted for rice in pilafs, soups, salads and side dishes. This versatile "mother grain of the Incas" cooks in only 15 to 20 minutes. Red quinoa can be cooked and used to add color, texture and flavor as a garnish or in a sauce. It looks like red caviar.

Spelt

Spelt's "nutty" flavor has long been popular in Europe, where it is also known as farro (Italy) and dinkle (Germany). Spelt is one of the oldest of cultivated grains and is a lesser-known cousin of wheat. It is processed into baking flour, cereals and an assortment of pastas including elbow macaroni, spaghetti and shells.

Kamut® (Khorasan Wheat)

Kamut is an ancient relative of modern durum wheat and is two to three times the size of common wheat with 20% to 40% more protein. It can be substituted for wheat in most products. Kamut is an important crop for sustainable, organic agriculture because of its ability to produce high-quality grain without artificial fertilizers and pesticides.

Teff

Teff was domesticated in Ethiopia between 4000 and 1000 BC. It is grown primarily as a cereal crop. One of the smallest grains in the world, most of a grain of teff consists of bran and germ, the most nutritious parts of any grain. Teff is high in protein, calcium and iron. Teff flour can be used in baked goods and the grains make a good thickener for soups, stews and puddings. Cooked teff can be used as a base to make grain burgers. Teff seeds can also be sprouted and the sprouts used in salads and on sandwiches.

Sustainable Agriculture and the Sustainable Foods Movement

Sustainable agriculture was addressed by the U.S. Congress in the Food, Agriculture, Conservation and Trade Act of 1990. [**16**] Under that law, the term "***sustainable agriculture***" is defined as: An integrated system of plant and animal production practices having a site-specific application that will, over the long term:

- Satisfy human food and fiber needs.
- Enhance environmental quality and the natural resource base upon which the agricultural economy depends.
- Make the most efficient use of nonrenewable resources and on-farm resources and integrate, where appropriate, natural biological cycles and controls.
- Sustain the economic viability of farm operations.
- Enhance quality of life for farmers and society as a whole.

According to the University of California Sustainable Agriculture Research and Education Program, sustainable agriculture integrates three main goals – environmental health, economic profitability, and social and economic equity. [**17**] Sustainability rests on the principle of meeting the needs of the present without compromising the ability of future generations to meet their own needs. Stewardship of both human and natural resources is of prime importance. Stewardship of human resources includes consideration of social responsibilities such as laborers' working and living conditions, the needs of rural communities, and consumer health and safety now and in the future. Stewardship of land and natural resources involves maintaining or enhancing this vital resource base for the long term.

Sustainable farming practices commonly include:

- Crop rotations that reduce weeds, disease, and insect and other pest problems; provide alternative sources of soil nitrogen; reduce soil erosion; and reduce risk of water contamination by agricultural chemicals.
- Pest control strategies that are not harmful to natural systems, farmers, their neighbors or consumers, including integrated pest management techniques that reduce the need for pesticides using practices such as scouting, use of resistant cultivars, timing of planting and biological pest controls.
- Increased mechanical/biological weed control; more soil and water conservation practices; and strategic use of animal and green manures.
- Use of natural or synthetic chemicals in a way that poses no significant hazard to humans, animals or the environment.

Purchasing local ingredients is an important part of the sustainable foods movement because it supports the local and regional community. According to the National Restaurant Association's 2016 Restaurant Industry Forecast, diners' desires for locally produced food items continues to grow. [**18**] In addition, a survey of more than 1,800 American Culinary Federation member chefs ranked hyper-local produce as the top food trend in 2018. [**2**]

Restaurants and college and university foodservice operations are leaders in the trend toward using local foods. Many chefs and restaurants support local farmers and farmers' markets, and some farms grow specific varieties for certain chefs. The local foods trend is particularly popular in fine-dining restaurants. Farm-to-foodservice programs such as National Farm to School (**www.farmtoschool.org**), Farm to College (**www.farmtocollege.org**) and Health Care Without Harm (**www.hcwh.org/us/food/issue**) have garnered national attention and are influencing the way commercial and noncommercial operators purchase products.

The ***local food*** movement – also called the ***locavore*** movement or food patriotism – builds more community-based, self-reliant food economies. Proponents of local eating often choose to limit their food purchases to only 100 to 150 miles from home, if possible. Certain foods like spices and coffee are not usually locally grown and are acceptable additions, particularly if sustainably grown. Local food networks include community gardens, food co-ops, community-supported agriculture, farmers' markets and seed-savers groups. The local foods movement recognizes the inherent connection among healthy soils, healthy foods, healthy communities and a healthy human society. Eating locally has become so popular that the term "locavore" was selected 2007 Word of the Year by the *Oxford American Dictionary*.

One challenge in using local products can be difficulty in locating local growers. Some restaurants (and even school foodservice districts) are hiring individuals who specialize in working with the grower producers.

casebycase | This Old Farm

Purdue graduate Jessica Roosa began her career in biochemistry, but it wasn't long before the land beckoned her. In 2001, Jessica launched This Old Farm near Lafayette, Indiana. "I started This Old Farm to feed our growing family with food that was not only organic, but safe and identifiable," explains Jessica, who is the mother, with husband, Lucas, of five children, all of whom work with her.

As a trained biologist and former vegetarian, Jessica saw an organic farm as a way to heal conventionally farmed fields that had been stripped of nutrients and could not support crops without large amounts of fertilizer. In 2009, This Old Farm incorporated with a mission to support family farms by processing, marketing and distributing locally raised, wholesome meat, produce, and value-added food such as cheese, honey and maple syrup.

Jessica transformed her original 88-acre organic farm into a food hub based on an alliance of local farmers and producers. A USDA-inspected meat processing facility was the centerpiece of the new enterprise. After a fire destroyed it, the company built an even bigger and better facility, which opened in June 2010. Now food service and retail customers can choose custom or packaged-to-order cuts of conventionally raised local, non-GMO, or organic meat beef, pork, lamb, goat, and poultry year-round. "Every package of meat or box of produce leaves our doors labeled with the name of the alliance farmer who put their heart into raising a product that first feeds family and then feeds the community."

Since 2012, This Old Farm has been an active participant in Indiana's farm-to-school network, working with school systems, state agencies, and other groups to introduce students to seasonal, Indiana-grown fresh vegetables and fruits they may have never experienced. For Jessica, teaching the next generation is a motivator. "Together," she notes, "we can make local, healthy, traceable food a reality for all Americans."

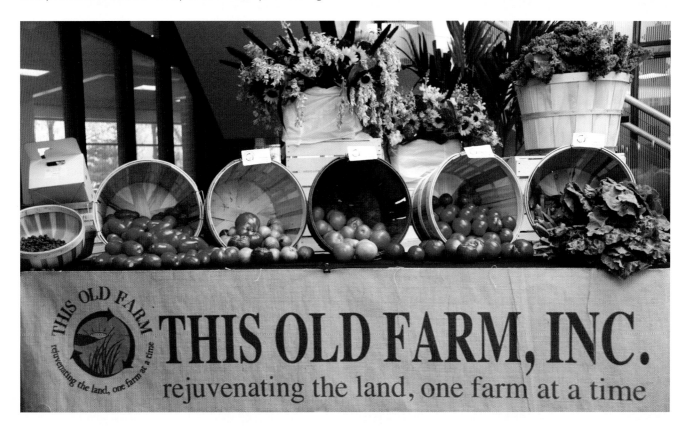

From the Kitchen
Max Knoepfel
Chef
Music City Center, Nashville TN

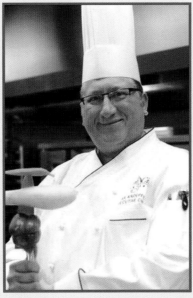

Nutrition is the key to joy, the key to a good life. Healthy food not only tastes and looks better, it also makes sense economically and environmentally. I believe it's important to pay attention to our carbon footprint, use sustainable ingredients, and also highlight the regional cuisine and flavor.

As a Chef, I get to plan and design a menu, inspire my culinary staff and my community, and show our guests a healthy, well balanced, amazing culinary experience. At home, I confess, my eating habits do not always live up, largely because of the demands of the job. I eat late into the night, and often skip breakfast. Butter, cheese, and artisanal bread are my weeks spots. I also love food that is healthy, simple, and fresh. Pho, Thai, tapas. It's all about balance.

Max Knoepfel traces his love of food and cooking back to his childhood. Raised by a Hungarian mother and a Swiss father, he grew up among gardens, learning all about gastronomy from his parents at an early age. His family canned fruits and vegetables for the winter months, composted food waste, and encouraged him to help tend the garden, picking cherries and shelling beans, digging up carrots and beets. At age 15, he started an apprenticeship with a 4-star restaurant and hotel, and his career took off from there.

Music City center is currently the only R.E.A.L. certified convention center in the country. It is also a L.E.E.D. certified Gold building, with four bee hives on the

roof, rainwater collection for irrigating outdoor plants as well as providing water for the buildings bathrooms.

As a chef for one of the biggest food operations in the south, Knoepfel is involved in the production of some 20,000 meals a day. What doesn't get eaten gets donated to local shelters and food banks. He and his team pride themselves on using local, sustainable ingredients, while reducing the carbon footprint of the meals they serve—in other words, using the food supply, not abusing it.

Sample Menu Highlighting Local Products at a Les Dames d' Escoffier Dinner

NAHA Restaurant
Chicago, Illinois

White Asparagus Soup, Door County Golden Caviar

Goujounettes of Great Lakes Whitefish
Saffron Aioli

Alaskan Sockeye Salmon Tartare on
Lebanese Farroush with Cilantro

Oxtail and Angel Food Goat Cheese Crostini and
"The Dames Royal" Cassis, Lillet, Cava and Raspberries

Salad of Nichol's Farm Organic Beets with Summer Farm
Greens and Stonefruit with Capriole Farm "Julianna" Herb
Crusted Goat Cheese, Cracked Hazelnuts, Apple Cider Syrup

Brioche Crusted Alaskan Halibut, Red Quinoa,
Medjool Dates, Shaved Radishes, English Peas
and Freshly Juiced Carrot Broth

Slow Roasted Wagyu "Kobe" Beef Brisket with a Cannelloni
of Green Acres Farm Asparagus and Magenta Swiss Chard,
White Beech Mushrooms, Housemade Buttermilk Ricotta
and French Black Summer Truffles

2008 Epiphany Camp Pour Vineyards
Grenache Blanc, Sta. Barbara 2008

Au Bon Climat Pinot Noir, Santa Barbara County

Lemon Nougat Glacé Madeleine Cake
Early Summer Sweet Michigan Cherries and
Lemon Balm Sorbet

Mignardises and Frivolities

*NAHA proudly supports Chicago's Green City
Market and The John G. Shedd Aquarium*

*Menu used with permission of chef-owner Carrie Nahabedian who notes that
Alaskan halibut is a sustainable fish but not local to Chicago.*

Quinoa and Butternut Stuffed Poblano Peppers

Serves: 10

Chef Max Knoepfel,
Music City Center, Nashville TN

This vegetarian dish is high in beta-carotene and fiber and makes an excellent vegan main dish.

Poblano peppers	10	large
Quinoa (blend of white, red and black)	2	cups
Vegetable broth	4	cups
Butternut squash, peeled and diced	4	cups
Olive oil	2	tablespoons
Canned kidney beans	2	cups
Tomatoes, diced	2	cups
Chili powder	2	tablespoons
Black pepper	¼	teaspoon
Salt	½	teaspoon

1. Roast the peppers in a 475° F oven until charred. Remove the charred skin. Cool. Cut off tops. Remove seeds.
2. In a sauté pan combine quinoa and vegetable broth, cook till al dente or crunchy 8-10 minutes.
3. Roast the diced butternut squash at 475° F with olive oil, salt and pepper, until tender.
4. Rinse canned kidney beans.
5. In a large bowl, combine the quinoa, butternut squash and kidney beans; add diced tomatoes and chili powder, salt and pepper to taste.
6. Spoon quinoa and vegetable mixture onto each pepper, packing gently. Place the peppers on a greased baking sheet and roast at 350 °F for 25 minutes
7. Serve with your favorite salsa or pico de gallo.

Per Serving

Calories	240	Cholesterol	0	mg
Fat	6 g	Sodium	320	mg
Saturated Fat	3 g	Carbohydrates	41	mg
Trans Fat	0 g	Dietary Fiber	9	mg
Sugar	6 g	Protein	9	g

Roasted Basil Pesto Salmon, Cauliflower Rice

Serves: 10

Chef Max Knoepfel,
Music City Center, Nashville TN

This "risotto" is made from finely chopped cauliflower that resembles rice, but without as many carbohydrates. Topped with a zesty pesto salmon, it is a perfectly balanced dish.

Fresh salmon filets, skinned	10 each	(6 ounces each)
Black pepper, freshly ground	¼	teaspoon
Salt (or smoked salt)	½	teaspoon
Cauliflower	4	heads
Olive oil	4	tablespoons
Basil, fresh	2	bunches
Garlic, peeled	4	cloves
Pine nuts, raw	1	cup
Parmesan cheese, grated	½	cup
Olive oil	3	tablespoons

1. Season salmon with salt and pepper, set aside. Preheat oven to 350° F. Convection setting if possible.
2. Wash and chop cauliflower and pulse in a food processor to achieve "rice" effect.
3. Spread cauliflower "rice" on a baking sheet, drizzle with olive oil. Bake at 350° F for 20 minutes.
4. To prepare the pesto, place basil, garlic, pine nuts, grated parmesan cheese, and olive oil in a blender. Pulse until paste-like consistency. Set aside.
5. Sear the salmon in a hot saute pan for 3 minutes, or until color is caramelized on the outside. Remove salmon from pan and let rest. Brush with pesto. Finish cooking the salmon in the oven at 350° F. for 8 minutes.
6. Place cauliflower "rice" on plate, top with salmon.

Per Serving

Calories	450	Cholesterol	110	mg
Fat	27 g	Sodium	340	mg
Saturated Fat	3.5 g	Carbohydrates	8	mg
Trans Fat	0 g	Dietary Fiber	3	mg
Sugar	3 g	Protein	45	g

Chefs Collaborative

The foodservice industry is an important participant in the sustainable agriculture movement. From fine dining establishments to college dining rooms, hospitals and schools, foodservice professionals can commit to purchasing, preparing and serving foods grown sustainably. The Chefs Collaborative (**www.chefscollaborative.org**) is a nonprofit network of chefs that fosters a sustainable food system through advocacy, education and collaboration with the broader food community. The collaborative inspires action by translating information about food into tools for making knowledgeable purchasing decisions that reflect seasonality, preserve diversity and traditional practices, and support local economies.

Mission:
Chefs Collaborative is a national nonprofit network with a mission to inspire, educate, and celebrate chefs and food professionals building a better food system.

Vision:
Sustainable practices will be second nature for every chef in the United States.

Chefs Collaborative Statement of Principles

1. Food is fundamental to life, nourishing us in body and soul. The preparation of food strengthens our connection to nature. And the sharing of food immeasurably enriches our sense of community.

2. Good food begins with unpolluted air, land and water, environmentally sustainable farming and fishing and humane animal husbandry.

3. Food choices that emphasize delicious, locally grown, seasonally fresh and whole or minimally processed ingredients are good for us, for local farming communities and for the planet.

4. Cultural and biological diversity are essential for the health of the earth and its inhabitants. Preserving and revitalizing sustainable food, fishing and agricultural traditions strengthen that diversity.

5. By continually educating themselves about sustainable choices, chefs can serve as models to the culinary community and the general public through their purchases of seasonal, sustainable ingredients and their transformation of these ingredients into delicious food.

6. The greater culinary community can be a catalyst for positive change by creating a market for good food and helping preserve local farming and fishing communities.

Sustainable Seafood

Poor fishing practices are destroying not only the population of some fish species, but also those of other marine animals caught and discarded as bycatch, including sea turtles, sharks and many thousands of seabirds. Several organizations monitor local and international waters and share their information with chefs and the public.

- The Smithsonian's National Museum of Natural History maintains a sustainable seafood website (**http://ocean.si.edu/sustainable-seafood**) that provides current information on suggested and problematic seafood choices.

- The National Oceanic and Atmospheric Administration (NOAA) maintains FishWatch (**www.fishwatch.gov**), which reports news on seafood and health.

- The Safina Center's Sustainable Seafood Program helps consumers, chefs, retailers and the medical community discover the connection between human health, a healthy ocean, fishing, and seafood. Their Healthy Oceans Seafood Guide (**http://safinacenter.org/seafoods/**) helps inform seafood choices.

- The Marine Stewardship Council (**www.msc.org**) certifies sustainable seafood.

BEST CHOICES

Abalone (farmed)
Arctic Char (farmed)
Barramundi (US & Vietnam farmed)
Bass (US hooks and lines, farmed)
Catfish (US)
Clams, Cockles, Mussels
Cod: Pacific (AK)
Crab: King, Snow & Tanner (AK)
Lionfish (US)
Lobster: Spiny (Mexico)
Oysters (farmed & Canada)
Prawn (Canada & US)
Rockfish (AK, CA, OR & WA)
Sablefish/Black Cod (AK)
Salmon (New Zealand)
Sanddab (CA, OR & WA)
Scallops (farmed)
Shrimp (US farmed)
Tilapia (Canada, Ecuador, Peru & US)
Trout: Rainbow (US farmed)
Tuna: Albacore (trolls, pole and lines)
Tuna: Skipjack (Pacific trolls, pole and lines)

GOOD ALTERNATIVES

Cod: Atlantic (handlines)
Cod: Pacific (Canada & US)
Grouper: Red (US)
Lobster: Spiny (Bahamas & US)
Mahi Mahi (Ecuador & US longlines)
Monkfish (US)
Octopus (Canada, Portugal & Spain pots and traps, HI)
Oysters (US wild)
Pollock (Canada longlines, gillnets & US)
Salmon (Canada Pacific & US)
Scallops: Sea (wild)
Shrimp (Canada & US wild, Ecuador & Honduras farmed)
Squid (Chile, Mexico, Peru & US)
Swordfish (US)
Tilapia (China, Colombia, Honduras, Indonesia, Mexico & Taiwan)
Trout: Rainbow/Steelhead (Chile farmed)
Tuna: Albacore (US longlines)
Tuna: Skipjack (free school, imported trolls, pole and lines, US longlines)
Tuna: Yellowfin (free school, trolls, pole and lines, US longlines)

AVOID

Basa/Pangasius/Swai
Cod: Atlantic (Canada & US)
Cod: Pacific (Japan & Russia)
Crab (Argentina, Asia & Russia)
Halibut: Atlantic (wild)
Lobster: Spiny (Belize, Brazil, Honduras & Nicaragua)
Mahi Mahi (imported)
Orange Roughy
Octopus (other imported sources)
Pollock (Canada trawls & Russia)
Salmon (Canada Atlantic, Chile, Norway & Scotland)
Sardines: Atlantic (Mediterranean)
Sharks
Shrimp (other imported sources)
Squid (Argentina, China, India & Thailand)
Swordfish (imported longlines)
Tuna: Albacore (imported except trolls, pole and lines)
Tuna: Bluefin
Tuna: Skipjack (imported purse seines)
Tuna: Yellowfin (longlines except US)

How to Use This Guide

Many seafood items appear in more than one column. Please be sure to check them all—beginning with Best Choices.

Best Choices
Buy first; they're well managed and caught or farmed responsibly.

Good Alternatives
Buy, but be aware there are concerns with how they're caught, farmed or managed.

Avoid
Take a pass on these for now; they're overfished, lack strong management or are caught or farmed in ways that harm other marine life or the environment.

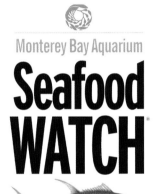

Monterey Bay Aquarium
Seafood WATCH®

YELLOWFIN TUNA

National Consumer Guide
January - June 2019

Your Choices Matter

Many of the fish we enjoy are in trouble due to destructive fishing and farming practices.

You can make a difference for our ocean by making responsible seafood choices.

Use these recommendations for popular seafood when dining and shopping. **For the full list, visit us online or download our free app.**

Take Action

ASK "Are you a Seafood Watch partner?" Let businesses know responsible seafood is important to you.

BUY Best Choices. If unavailable, look for Good Alternatives or the eco-certified options found on our app and website.

CHOOSE Seafood Watch partners from our app or website when dining and shopping.

DOWNLOAD Our free app.

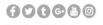

SeafoodWatch.org

Seafood Watch

The Monterey Bay Aquarium Seafood Watch program helps consumers and businesses choose seafood that's fished or farmed in ways that support a healthy ocean, now and for future generations.

Monterey Bay Aquarium
The seafood recommendations in this guide are credited to the Monterey Bay Aquarium Foundation ©2018. All rights reserved. Printed on recycled paper.

Reprinted with permission from Monterey Bay Aquarium, www.seafoodwatch.org or www.montereybayaquarium.org

- The Monterey Bay Aquarium Seafood Watch® (**www.seafoodwatch.org**) empowers consumers and businesses to make choices for healthy oceans. The aquarium's Seafood Watch Pocket Guide assists consumers and foodservice professionals in identifying the most environmentally responsible sources of seafood. The guide is available in a national version as well as in six regional versions. Seafood Watch suggests that food buyers gather details on where fish comes from, whether it was farmed or wild caught, and how it was farmed or caught.

- The Environmental Defense Fund states that of all the threats facing the oceans today, overfishing takes the greatest toll on sea life and people. Their Seafood Selector (seafood.edf.org) guides best and worst choices.

Organic Foods

Organic foods have outgrown specialty markets and have taken their place on mainstream American tables. The Hartman Group, a market research company, reports several groups of users of organics. "Core" organic consumers tend to be deeply entrenched in organic lifestyles and environmental concerns; most of them buy organic products weekly. A larger group of consumers selectively choose organic products, particularly foods, where they feel that freshness and health are most important. As many consumers consider organics, there is less interest in organic sweets and snacks than fresh foods.

Since 2000, organic foods have been increasingly available in the U.S. food supply. According to industry reports, organic food sales were 1.2% of total food sales in 2000 and now account for 5.3 % of total food sales in this country. The majority of our organic purchases are fruits, vegetables and dairy products. [19] The Hartman Group reported that 82% of Americans buy organic products occasionally and that about 40% use some organic products regularly, citing health benefits as their primary motivation. [20]

Are organic foods healthier? Stanford's Center for Health Policy did not find strong evidence that organic foods are more nutritious or carry fewer health risks than conventional alternatives, though consumption of organic foods can reduce the risk of pesticide exposure. No consistent differences were seen in the vitamin content of organic products, and only one

Resources for Sustainable Foods

- American Farmland Trust, **www.farmland.org**
- Animal Welfare Approved, **www.animalwelfareapproved.us**
- Center for Integrated Agricultural Systems, **www.cias.wisc.edu**
- Land Stewardship Project, **www.landstewardshipproject.org**
- Marine Stewardship Council, **www.msc.org**
- Monterey Seafood Aquarium, **www.montereybayaquariaum.org**
- National Oceanic and Atmospheric Administration, **www.fishwatch.gov**
- National Sustainable Agriculture Coalition, **www.sustainableagriculture.net**
- National Sustainable Agriculture Coalition, **www.attra.ncat.org**
- Organic Trade Association, **www.ota.com**
- The Safina Center, **safinacenter.org**
- Smithsonian National Museum of Natural History, **http://ocean.si.edu/sustainable-seafood**
- Sustainable Agriculture Research and Education, **www.sare.org**
- USDA, Agricultural Marketing Services, Farmers' Market Locator, **https://www.ams.usda.gov/local-food-directories/farmersmarkets**

Hartman Group's Organic & Natural Report 2016

Primary Reasons for Buying Organic Food and Beverages (by organic purchasers)

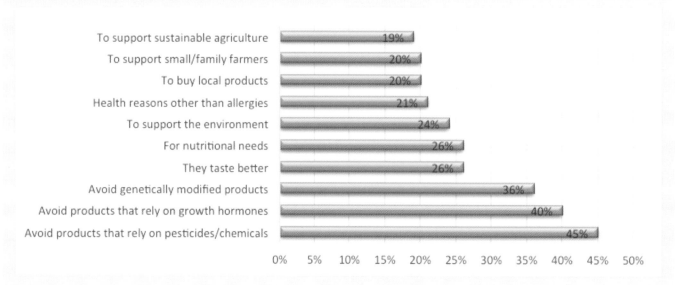

nutrient -- phosphorus -- was significantly higher in organic versus conventionally grown produce (and the researchers note that because few people have phosphorous deficiency, this has little clinical significance). [21] Another major review of studies concluded that there is little evidence to support any nutrition-related health effects resulting from the consumption of organically produced foodstuffs. [22] Both of these reviews looked at findings from well-controlled and peer-reviewed research studies worldwide.

According to Charles Benbrook, Ph.D., chief scientist of The Organic Center, however, well over 100 published studies compare the nutrient content of organic and conventional food grown in similar soils in the same region. These studies show that organic foods are nutritionally superior in about two-thirds of the "matched pair" cases. Moreover, the magnitude of the differences clearly favors organic production systems. [23]

And while several major reviews of the scientific literature prior to 2001 found that vitamin and mineral levels of conventionally grown and organic produce were quite similar, Benbrook and other more recent studies measuring levels of health-promoting phytochemicals found about two-thirds of the organic samples had higher amounts of phytochemicals, and many were also higher in vitamins C and E.

Much support for the nutritional superiority of organic foods is available on websites and in the media, but relatively little evidence of this is found in peer-reviewed scientific journals. Organic products are an optimal choice for many environmental reasons, including support of farms and farmland. Certainly there are advantages to consuming foods without pesticides, herbicides, growth hormones, artificial flavors and colors, and antibiotics, but these advantages do not directly affect the nutrient composition.

Organic produce is less available in some geographic areas and costlier in some locales and seasons. Many people and foodservice operators simply cannot afford the increased cost of organic foods. Very limited food dollars are better spent on purchasing enough basic healthful foods. Small farmers may not be able to afford organic certification, even though they follow organic methods. An "organic only" philosophy may be appropriate for some foodservice operations, but not feasible for others.

Locally grown seasonal produce is generally available and often a healthful choice. As the number of farmers' markets and community-supported farms increases and demand grows for locally grown and organic foods, prices should come down. The *Dietary Guidelines* encourage local foods and farmers' markets and gardens.

Functional Foods

The term "functional food" currently has no legal meaning in the United States. All foods are functional at some physiologic level.

In 2009, two leading food and nutrition organizations put forth definitions of **functional foods**:

- The Institute of Food Technologists: "Foods and food components that provide a health benefit beyond basic nutrition (for the intended population). These substances provide essential nutrients often beyond quantities necessary for normal maintenance, growth and development and/or other biologically active components that impart health benefits or desirable physiological effects." [24]

- The Academy of Nutrition and Dietetics: "Foods defined as whole foods along with fortified, enriched, or enhanced foods that have a potentially beneficial effect on health when consumed as part of a varied diet on a regular basis at effective levels." [25]

Because functional foods are an emerging area of food and nutrition science, The Academy of Nutrition and Dietetics supports research to further define the health benefits and risks of individual foods and their physiologically active compounds. The Academy states that any health claims on food products, including functional foods, should be based on significant evidence and scientific agreement. Unfortunately, some producers and manufacturers use testimonials, limited and biased research studies, and aggressive sales and marketing techniques to promote functional foods. Many of their health-related claims are not based on sound research. At best, such claims can be confusing and misleading; at worst, they may rise to the level of fraud.

The Evolution of Functional Foods

Conventional foods with specific health benefits ⇨ Enriched and/or fortified foods ⇨ Special medical foods for treating specific intolerances or needs ⇨ Enhanced foods with bioactive ingredients or amino acids

A functional food should be healthful before extra nutrients are added and its health benefits are extolled. Adding something or putting a "healthful" ingredient in a high-fat or high-sugar food does not make that food a good choice. For example, some grain bars are essentially candy bars with added nutrients.

Functional foods emerged as food and nutrition science evolved from a focus on treatment of deficiency diseases to a focus on disease prevention and health promotion. Foods are no longer evaluated in terms of energy, nutrients, vitamins and minerals alone. Other components that influence physiologic functioning and ultimately health are also important. Today, the government regulates many functional foods because health claims, nutrient content claims and/or structure/function claims are made on food labels. (See Chapter 2.)

Consumer interest in health and longevity has created a demand for cost-effective, diet-based approaches to preventing chronic diseases like heart disease, preserving bone and joint health, promoting cognitive function and memory, and protecting eye health. Some enhanced foods are useful for particular segments of the population with unique nutritional needs – for example, vegans who do not drink milk and need to find their calcium elsewhere. In addition to calcium-fortified fruit juices, other commonly used functional foods are margarine with stanols, omega-3 eggs, fat-free half-and-half, gluten-free baking mixes and juices with added fiber or citrus pulp.

As functional foods become even more prevalent and popular, it becomes increasingly challenging to evaluate them. Here are some basic questions to ask before depending on a functional food:

- Does it work? Is there a true scientific basis for its health claims?
- How much of the functional ingredient(s) does the food contain?
- Is the food safe? Are there risks associated with consumption?
- Is the food healthful? Is there a more cost-effective source of the same functional ingredients?

Probiotics and Prebiotics

Probiotics are live microorganisms added to food to convey health benefits. For example, "friendly bacteria" that normally occur in the digestive tract ferment milk into yogurt and other cultured products. Providing additional bacteria helps keep the digestive tract healthy. When antibiotics destroy normal digestive tract bacteria, the "active culture" in yogurt restores the digestive tract function and boosts the immune system.

Eating foods with probiotics also aids digestion and absorption and helps treat irritable bowel syndrome, some ulcers, colitis, other intestinal diseases and some allergy conditions. Although fermented dairy products such as yogurt and kefir are typically associated with "beneficial cultures," the types of foods claiming to deliver probiotics have expanded to include granola and candy bars, frozen yogurt, cereal, juice and cookies. Whether or not any given product, even ones that claim to contain probiotics, actually delivers useful amounts of probiotic strains cannot be determined from just looking at the product.

In food products, the probiotics added are primarily species of *Lactobacillus* or *Bifidobacterium*, or *Streptococcus thermophilus*. For example, in the United States, yogurt must be produced by the fermentation of *Lactobacillus bulgaricus* and *Streptococcus thermophilus*; however, post-fermentation heat treatment of yogurt, which kills all live cultures, is allowed. The National Yogurt Association established a Live Active Culture seal to help consumers distinguish between yogurts that contain live active cultures and those that do not. Look for the words "live culture" or the Live Active Culture seal.

Particularly popular in the past couple years are fermented foods, such as kimchi and sauerkraut, and beverages such as Kombucha.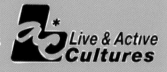

Prebiotics are nondigestible food ingredients that are helpful in stimulating the growth or activity of beneficial bacteria in the colon. Prebiotics, sometimes known as fermentable fiber, are found in artichokes, bananas, barley, berries, chicory, flax, legumes and oatmeal. Prebiotics are also added to foods such as yogurt, drink mixes and meal-replacement bars.

Functional Foods

Category	Description	Example
Conventional Foods	Foods with naturally occurring beneficial compounds. These foods may have an FDA health claim on the label	Fish high in omega-3 fatty acids that reduce risk of heart disease; fruits or vegetables high in phytochemicals that reduce risk of certain diseases; cruciferous vegetables that may reduce risk of several types of cancer; fermented dairy products that may improve irritable bowel syndrome; cranberry juice that may reduce urinary tract infection
Modified Foods	Foods that have been modified through fortification, enrichment or enhancement	Calcium-fortified fruit juice for bone health; margarines with plant stanols or sterols to lower cholesterol; no-trans-fat oils for heart health
Medical Foods	Foods that are specially formulated and intended for the dietary management of a disease that has distinctive nutritional needs that cannot be met by normal diet alone. Medical foods must be administered under the supervision of a physician	Tube feedings; specialized formulas; shakes and puddings
Foods for Special Dietary Use	Foods that: • Meet a special dietary need • Supply a vitamin, mineral or other ingredient to supplement the diet • Meet a special dietary need and are used as the sole item of the diet (infant foods)	Foods for weight loss; vitamin water; lactose-free foods; gluten-free ingredients or foods; baby formulas

Source: Position of The American Dietetic Association (now Academy of Nutrition and Dietetics): Functional Foods, Journal of The American Dietetic Association, April 2009, **www.eatright.org/About/Content.aspx?id=8354**

Super Foods

"*Super foods*" is a term used to describe foods such as leafy greens, berries, winter squash, red grapefruit, pumpkins, avocados, seaweed, kamut, almonds and dried plums that have relatively high amounts of many phytochemicals and nutrients. Unique or rare super foods – acai or chia seeds, for example – are very expensive. Many super foods are highly publicized as having unique health benefits; most of this publicity is hype. A small amount of the food used as an ingredient often comes at a high cost. For example, a very small amount of acai juice, high in phytochemicals, may be added to a food and the resulting product is publicized as especially healthful. Consider more common food sources of the same phytochemical or other phytochemicals with similar biologic functions.

Fermented and Pickled Foods

Naturally fermented foods and beverages, such as kimchi, kefir, miso, and kombucha, have stepped into the spotlight over the past couple years. Our interest in health and fermented foods' ability to provide the good bacteria that the gastrointestinal tract needs has proven irresistible for the public. The intrigue with ethnic foods that use these ingredients has also propelled them.

Fermentation is a process for preserving foods using particular types of microbes – bacteria, yeasts and molds. Vegetables, fruits, beans, grains, meats, fish, honey, tea and dairy products can be fermented. Yogurts, cheese, sauerkraut, beer and wine are common examples of fermented foods.

Pickling is the practice of adding enough vinegar or lemon juice to a low-acid food to lower its pH to 4.6 or less. Examples of commonly pickled foods include fruits, vegetables, meats and eggs. Fresh-pack or quick-process pickles are not fermented. Sometimes salt, sugar and seasonings are added to pickling liquids.

Fermentation and pickling can intersect. Fermented pickles undergo a curing process for several weeks in which fermentative bacteria produce acids necessary for the preservation process. These bacteria also generate flavor compounds which are associated with fermented pickles. Other vegetables may be fermented, such as using cabbage to produce sauerkraut.

A staple element of many cultures' culinary traditions, fermented ingredients are making their way into a wide range of restaurants and foodservice operations. For example, kimchi has seen a dramatic rise in its popularity and profile to the everyday consumer. Celebrity Korean-American chefs, including Roy Choi (Kogi BBQ Food Truck), David Chang (Momofuku), and Hooni Kim (Danji in Hell's Kitchen), have pushed Korean cuisine forward. As an integral element of Korean cuisine, kimchi has nearly 200 hundred varieties and has clearly benefited from this trend.

Examples of fermented foods and beverages include:

Foods	Beverages
• Yogurt	• Wine
• Cheese	• Beer
• Kimchi	• Sake
• Sauerkraut	• Kombucha
• Chutney	• Kefir
• Some pickles	• Lassi
• Miso	• Kvass
• Tempeh	• Vinegars
• Sourdough bread	
• Natto	

Wild Mushroom Farrotto

Yield: 10 servings

Chef Jeremy Bearman, Rouge Tomate
New York City, New York

This is a variation of the classic risotto using farro, a whole grain from the wheat family. The hearty, nut-like flavor complements the wild mushrooms.

Farro:

Farro	1 ½	cup
Mushroom stock, unsalted	5	cups

Mushroom puree:

Olive oil	¼	cup
White mushrooms, diced	2	cups
Oyster mushrooms	1	cup
Hen of the woods mushrooms	1	cup
Other wild mushrooms such as chanterelle, king oyster, or porcini	1	cup
Shallots, sliced	1	cup
Garlic, chopped	3	cloves
Salt	½	teaspoon
Madeira wine	1	cup

Sautéed mushrooms:

Hen of the woods mushrooms	2	cups
Oyster mushrooms	2	cups
Other wild mushrooms	2	cups
Canola oil for sautéing	¼	cup
Thyme leaves, fresh	1	tablespoon
Garlic	4	cloves
Salt	¼	teaspoon
Black pepper, ground		to taste
Parmesan, grated	1	cup

Per Serving

Calories	270	Cholesterol	6	mg
Fat	13 g	Sodium	470	mg
Saturated Fat	3 g	Carbohydrates	34	mg
Trans Fat	0 g	Dietary Fiber	4	mg
Sugar	3 g	Protein	9	g

1. **For the farro**: Soak the farro in cold water for 12 to 24 hours and drain. Place the farro and the mushroom stock into a small stock pot. Simmer until tender, approximately 45 to 60 minutes. Keep the stock covering the farro at all times. Strain residual liquid from the farro and reserve. Spread the farro on a sheet tray to cool.

2. **For the mushroom puree**: In a large sauce pot, heat the olive oil until just before smoking. Add all of the mushrooms, season with salt and cook on high heat constantly stirring until all of the moisture has been released. Once they have begun to brown, turn the heat down to low and add the shallots and garlic. Sweat the shallots and garlic for about 5 minutes and add the Madeira. Cook on medium heat until all of the liquid is evaporated and the mixture is dry. Transfer the mixture to a blender and blend until smooth. Reserve.

3. **For the sautéed mushrooms**: Heat the canola oil in large saute pan until just before smoking. Add the mushrooms and pieces of garlic and saute until nicely browned. Just before removing, add the thyme and saute with the mushrooms. Season the mushrooms with salt and pepper, place the mushrooms on a dry towel to drain any excess oil.

4. **For the farrotto**: In a sauce pot, add about 5 cups of the cooked farro and about 1 cup of the reserved liquid. Heat the mixture constantly stirring. Add about 2 cups of the puree, along with the parmesan and stir until mixture hot. It should be the consistency of a risotto. Add more liquid or stock and if you want it creamier. Check the seasoning and adjust if necessary.

5. Serve farrotto immediately as the mixture will tend to tighten up as it sits. Garnish with the sautéed mushrooms.

Opportunities for Chefs

Applying the basic principles of adequacy, balance, moderation and variety to menu planning is the fundamental approach to planning healthful menus. Menu trends indicate that consumers are increasingly interested in healthful menu options. Increasing whole grains, legumes, fruits and vegetables and using healthful cooking techniques makes menus more healthful. Among the food trends that foodservice operators need to consider in planning healthful menus is the use of sustainable, organic and local products. By moderating portions and incorporating a variety of healthful menu options, the foodservice industry has a great opportunity to have a positive impact on our nation's health.

Learning Activities

1. Design a healthful menu with at least four items in each of five categories: appetizer, salad, soup, main course, dessert, breakfast, sandwiches, etc.

2. Using a menu from a favorite foodservice operation, develop 10 healthful items that can be added to increase the healthfulness of the total menu.

3. Create four children's menus (one for each season) focusing on seasonal produce.

For More Information

- *Chemical Cuisine*, a guide to food additives when packaged foods are a more convenient choice, **www.cspinet.org**

- Environmental Defense Fund, for information about sustainable seafood and issues, **www.edf.org/seafood**

- Environmental Working Group, for information on produce handling, safety and pesticide use, **www.ewg.org**

- Food label information and current food product and eco-labeling advice from Consumer Union, **www.consumerunion.org/**

- Guide to grass-fed and organic meat, poultry and dairy products with a list of suppliers of pasture-raised products, **www.eatwild.com**

- International Scientific Association for Probiotics and Prebiotics, **https://isappscience.org/**

- Monterey Bay Aquarium, for information on seafood, **www.seawatch.com**

- Produce for Better Health Foundation, **www.fruitandveggiesmorematter.org**

- Smart guides to healthy choices from Institute for Agriculture and Trade Policy, **www.iatp.org**

- Sourcing local foods and community-supported agriculture, **www.localharvest.com**

- US Probiotics, **www.USProbiotics.org**

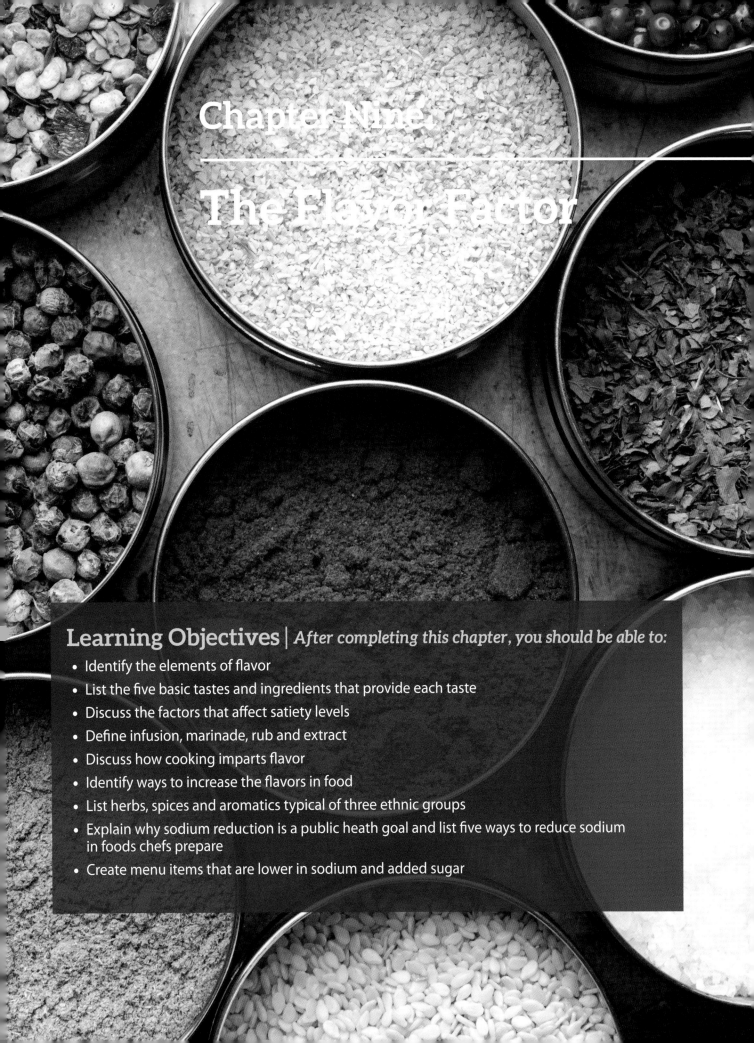

Chapter Nine

The Flavor Factor

Learning Objectives | *After completing this chapter, you should be able to:*

- Identify the elements of flavor
- List the five basic tastes and ingredients that provide each taste
- Discuss the factors that affect satiety levels
- Define infusion, marinade, rub and extract
- Discuss how cooking imparts flavor
- Identify ways to increase the flavors in food
- List herbs, spices and aromatics typical of three ethnic groups
- Explain why sodium reduction is a public heath goal and list five ways to reduce sodium in foods chefs prepare
- Create menu items that are lower in sodium and added sugar

Survey after survey, year after year, shows that flavor is the biggest factor influencing food choice. Consumers are not willing to, nor should they have to, sacrifice flavor for nutrition. Healthful foods taste good, too. According to the International Food Information Council Foundation's *2017 Food & Health Survey*, taste continues to drive food and beverage choices. In 2017, 84% of those surveyed rated taste as most important, up from 83% in 2015. [1]

A longstanding criticism of healthy foods is that taking out fat, salt and sugar results in foods that are bland, boring and lacking in flavor and texture. Many times, that criticism is justified. It is true that the omission of key flavor-enhancing ingredients does make creating wonderful flavors and textures more challenging. A goal of this book is to help chefs meet that challenge.

The unlimited availability and over-consumption of foods high in fat, salt and sugar has led to weight and health problems. This has created an increased public awareness of the need to make some dietary changes. In his 2013 book, *Salt Sugar Fat*, Pulitzer Prize winning investigative reporter Michael Moss takes readers on a tour of the $1 trillion processed food industry, showing how much effort and how many dollars are put into finding the magical formula of sugar, salt and fat to addict consumers. But many Americans, of all ages and economic status, want to eat more healthful foods in order to control weight and reduce health risks. That desire does not always transfer into behavior. The degree to which individuals are willing to make changes varies, but the desire for delicious foods remains. While foodservice operations will continue to offer some traditional and popular high-fat-sugar and -salt menu items, an abundance of healthier items should be offered to meet the needs of the growing number of guests who seek delicious and healthful foods.

Getting a Sense of Taste

"As soon as an edible body has been put into the mouth, it is seized upon – gases, moisture and all – without possibility of retreat. Lips stop whatever might try to escape; the teeth bite and break it; saliva drenches it; the tongue mashes and churns it; a breathlike sucking pushes it toward the gullet; the tongue lifts up to make it slide and slip; the sense of smell appreciates it as it passes the nasal channel, and it is pulled down into the stomach to be submitted to sundry baser transformations without, in this whole metamorphosis, a single atom or drop or particle having been missed by the powers of appreciation of the taste sense."

Source: Jean Antheime Brillat-Savarin, *The Physiology of Taste*, Kessinger Publishing, LLC 2010

Nutrition is not first and foremost with customers. Flavor is. As a chef, I was hired to create delicious food – not spa food that is "pretty good," but WOW! Food that is amazing.

Scott Uehlein
Former Corporate Chef
Canyon Ranch

Flavors are difficult to describe because each ingredient in a dish provides an array of tastes that cooking blends. Flavor is also influenced by aroma. Consider a ripe strawberry: Smell, flavor, texture and intensity of color all influence the perception of taste.

The American palate has grown bolder over the years. Today's recipes have more intensely flavored ingredients, spices and herbs than recipes in cookbooks of 25 years ago. Bold, ethnic flavors – hot and spicy, sweet and sour – have been an important trend since about 2003. Flavor and healthful cooking are clearly bound together. Consumers are transitioning away from low-calorie, low-fat foods and moving in the direction of fresh, less-processed foods with an emphasis on flavor. Similarly, the traditional indulgence foods from years past (candy, desserts, fried foods) will gradually transform into more complex, comfort experiences driven by higher-quality ingredients and flavors.

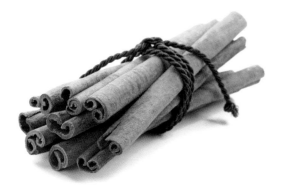

The Physiology of Taste

According to *Larousse Gastronomique*, **flavor** is "the sensation produced when food comes into contact with the taste buds on the tongue." [2] The fact is, however, that it is taste, not flavor, that we experience as our taste buds detect bitter, sweet, sour, salt and umani. All of the senses – smell, touch, taste, sight and sound – work together to create the far more complex sensation we call flavor.

How well you control the interaction of factors that comprise flavor defines your ability to produce food that is as tasty as it is healthy. Like any "good cooking," good healthy cooking balances the five tastes by mixing and matching ingredients to produce taste, aroma, texture, temperature and visual impact. Whether you are offsetting the richness of a steak with the bitterness of grilled radicchio; sweetening a tomato sauce with basil or a bit of sugar; adding lime juice instead of salt to bring out the flavor of a black bean soup; or serving coffee to enhance the sweetness of a dessert, you are orchestrating the components that determine the success or failure of your dish. The following information is offered to assist you to better understand these components.

Taste

The top of the tongue is covered with a layer of bumps called **papillae** that help grip food and move it around while chewing. Papillae contain the **taste buds**. Humans are born with about 10,000 taste buds, each made up of 50 to 150 receptor cells. These cells live for only one to two weeks and then are replaced. Each receptor in a taste bud responds best to one of the basic tastes: sweet, salty, sour, bitter or umani.

When taste buds are stimulated, nerves send a signal to the brain for processing and interpretation. Different parts of the brain process information about flavor, pleasure, temperature and texture. Older studies maintained that different regions of the tongue detected different tastes. In fact, taste buds detect multiple tastes, and the classic "tongue map" is no longer used. Taste buds are also on the soft palate at the top of the mouth and on the upper esophagus.

Because children have more taste buds than adults, they are often very sensitive to flavor and may intensely dislike some vegetables and other foods that they perceive as bitter or sour. An elderly person, however, may have only half as many taste buds as a child. Years ago, it was thought that elderly people preferred soft, bland foods. While some texture modifications may be necessary if there are problems with chewing, most seniors actually prefer more intensely flavored foods to compensate for decreased taste sensitivity. Because people have varied numbers of taste buds and different sensitivities and flavor intensity preferences, chefs should be mindful that their customers may have different taste tolerances than they do. Additionally, lifestyle factors such as cigarette smoking and health issues such as colds or respiratory problems will decrease the perception of flavor. Chefs who smoke or have a cold should be careful of seasoning "to taste" to avoid over-salting or over-seasoning foods. Dental surgery, Alzheimer's and Parkinson's diseases, and deficiencies of folacin, thiamine, zinc or vitamin B12 also can contribute to a reduced ability to taste.

Medicines, particularly antibiotics, antifungals and chemotherapy, can alter flavor perception. Some even create persistent bad tastes by changing the chemical composition of saliva. Surgery, injury or radiation to the head or neck can damage nerves that affect taste messages sent to the brain, resulting in a perception of unpleasant flavors or odors or an inability to perceive taste.

Super Tasters

According to our ability to taste, we can be categorized as super tasters, average tasters or nontasters. **Super tasters** experience taste with far greater intensity than average people. About 25% of Americans are super tasters. They have an unusually high number of taste buds – at least twice as many as normal. Evidence suggests that super tasters are genetically predisposed to be more sensitive to bitter tastes and fattiness in food. They tend to dislike strong, bitter foods like raw broccoli, kale, grapefruit juice, coffee and dark chocolate as well as paprika, celery powder, smoked flavors and almond extract. They are often picky eaters who readily identify food flavors but dislike very intensely flavored foods. About 30% of women and 15% of men are super tasters. A simple chemical test can determine whether or not a person is a super taster, but most super tasters know without having the test.

Salty

Salt (sodium chloride) is one of the most used and, from a health point of view, most overused flavor enhancers. Although salt improves the flavor of food by stimulating the taste buds and by balancing the effects of sweet, sour and bitter, we are becoming increasingly aware of salt's potentially negative effects on health. (See pages 230-233 for more information on salt.)

The preference for saltiness in foods, although partially genetic, is strongly influenced by environmental factors and varies a great deal from person to person. In other words, it's an acquired taste. Infants develop a taste for salt at 4 to 6 months of age based on how much salt is in their diet. At any age, however, a gradual reduction in sodium intake over 8 to 12 weeks can retrain the palate and increase acceptance of foods with less salt. [3] Super tasters commonly require more salt, not to intensify flavor but to counteract their super-sensitivity to bitter taste.

One way to reduce salt in recipes is to use flavor enhancers such as yeast extracts, yeast-based ingredients or monosodium glutamate (MSG). These ingredients activate taste receptors in the mouth and throat to amplify flavor and compensate for less salt. MSG, for example, contains about one-third the sodium found in salt.

When trying to cut back on salt in your cooking, be aware of salty ingredients already in a recipe such as soup bases, soy sauce, anchovies, prosciutto, olives, fish sauce, capers, bacon, mustard, oyster sauce and Parmesan cheese. Reduced-sodium soy sauce can be substituted for regular soy sauce for a moderate reduction in salt without a significant change in flavor. Rinsing canned vegetables, particularly beans, before adding them to a recipe can reduce sodium content by 40%.

Another approach to reducing sodium is to take advantage of the importance that smell has on flavor by increasing aromatic ingredients and assertive flavors to replace the taste lost when cutting down on salt. Today's diners are receptive to more intense flavors from spices and herbs as well as to the sensation caused by chili peppers.

Unfortunately – from a health point of view – salt also has become a popular addition to many desserts that are already high in fat and sugar, including salted caramel, salted chocolates and salted pralines. Many desserts, however, do have fruit to their credit!

Bitter

Bitter is defined as an acrid, sharp and unpleasant taste. Many people avoid the taste of bitterness. Poisonous foods are often bitter, so from an evolutionary point of view, bitterness helped early humans avoid natural toxins.

The taste of bitterness stimulates the appetite and cuts through the richness of some foods. Chefs typically balance bitterness with salt and sugar or with flavorful sauces and fats. This approach is important because even though many poisonous plants are bitter, other plants that are healthful to eat also have a bitter taste. In fact, many edible plants protect themselves against insects by secreting natural pesticides that are not harmful to humans when consumed in small amounts. Although plants are being engineered to remove these substances through selective breeding, many phytonutrients thought to reduce cancer risk and heart disease are being removed at the same time.

More recently, chefs have been highlighting bitter taste as a way to balance the richness of some foods while cleansing the palate between bites. Small amounts of bitterness can be pleasant and provide flavor contrast. Salads made of bitter greens, such as chickory, frisee, endive, watercress, radicchio and arugula, are commonly served with fatty steaks and fish. Cooked collards, Swiss chard, kale and other bitter nutrient-rich vegetables are popular side dishes. Bitterness is sometimes considered a positive attribute in products like coffee, strong tea, beer, wine and many mixed cocktails that contain tonic or bitters as a main ingredient. Although bitterness is not prized in most Western cultures, it is considered a key component of a balanced dish in much of India and Asia.

Monosodium Glutamate Explained

Glutamate, or glutamic acid, is one of the most common amino acids. It is found in all proteins and many other foods. In its bound form, glutamate links to other amino acids to make proteins. In its free form, it is a single amino acid that affects the flavor of food. Foods high in free glutamate, such as fermented fish sauces, seaweed products, meat extracts, tomato products and shiitake mushrooms, have been used for centuries to enhance flavor.

Monosodium glutamate (MSG) is a combination of glutamate, sodium and water. It acts like free glutamate and adds umami – a savory, broth-like or meaty taste– to foods. The body metabolizes glutamate, including that in MSG, the same way that it metabolizes glutamate found naturally in foods and the glutamate made in the body.

MSG Benefits

MSG has about one-third as much sodium as salt. MSG contains 12% sodium by weight, while salt contains 40% sodium. Some professionals suggest substituting small amounts of MSG for salt to reduce sodium while preserving a flavoring-enhancing effect. This approach is particularly useful when amplifying flavors for people who have a reduced ability to taste or poor appetite or for those who cannot tolerate large amounts of salt. MSG works by sensitizing taste buds to spread pleasing sensations throughout the mouth and by activating umami sensors.

MSG is most effective in recipes containing meat, poultry, seafood and vegetables and in combined dishes. MSG does not enhance the flavor of highly acidic foods, milk products or sweet foods such as pastries and desserts. It can added before or during cooking; MSG is not destroyed by heat.

Chinese Restaurant Syndrome

The term *"Chinese restaurant syndrome"* was first used in 1968 in the *New England Journal of Medicine*.

The author, a physician, described pain in the back of his neck, heart palpitations and other symptoms after eating in a Chinese restaurant. Others confirmed that they had had similar experiences, and a syndrome was born. While a significant number of Americans report symptoms of what is now called *MSG symptom complex*, virtually all cases have been anecdotal. Due to public concern that MSG causes headaches, facial flushing, chest tightness, nausea, weakness and neurologic problems and contributes to asthma, it is one of the most studied food additives. The American College of Allergy, Asthma and Immunology states that MSG is not an allergen. The European Union, the United Nations Food and Agriculture Organization, and the World Health Organization place MSG in the safest category of food additives. The Food and Drug Administration lists MSG as Generally Recognized as Safe (GRAS). MSG is used in greater amounts in China than in Chinese foods in America and Chinese people do not report Chinese Restaurant Syndrome.

What the Research Says

Many well-designed scientific studies have recorded no symptoms when people with reported sensitivities were given MSG under controlled conditions. Some research indicates that individuals who think that they have MSG sensitivity are actually having an allergic reaction to shellfish, soy, peanuts or other ingredients in Chinese cuisine.

Some people may in fact be sensitive to MSG, just as some individuals are sensitive to other foods and food ingredients. They may experience mild, transient symptoms such a facial flushing and rapid heartbeat that do not require treatment. Research continues, but today there is considerable scientific consensus that MSG, as normally used, poses no significant health risk and that MSG in food has no discernible effect on healthy people. Despite this consensus, a number of individuals and advocacy organizations continue to promote the belief that MSG is a dangerous food additive.

According to Food and Drug Administration regulations, when MSG is added to a food, it must be included in the ingredient list. When glutamate-containing ingredients are products' components, they are listed by their common name – for example, Parmesan cheese, tomatoes, shiitake mushrooms, Worcestershire sauce, hydrolyzed protein or yeast extract.

Sources:
Federation of American Societies for Experimental Biology. *Executive Summary from the Report: Analysis of Adverse Reactions to Monosodium Glutamate (MSG).* Available at http://jn.nutrition.org/cgi/reprint/125/11/2891S.pdf.

Walker R, Lupien JR. The safety evaluation of monosodium glutamate. *J Nutri*.2000;130:1049S-52S Available at http://jn.nutrition.org/cgi/reprint/130/4/1049S.

Food and Drug Administration. Questions and Answers on Monosodium glutamate (MSG). https://www.fda.gov/Food/IngredientsPackagingLabeling/FoodAdditivesIngredients/ucm328728.htm.

Sweet

While our tongues are hard-wired to be cautious of bitter taste, we are born with a strong desire to search out sweet taste. This phenomenon is also thought to be a survival mechanism because sweet foods usually contain energy-rich nutrients. In addition, in response to sweet flavors, the brain releases **endorphins**, which are neurotransmitters that reduce pain and create a feeling of well-being.

Health problems arise when we over-consume refined sugars, which are simple carbohydrates that provide calories but no other nutrients. (See Chapter 3 for a complete discussion of sugar.)

Some chefs are substituting brown sugar, honey, palm sugar, molasses, agave or maple syrup to add flavor. From a nutrition point of view, however, these sweeteners are not significantly different from refined sugar. Dates and fruit purees are popular nutrient-rich substitutions for sugar. Some spices, such as cinnamon and cardamom, have a sweet note that makes it possible to cut the amount of sugar used.

Sugars are not the only source of sweetness. Sugar alcohols and artificial sweeteners are also available. Some sugar alternatives are available in combination with sugar for use in baking. Diners limiting calories and sugar intake may want "diet" soda as well as alternative sweeteners to use in coffee and other beverages. Some alternative sweeteners, also called sugar substitutes, taste sweet at first but have a metallic, licorice-like or chemical aftertaste for certain individuals.

Non-nutritive sweeteners or artificial sweeteners can be used in cooking but generally are not popular with chefs, except those cooking for people with diabetes or specific health conditions. Although they add sweetness, most don't act like sugar. Non-nutritive sweeteners don't caramelize, add volume, cream well with fat or perform well in baking. Some are not stable when heated. In addition, non-nutritive sweeteners are more expensive than sugar. Because of the intensity of sweetness, small amounts of these sweeteners are used to provide sweetness.

Relative Sweetness of Sugars

Sugar sweetness is measured by comparison to the sweetness of sucrose, which is assigned a value of 100.

Sweetener	Sweetness Value
Sucrose (table sugar)	100
High-fructose corn syrup	100 - 130
Fructose	120
Honey, liquid	100
Invert sugar syrup	95
Glucose	70
Dextrose	60 - 70
Maltose	45
Lactose (milk sugar)	40
Corn syrup	30 - 50

Source: Adapted from: McGee H. *On Food and Cooking. 2nd ed.* New York: Scribner; 2004

Relative Sweetness of Sugar Substitutes

The sweetness of sugar substitutes is measured by comparison to the sweetness of table sugar, which is assigned a value of 100.

Sugar Substitute	Sweetness Value
Sucrose (table sugar)	100
Sugar alcohols	
Erythritol (Zsweet®)	70
Sorbitol	60
Mannitol	70
Maltitol	90
Xylitol	100
Aspartame (Equal®, NutraSweet®)	18,000
Acesulfame K (Sunnet®)	20,000
Saccharin (Sweet'N Low®)	30,000
Stevioside (Truvia®, Pure Via®, Sweet Leaf®)	30,000
Sucralose (Splenda®)	60,000
Neotame	800,000

Source: Adapted from: McGee H. *On Food and Cooking. 2nd ed.* New York: Scribner; 2004

Sour

The basic taste of *sour* comes from acidic ingredients. Acidic foods provide bright, sharp flavors that can reduce the need for salt. For example, a small amount of lime juice enhances the flavor of a black bean soup. The most fruit group contains naturally sour foods, particularly citrus fruits, including lemon, lime, orange, grapefruit, kumquat, tangerine, mandarin, tangelo and Meyer lemon. Vinegars, such as malt, cider, balsamic, champagne, fruit, herb, rice, wine and garlic, also add sourness.

The popularity of international cuisines, particularly Asian cooking, has introduced many new sour ingredients to the chef's pantry – kaffir lime, tamarind, sumac, lemon grass, ponzu, galangal and powdered pomegranate seeds, to name a few.

Just as the American palate embraced the fiery excitement of hot chilies, diners have now turned their attention toward sour taste in food. From green apple martinis to Japanese yuzu to Indian vindaloo, sour is in demand and presents new opportunities for chefs to expand their menus. Sour is a perfect accompaniment to spicy hot food because it cuts the heat and freshens the palate for the next fiery bite.

Americans have a long history of combining sour with sweet as in lemonade and strawberry-rhubarb pie. The growing popularity of a simple squeeze of citrus into soups and salads as well as on grilled meats, seafood and even sweet corn is evidence of a new appreciation of tartness. As diners continue to explore and experience the sour aspect of various cuisines, chefs can use this taste to offer healthier options that cut sodium, sugar and fat from recipes.

Umami

Umami is a Japanese word meaning delicious. Sometimes described as savory, brothy or meaty, the sensation of umami is conveyed by several substances, including the amino acid glutamate. Glutamate is found naturally in many foods, including fish, meat, cheese, tomatoes, mushrooms, peas, corn, seaweed and human milk. Foods that are ripe and at their flavor peak have more umami. Deep red, ripe tomatoes have five times the glutamate of unripe early tomatoes. Monosodium glutamate (MSG branded as Accent®) is often used to enhance and harmonize the flavor of food. Many Asian cuisines routinely use MSG in cooking.

The Monell Chemical Senses Center in Philadelphia specializes in the study of taste and smell and the treatment of taste and smell disorders. Scientists at Monell confirmed the presence of specific taste receptors for umami in 2009. The landmark study found the genes associated with umami perception along with various levels of umami sensitivity. [4]

Taste Interactions

The flavor experience is a mixture of taste, aroma and texture with limitless possibilities. The five basic taste sensations work together to highlight, offset, complement and balance each other. Desserts taste sweeter with a bitter caffeine beverage than with water; acids taste even more sour with salty foods and cut the fiery effects of hot peppers.

"I have a cupboard full of acids! Everyday culture is doing the same thing when it comes to using acid in its food: it is all about enhancing flavor without adding salt. When I lived in England, they joked with me because I would add orange juice to almost everything, especially vinaigrettes. I really like its acidity and the light fruity flavor it adds. On a totally different end of the spectrum is tamarind. We always have tamarind water in our refrigerator and use it to finish sauces. Depending on the country of inspiration, I will use a different acid: for India, tamarind; Japan, ponzu, yuzu; Middle East, sumac, preserved lemon, and yogurt; and for Southeast Asia, lemon, lime and tamarind."

Chef Brad Farmerie as quoted in Karen Page and Andrew Dornenburg's *The Flavor Bible* Little, Brown and Company, New York 2008

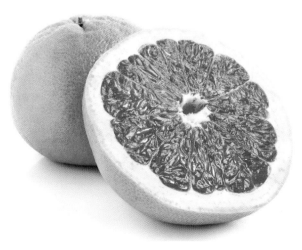

Smell

The classic saying "we eat with our eyes" gives short shrift to the power of aroma. The nose often sets up tasting expectations; in fact, the perceived flavor of food is primarily influenced by smell. An excellent example of this is cocoa powder. When you smell it, a chocolate expectation is triggered, but when you taste it, it is extremely bitter and unpalatable. Aroma may be responsible for as much as 80% of flavor perception, which is why foods seem to taste bland when the nose is blocked by a cold. It's not the sense of taste that changes; rather, it's a failure to sense aroma.

Aromatic ingredients such as fresh herbs, garlic and lemon zest enhance flavor. The aroma of onions sautéing or bacon broiling can trigger the appetite before the menu is presented. Of the five senses, smell is the most acute. It is a thousand times more sensitive than the sense of taste. Consider vanilla, the most popular flavor in the world, and how aroma adds to its flavor.

The sense of smell is tremendously complex. Scientists estimate that the human nose can detect nearly 10,000 distinct scents. Scientists Richard Axel, MD, and Linda Buck, PhD, won a joint Nobel Prize in 2004 for their work studying the olfactory process and identifying 1,000 olfactory genes.

There are six fundamental aromas: spicy, flowery, fruity, resinous, foul and burned. With age, sensitivity to aroma and taste decreases. As powerful as the sense of smell is, it is also very fragile. For example, when walking into a cinnamon bun shop the smell of cinnamon is very strong, but after a few minutes the aroma may no longer be noticeable. This is called **sensory adaptation**.

Mouthfeel

The **mouthfeel** of foods can affect the flavor experience. For example, people expect chips and crackers to be crisp. Crunchiness and crispiness contribute sound as well as textural appeal. If a mousse is gritty when it should be smooth or if a crust is chewy when it should be flaky, the flavor experience is adversely affected. A variety of textures enhances the enjoyment of food. Many creamy soft foods (soups, mashed potatoes, macaroni and cheese, puddings and ice cream) are considered comfort foods and are often preferred in times of stress or illness. Different people have different comfort foods based on their personal food histories. Crispy, crunchy foods (chips, French fries, popcorn and nuts) are often "fun" foods.

Dehydration, the removal of water, also concentrates flavor. Thin slices of fruit and vegetables can be made into wafers, chips or crisps in a dehydrator or in an oven set at a very low temperature. Carrots, potatoes, sweet potatoes, parsnips, squash and other vegetables make healthful, delicious chips when dehydrated. Apples, beets, pineapples and pears make wonderful crisps to add crunch, flavor and visual appeal. Thin slices of tart or sour fruits, such as lemons and kumquats, can be dehydrated with a sprinkle of sugar to caramelize the crisp. Dried fruits, such as raisins, cranberries, apricots or prunes, have concentrated flavor and sweetness from dehydration. They add color, texture and sweetness to many cooked foods and salads. Nutrients and added fiber are a bonus!

Temperature

Temperature also affects the flavor experience. An ice cream base will taste very sweet at room temperature but not so sweet when it has been frozen. Beer is quite bitter at room temperature but just fine when chilled. A contrast in temperatures adds to the enjoyment of eating – for example, a hot fudge sundae, grilled chicken Caesar salad or warm pie a la mode.

How Hot Is Hot?

Diners will find varying degrees of spiciness or piquancy desirable. Piquancy of peppers is measured by the **Scoville scale**, which is based on the amount of **capsaicin** (a chemical compound that stimulates nerve endings in the skin) present. Wilbur Scoville first rated the "heat" of peppers in 1912. Until recently, the Trinidad Moruga Scorpion was known as the world's hottest chile pepper. But according to the 2013 Guinness Book of World Records, it's now the

Scoville Rating	Type of Pepper
100,000–350,000	Habanero chili, Scotch bonnet pepper, Jamaican hot pepper
50,000–100,000	Thai pepper, Pequin pepper
30,000–50,000	Cayenne pepper, Tabasco pepper, some chipotle peppers
10,000–23,000	Serrano pepper, some chipotle peppers, some jalapeño peppers
2,500–8,000	Some jalapeño peppers, sharp paprika pepper
500–2,500	Anaheim pepper, guajillo pepper, poblano pepper
100–500	Pimiento, pepperoncini
0	Bell pepper, sweet paprika pepper

Carolina Reaper grown by Ed Currie of PuckerButt Pepper Co. in South Carolina. The pepper rates an average of 1,569,300 Scoville heat units, as tested by Winthrop University in South Carolina throughout 2012, says the Guinness entry. [5]

Astringency

The dry, puckery sensation caused by **tannins** also contributes to the flavor of foods. This **astringency** is desirable in some red wines, strong tea, walnuts (especially black walnuts), rhubarb and cranberries. But it can also be unpleasant, such as in an unripe banana or persimmon. Acids and salts can increase astringency; sugar will reduce and balance it.

Pungency

Pungency refers to the combination of taste and aroma from ingredients containing chemicals that irritate taste buds. Some stimulation can be pleasant; too much can be unpleasant or even slightly painful. Hot mustards, spices, sauces and horseradish provide pungency, which creates flavor contrasts in dips and sauces.

Chemesthesis

Chemesthesis refers to other sensations that tickle or play tricks on the senses and happens when chemical compounds activate sensory receptors. Membranes in the mouth, nose and eyes are particularly susceptible to chemesthesis stimuli. The tickle of carbonation in a soft drink, sparkling wine or juice; the "cool" of peppermint and the "burn" of chili peppers; and mouthfeel surprises such as foams and flavor wafers created by molecular gastronomists are examples of chemesthesis.

Sight

The rich redness of strawberries indicates ripeness and sweetness. A uniformly brown skin on roast chicken suggests crispness. Moisture in a properly cooked piece of fish indicates tenderness. Color and moistness suggest the flavors to come. Learned associations like these may alter perceptions and create expectations about how food should smell and taste; cherry flavors are supposed to be red and lime is meant to be light green. The overall visual appeal of a dish – shapes, colors and plate presentations – also plays a role in stimulating the appetite and preparing the diner for flavorful foods. The combination of these perceptions leads to a decision about whether a food is delicious or not, even before the first bite.

Over the past 20 years, beautiful food styling and photography have become common in magazines and newspapers, in cookbooks, on the Internet, on television cooking shows, and in food advertising. The visual presentation of a dish can greatly enhance enjoyment of it. Colorful fruits and vegetables and fresh herbs are healthful ways to add visual interest. Plate presentation is discussed in Chapter 10.

Sound

Even the sounds of foods as they are being prepared or eaten can influence flavor perception. The crunch of radish, celery or jicama, the crack of a flatbread and the slurping of noodles are sounds that stimulate appetite and promise satisfying food.

Modern Cuisine

Modern cuisine, also called experimental cuisine or culinary physics, uses food science to create innovative food flavors, textures, aromas, mouthfeel and presentations. While specific techniques are beyond the scope of this book and involve specialized equipment, ingredients and skills, chefs may view an excellent video discussing and demonstrating techniques used at the renowned Alinea Restaurant in Chicago. Chef Grant Achatz presented the lecture, "Reinventing Texture and Flavor," at the Harvard University School of Engineering and Applied Sciences in 2010 (**www.youtube.com/ watch?v=dYDe3RASpa0**).

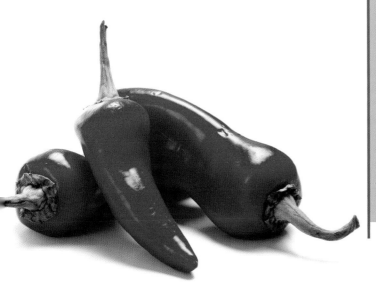

What Makes Us Feel Full?

The main role of food is to satisfy hunger and to provide essential energy, nutrients, and other substances for growth and maintaining health. Much of what we choose to eat is influenced by the palatability of foods, including the taste, smell, texture and appearance. Of course, social setting, personal preferences, habits, mood and other environmental factors also influence food intake.

Appetite can be divided into three components: hunger, satiation and satiety. *Hunger* is the sensation that causes us to seek and eat food. As eating proceeds, hunger subsides while satiation, the feeling that governs how much and how long we eat, takes over. Eventually, the feeling of *satiation* (when hunger ends) ends eating, and a period of not eating begins. *Satiety* refers to the sensations that determine the time between meals. [6] Regulation of appetite – including the hunger, satiation and satiety that influence what we eat – has both a physiological and psychological basis.

Satiety describes the effects of a meal after it has ended. The mechanisms involved in controlling satiety range from those involved with digestion, such as gastric distention and emptying, to more complex hormonal effects. In addition, people do not always eat when they are hungry, possibly due to lack of food or social constraints, and they do not always stop eating when satiated, perhaps because of boredom or stress. Oversized portions can also encourage overeating beyond satiety.

The macronutrients – protein, fat and carbohydrates – affect the feeling of satiety. Protein is the most satiating of the three. Increased satiety can come from foods high in fiber or water, too. Fats and carbohydrates are less satiating. It appears that taste, palatability and caloric value greatly influence the degree to which macronutrients promote or reduce appetite. *Palatability*, the measure of a food's pleasantness, and energy-density also influence satiety and therefore hunger. People prefer foods that are energy dense because they are more palatable. Less-caloric foods typically contain more water and less fat. They tend to be more physiologically satiating but generally less palatable. [7] Barbara Rolls, PhD, a professor at Pennsylvania State University and author of the popular book *Volumetrics* has studied how energy density affects satiety. She states that "satiety is the missing ingredient in most weight-loss programs." [8] People need to eat more foods that are higher in water and fiber to create a feeling of fullness. In other words, low-energy dense foods with high palatability mitigate overconsumption and create a high satiety level. These foods include those with protein and fiber, including plenty of fruits, vegetables, whole grains and water. [9]

Flavors Imparted by Cooking

Raw food will taste completely different when cooked, and flavor may vary according to cooking technique. Compare the taste of a raw onion with one that is sautéed or caramelized. Does a hot smoked chicken breast taste different from one that is poached, sautéed or grilled? Think about how simply toasting nuts and seeds such as sesame seeds changes and intensifies their flavors and aromas. Heat can enhance or destroy flavor, depending on how it is used. Many flavors can be developed through proper execution of various cooking techniques, often without adding extra calories, fat or salt.

The Heat Is On

A *Maillard reaction* occurs when heat is applied to a food that contains both carbohydrate and protein. This reaction is identified by browning and development of flavor. Examples of the Maillard reaction can be seen in bread crusts and roasted meats. The browning of sugar is a reaction called *caramelization*.

The transformation of sugar results in a rich aroma, color and taste. Caramelizing a simple sweet food can change it into something more complex and rich with a nutty or toasty flavor. Browning onions is an example of caramelization; sautéed, browned onions are more fragrant and sweeter than raw onions.

From the Kitchen
Justin Dean
Co-Owner
Madhouse Vinegar Co.

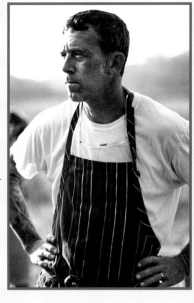

My food philosophy is simple. I like it. Food makes people smile and I like smiles. Healthy, local, and fresh are my top priorities. Personally, I make every effort to eat as close to the source as possible. Basically, if it's fresh, local, and in season, I'm a fan.

This extends to my professional life as well. At Madhouse Vinegar Co., we pride ourselves on using locally sourced, locally foraged and locally recycled products to make top quality vinegars with unique and wholesome flavors like persimmon, paw paw, spicebush berry and coffee, to name a few.

The truth is what we put into our bodies is what we put out. But also? Healthy food tastes good. Respect your body, your community, and the environment by eating close to the source. The rest is gravy.

Justin Dean grew up working on his parents' farm in Kentucky. He later moved to Providence, Rhode Island to pursue a degree in Food and Beverage Management, and from there landed at a restaurant called Maisonette, which boasts the longest running streak of five-star awards from the Mobil Travel Guide.

Over the span of his 30-year career, Jason has consulted on dozens of concept restaurants and side projects, including stints at Woodlands Pork and Black Oak Holler Farm in the backcountry mountains of West Virginia. It was there where he learned to carve up a pristine hog.

When he's not in the kitchen, he's out in the schools, educating folks about ways to improve the quality and nutrition of the meals our kids are eating. He believes in giving new life to food waste whenever and however possible, and he always keeps the vinegar bubbling.

Caramelized Brie, Grilled Figs, Ham, and Kentucky Bibb Lettuce with Fig Vinaigrette
Serves: 10

Justin Dean
Founder and Co-Owner Madhouse Vinegar Co.

Vinaigrette:

Shallots, diced	4	small
Madhouse barrel aged fig vinegar	4	tablespoons
Dijon mustard	2	teaspoons
Carriage house farms wildflower honey	2	tablespoon
Extra virgin olive oil	6	tablespoons

Caramelized Brie:

Triple cream brie	10	wedges
Sugar	1	tablespoon
Fresh figs, cut in half	30	
Kentucky limestone bibb lettuce	2	heads
Country or Serrano ham or prosciutto	6	ounces

1. For the vinaigrette, mix shallot, vinegar, mustard and honey to combine. Whisk in olive oil. Season with salt and pepper.

2. For the brie, sprinkle brie with sugar and caramelize with propane torch or under the broiler.

3. Brush figs with olive oil. Grill just until colored and warm throughout.

4. Wash and dry bibb lettuce. Toss lettuce with vinaigrette. Serve with the grilled figs, caramelized brie and ham.

Per Serving

Calories	350	Cholesterol	40	mg
Fat	18 g	Sodium	670	mg
Saturated Fat	4 g	Carbohydrates	37	mg
Trans Fat	0 g	Dietary Fiber	5	mg
Sugar	31 g	Protein	12	g

What Today's Chef Needs to Know about Flavor

Chef Brad Farmerie offers these flavorful tips.

- Build a great dish by developing richness then cutting it with acidity. Add complex but subtle spices and season with salt, soy or miso as needed.

- Analyze the taste experience of every ingredient and use what you learn to lengthen the taste experience.

- Spice is nice; just use a variety. For example, if you put black pepper in every dish, they all taste like black pepper. Why not use fresh or dried chilies to create a similar effect but a broader palate of flavor and nuance.

- Bitter is not a bad thing if it is in balance with other flavors.

Woods Add Flavor in Grilling and Smoking Foods

The best woods for grilling and smoking are hardwoods from certain fruit and nut trees. Grilled foods cook more quickly and thus require a strongly flavored smoking wood in order to pick up the wood flavors. Herbs, such as oregano, sage, thyme, marjoram, rosemary and basil, used both dried and fresh, will permeate meat being smoked with their own particular flavors. Use the woody stems of rosemary and sage as well as the branches and leaves. Place herbs over smoldering wood.

Types of Wood	Characteristics and Typical Use
Alder	This tree originates on the West Coast of the US and generally produces wood that imparts a light, delicate-to-sweet-mild taste. It is the traditional wood used for smoking salmon, particularly in the Pacific Northwest.
Apple	This tree produces wood that imparts a mild and fruity, slightly sweet, taste. Use with sausages, poultry, fresh pork, bacon and ham.
Cherry	Often used with lamb, game birds and venison, cherry wood imparts a taste similar to apple but with a slightly tart finish.
Hickory	The so-called king of woods, hickory trees are prevalent in the South. The wood imparts a sweet-to-strong, hearty taste but is milder than mesquite. Hickory is often used with barbecued steaks, chops and spicy foods and to smoke bacon.
Maple	Maple trees are generally found in the Northeast. Maple wood imparts a sweet and light taste that complements poultry, ham, game and vegetables.
Mesquite	Mesquite flavor can become strong very quickly. Small amounts of mesquite may be added when smoking other woods as the primary heat source. Mesquite is used in Southwestern cooking and with spicy foods.
Oak	Oak, an excellent wood for smoking large pieces of meat for several hours, is also great for steaks, duck and burgers.
Peach	Peach wood chips, which impart a sweet, fruity flavor and leave a nice mellow hint of smoke, are great for poultry or pork.
Pecan	Abundant in the Southwest, pecan wood imparts a medium fruity taste. It will burn cool and offers a richness of character. Pecan is most often used with chicken, duck and game birds.

Other less common woods used for grilling and smoking include guava, almond, walnut, apricot, lemon, orange, bourbon barrel wood chips, wine barrel wood chips and juniper, which is slightly resinous.

Flavor from Processes

Using processes that capture flavor is essential to maximizing the appeal of healthful foods. Easy flavor boosters – lots of fat, sugar and salt – should be limited in healthful cooking, but chefs can meet the flavor challenge by mastering other techniques and processes.

Infusion and Extraction

Pulling flavor out of ingredients and infusing it into liquids used in food preparation adds flavor to dishes. **Infusion** means steeping a seasoning or food in a hot liquid until the liquid absorbs the item's flavor. Solids are then strained out. Herbed oils and vinegars are common infusions.

Extracts

Extracts, also called essences, are concentrated liquids used to enhance or flavor foods. Plant extracts are obtained by distillation or infusion and include essences of vanilla, almond, orange, lemon, cinnamon and other plants and flowers. Some essences are reductions of a cooking liquid such as mushroom, tarragon, tomato or stock or are made by marinating truffles, garlic, anchovies or other items in wine or vinegar and concentrating that liquid to intensify flavor.

Essential oils are strongly flavored fragrant substances extracted from the flowers, fruit, leaves, seeds or roots of plants. Most essential oils are used to make perfumes and scented and aromatherapy products, but citrus oils, peppermint and almond oils are sometimes used in small amounts to flavor foods.

Extraction and concentration are taken to new levels by some chefs who use specialized techniques and equipment to extract and concentrate all manner of foods and serve them in unique ways. The flavors, aromas, temperatures and textures created through the discipline of molecular gastronomy make it an art form in cuisine.

Juice

A fruit and vegetable juicer is a valuable piece of equipment in the healthful kitchen. Use a concentrated or reduced juice instead of water to add nutrients and flavor. Adding vegetable juice to poaching liquid, sauce or soup boosts nutrients, flavor and color. Juices can be infused with herbs or spices – for example, apple juice infused with rosemary, zucchini juice with thyme and carrot juice with ginger. Fruit juice will also help sweeten a cooked whole-grain cereal such as oatmeal. Grains such as couscous can be cooked in carrot juice. While juicing concentrates some nutrients and phytochemicals, the fiber strained out during juicing is lost.

Stocks and Broths

Stocks are clear, flavorful liquids prepared by simmering bones (with some adhering meat) in water with aromatics until their flavor is extracted. Stock is used as a base for soups, sauces, stews and other preparations. A **broth** is a flavorful, aromatic liquid made by simmering meat or poultry for a long time. Both stocks and broths have an important role in healthy cooking. A good stock is fat free, flavorful, low in added salt, clear and versatile. Many healthful stocks and broths are cooked ahead, concentrated and defatted. Some excellent quality stocks and broths are available, but look closely at the sodium content. Cooking grains in stock instead of water adds flavor and nutrients. Stock reduced down to a paste consistency is called a **glacé** (gla-say).

Stocks and Broths		
Fundamental Stocks	**Other Stocks**	**Broths**
Chicken	Lamb	Shallot
Brown (beef or veal)	Pork	Mushroom
Fish	Game	Lemongrass
Shrimp	Turkey	Onion
Vegetable	Lobster	

Vinegars and Oils

Oils can be infused with garlic, horseradish, citrus zest, shallots, fresh herbs, dried herbs, hot peppers or spices. Infused oils can be used in dishes such as shrimp salad with curry oil or chilled cucumber soup with dill oil. Vinegars can be infused with fresh herbs, dried herbs or fruits and used in salad dressings as well as dressings for vegetables and meat. A small amount of infused oil or vinegar sprinkled over a vegetable can have great flavor impact.

Marination

A ***marinade*** is an intensely flavored liquid or dry mixture applied to foods before cooking to impart flavor and to tenderize tougher cuts of meat. The marinating process may last seconds or days. A liquid marinade is used to soak foods and is typically made of oils, acids and seasonings. Plain yogurt can be used as the base, as in an Indian Tandoori marinade. The acid in a marinade (wine, beer, vinegar or citrus juice) can also "cook" a food by denaturing its proteins, as in fish or seafood ceviche. A ***dry marinade*** or rub is a mixture of herbs, spices, citrus zests or salt. In some cases, oil or mustard is used to make a paste, which is rubbed over a food. The coated item will absorb the rub's flavors. Adding pineapple or papaya to a marinade helps soften meat fibers because they contain enzymes that tenderize muscle fiber.

Reduction

Fruit juices, vegetable juices, stocks, broths, wine, spirits and vinegars can be reduced, thus enhancing their flavor through concentration. Aromatics can be added to further develop the flavor. Common reductions include:

- Balsamic vinegar
- Cabernet wine
- Raspberry-Riesling wine
- Port
- Apple cider
- Pomegranate molasses
- Pure maple syrup
- Agave nectar/syrup

Reduced balsamic vinegar or pomegranate molasses can be drizzled over a salad, meat, fish or a dessert for both flavor and visual effect.

Flavor from Ingredients

Who cannot wait for the first asparagus of spring or the juiciest strawberries from the June farmers' markets? Does tomato salad taste better in the middle of winter or at the height of the season in August? Creating a dish with the best flavor means starting with the best ingredients available. This does not mean flying in exotic items from around the world – although a chef can get almost any ingredient from somewhere year-round. Rather, it means developing menus or special promotions to reflect the seasons and working with local purveyors to get the freshest local products. Freezing or canning can capture seasonal flavor at its peak for use all year, but generally fresh is best. The "farm-to-fork" trend toward sustainable farming and focus on using local products in season has changed how many consumers think about flavor and fresh ingredients. We have come to expect seasonal products, sourced within a 200-mile radius, that taste great.

Many ingredients add flavor during cooking. Plants in the allium family – garlic, leeks, onion, ramps, scallions and shallots – add pungent, spicy flavors and aromas that enhance eating pleasure. Sweet or hot peppers are used in a variety of dishes to add piquancy and depth. They can be raw or cooked, fresh, dried, flaked, powdered, pickled, smoked or in extract form (think hot sauce). Peppers are frequently used raw and chopped in salads or cooked in stir-fries or other mixed dishes. They can be sliced into strips and fried, grilled, roasted whole or in pieces, or chopped and incorporated into salsas or other sauces. Favorite hot pepper varieties include chipotle, jalapeno, serrano, habanero and Scotch bonnets. Sweet peppers include ancho, poblano, and green, red, yellow, orange and purple bell peppers.

Prepared condiments can be used in sauces, dressings, soups, stews, stuffings and main items as flavor enhancers. Examples include horseradish, wasabi, ginger, mustards, pickle relishes, soy sauce, olives, capers, salsas (fruit and vegetable), chutneys, catsup, Worcestershire sauce, chimichurri sauce and chili sauce. Light or reduced-sodium soy sauce has good flavor and is easily substituted for regular soy sauce or tamari sauce in a health-conscious kitchen.

High-sodium or high-fat ingredients such as cheese, pickles, capers, anchovies and fried onion straws have bold flavors. Sometimes just a small amount can create a big impact. Using a small amount on top, rather than mixed into a dish, creates maximum visual and flavor impact while limiting salt and/or fat.

Herbs and Spices

Herbs and spices create wonderful opportunities for chefs to express their creativity. The flavor lost when fat, salt and sugar are reduced can be replaced with seasonings. Spices and herbs add flavor without calories and many also provide antioxidants and phytochemicals.

Most **herbs**, which are the leaves of aromatic plants, are available fresh, dried and, in some cases, frozen. Some herbs dry more successfully than others. Aroma is a good indicator of quality in both fresh and dried herbs. Some herbs, such as fresh basil, mint and dill, are delicate; others, such as rosemary and thyme, are more assertive. Herbs also can be purchased as pastes or made into pestos. Herbs are generally added toward the end of cooking because their flavor and aroma are more delicate. Many chefs have kitchen gardens that provide fresh herbs for cooking and garnishing.

Spices are aromatics prepared from the roots, buds, flowers, fruits, bark or seeds of plants. Cinnamon comes from a bark, pepper from a berry, ginger from a root and nutmeg from a fruit. Most spice flavors are intense and powerful. Spices are usually dried and available whole or ground. Whole spices will retain flavor longer than ground spices.

Some spices and seeds used for seasoning can be toasted to make them more aromatic. A few spices, such as cayenne pepper, intensify in flavor during cooking. When changing the yield of recipes, the amount of spices and herbs should be adjusted by taste. A recipe increased from 10 to 50 servings will not need five times the amount of herbs and spices.

Many herbs and spices are now believed to have health benefits, such as turmeric as an antioxidant. Since the amount of an herb or spices used in a single serving is relatively small some spices are sold for theraputic uses in tablets and capsules.

Herb Equivalents

- 1 tablespoon finely cut fresh herbs
- 1 teaspoon crumbled dried herbs
- ¼ to ½ teaspoon ground dried herbs

casebycase | Spice: The Proof in the Pudding

At Chicago's renowned Spice House (**www.thespice-house.com**), spices from around the world are ground and blended by hand in small batches on the store premises. Owners Patty and Tom Erd, and Patty's parents before them, have spent six decades finding the best sources and countries of origin for each spice. The Erds are slowly easing into retirement now, but CEO Charlie Mayer is on board to help ensure that Spice House operations never skip a beat.

Over the past few years, the enterprise has expanded, adding two Milwaukee, WI, locations to its flagship Chicago shop and its Evanston, IL, satellite. Spice House also has increased its presence on social media. But the company's growth has not distracted from its mission to bring its customers the freshest possible products – such as cinnamon from Ceylon and Tahitian vanilla.

Patty and Tom are members of several culinary arts organizations and have participated in many educational programs for restaurateurs and chefs. Here is a quick tip from flavor guru Patty Erd: "Add dried herbs to a recipe toward the end of cooking, rather than early on, as is the conventional approach. In most cases," she explains, "prolonged cooking will diminish dried herbs' essential oils. Compared to spices, herbs have a very low percentage of essential oils." Sooner v. later? Try it both ways. As the old proverb goes, "the proof of the pudding is in the eating."

Cilantro Warning

Be careful with cilantro: It looks tame but can elicit very strong reactions. Some find it refreshing and lemony or lime-like and enjoy it in ethnic cuisines such as Mexican, Indian, Thai and Chinese. Others perceive it as soapy, bitter and foul smelling. If you use cilantro as an ingredient, let it be known so it is not a surprise to those who will reject any food containing it – or simply substitute Mexican (not Greek or Italian) oregano instead.

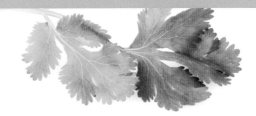

Storing Spices and Herbs

Fresh Herbs

- Refrigerate cut fresh herbs to prevent spoilage. Fresh herbs will keep up to four days in the refrigerator.

- Put fresh herb bouquets in containers, with stems down like cut flowers, and place in the refrigerator. Change the water daily.

- Loosely wrap the herb bouquet in film wrap or perforated plastic bags to extend shelf life. Smaller sprigs and individual leaves should be wrapped in a paper towel or placed in a food-safe plastic bag.

- Wash herbs and slice them into fine strips (chiffonade). Fill an ice cube tray halfway with water. Place a teaspoon or so of the herbs in each square of the tray. Make sure the leaves are down in the water. Place the half-filled tray in the freezer. When the ice cubes are almost frozen, finish filling the tray with water. Place the tray back into the freezer to freeze solid. Once the ice cubes are frozen, remove from the tray and store in zip-closure plastic bags. Use a cube as needed to flavor soup, stock, pasta, sauces or stew.

Dried Herbs and Spices

- Store dried herbs and spices in a cool, dry place in an airtight container. Do not keep containers of herbs near a hot stove. Dried herbs and spices provide flavor because they contain oils that break down faster if they are exposed to air, light and warm temperatures.

- Dried herbs and spices will retain their flavor for about six months. Record the date of delivery on all dried spice and herb containers. Discard a dried spice or herb that has lost aroma or faded in color.

- Avoid buying dried herbs in powdered form. They lose their flavor in a matter of weeks.

We frequently associate specific grapes with their microclimate and the characteristics of the soil in which they grow. Spices also will acquire different flavor spectrums based on growing conditions. For example, vanilla beans grown in Madagascar display a very pure, clean essence of vanilla. The same plant grown in Mexico has a much spicier bouquet, and vanilla beans grown in Tahiti have an extremely complex floral flavor profile.

Patty Erd, Owner
The Spice House
Chicago, Illinois

Seasoning Tips

The possibilities for using herbs and spices, alone or in combination, are infinite. Creative chefs develop unique balances and flavor contrasts through innovative use of seasonings. Many cookbooks and resources describe flavoring philosophies and provide recipes. The International Association of Culinary Professionals' award-winning book *The Flavor Bible: The Essential Guide to Culinary Creativity, Based on the Wisdom of America's Most Imaginative Chefs* is among the best resources a chef can use. [10] Learning to use a wide variety of seasonings requires experience. Here are some seasoning tips.

- Sweet herbs like mint, nutmeg, ginger or anise complement citrus fruits.

- Fresh herbs like savory, dill, basil or cilantro can be added directly to a green salad.

- Salads with strong-flavored ingredients call for peppery dressings. Try some of these additions to a basic dressing:
  - Peppery herbs: red pepper, black pepper, mustard, chives and paprika
  - Strong herbs: oregano, tarragon and dill

- For delicately flavored vegetables such as mashed sweet potatoes, add a sweet spice such as nutmeg to complement the flavor; add a savory spice such as oregano, chives or dill to totally change the flavor.

- Freshly grated cheeses and freshly ground herbs and spices have more flavor, pungency and aroma. When possible, use freshly grated nutmeg, ground pepper and other spices and seeds.

- For strong-flavored vegetables, use peppery spices like basil, black pepper and savory.

- For baked fruits, use spices such as nutmeg, cloves or cinnamon.

- Dry spice blends can be rubbed into cuts of meat the day before cooking as a dry marinade. The flavors are absorbed into the meat before and during cooking.

- The ingredients in seasoning blends may age differently, so taste before seasoning. In lemon-pepper, for example, the pepper fades first, leaving much more lemony flavor.

- Herbs and seeds like caraway, dill, poppy and sesame can be baked into bread or sprinkled on top of breads or vegetables for a nice accent.

- The flavor of ground herbs can be lost quickly. Ground herbs should be added just before the cooking is complete. Adequate time should be allowed for the dried herb to absorb enough moisture to release its flavor.

- Whole spices are best suited to long-cooking recipes. Whole spices should be added as soon as cooking begins for maximum flavor. Whole spices and herbs (fresh and dried) should be removed before the food is served. The use of a **sachet d'epices**, small spice bag, makes removal of whole herbs and spices easy.

- Toast whole spices, like fennel, star anise or coriander, and mustard or sesame seeds before adding them to a dish for more depth in flavor and to release oils.

- In a fruit recipe, a general rule is to increase the spice by 50% and decrease sugar by 50%. The spice enhances the flavor, reducing the need for sugar.

- Dry mustard as well as horseradish and wasabi powder have no odor. The aroma develops when they are mixed with a cold liquid. Allow 10 to 15 minutes for the full flavor to develop. Mixing with an acid such as vinegar brings out more heat.

- The flavor of spices tends to become more intense in a food over time. If a food such as tomato sauce is cooked the day before and reheated for serving, this timing should be taken into consideration when deciding how much seasoning to use. The longer a food is held after preparation, the more opportunity flavors have to fuse, mellow and develop a full, rich taste.

- For cold foods such as salad dressings and chilled salads, add the seasoning at least several hours in advance to allow the flavors to develop.

- In quick-cooking foods such as vegetables, add herbs at the start of cooking.

- In slow-cooking foods such as soups or stews, add herbs in the final 15 to 20 minutes.

- To prepare fresh herbs for use in a bouquet garni, wash in cool water and discard any blemished leaves. If the fresh herbs are to be chopped, the woody stems should be removed and the herb should be chopped to the size appropriate for the food.

- Black sesame seeds, black or red salts, and other colorful seasonings, such as chopped chives, add color and drama to plate presentation.

Traditional Herb and Spice Uses

Meat, Poultry, Fish and Eggs

Beef	Bay leaf, marjoram, nutmeg, onion, garlic, pepper, sage, thyme
Lamb	Curry powder, garlic, rosemary, mint, thyme, garlic
Pork	Garlic, onion, sage, pepper, oregano, chiles
Veal	Bay leaf, ginger, marjoram, oregano
Chicken	Ginger, marjoram, oregano, paprika, poultry seasoning, rosemary, garlic, sage, tarragon, thyme
Fish	Curry powder, dill, dry mustard, lemon juice, marjoram, paprika, pepper, celery seed
Eggs	Chives, parsley, thyme, paprika, freshly ground pepper, mustard powder, chervil

Vegetables

Carrots	Cinnamon, cloves, marjoram, mint, nutmeg, parsley, rosemary, sage, allspice, ginger
Corn	Cilantro, cumin, curry powder, onion, paprika, parsley, chile powder
Green beans	Curry powder, dill, lemon juice, marjoram, oregano, tarragon, thyme
Greens	Onion, pepper, nutmeg with spinach, garlic
Peas	Ginger, marjoram, onion, parsley, sage, mint
Potatoes	Dill, garlic, onion, paprika, parsley, sage, rosemary
Summer squash	Basil, cloves, curry powder, marjoram, nutmeg, rosemary, sage, thyme
Winter squash	Cinnamon, ginger, nutmeg, onion, allspice, mace
Tomatoes	Basil, bay leaf, chives, cilantro, dill, marjoram, onion, oregano, parsley, pepper, thyme

Traditional Herb and Spice Blends

Bouquet garni is a small bundle of fresh herbs such as parsley, thyme, celery leaf, fennel fronds or marjoram, and fresh or dried bay leaf tied with a string or enclosed in cheesecloth to make a sachet. It is used to flavor stocks, braises, stews and other slowly cooked meat dishes. Remove the herb bundle after cooking, before the food is served.

Fines herbes is a time-honored French seasoning composed of fresh minced parsley, tarragon, chervil and chives. It is often used in omelets, on grilled meats and in marinades. The blend is added toward the end of cooking or used fresh in a salad dressing. Try mixing fresh fines herbs into bean spread, lowfat mayonnaise, sour cream and cottage cheese or use it as a spread for sandwiches.

Quatre-epices, traditionally used in charcuterie, is a mixture of fresh ground black or white pepper, nutmeg, cloves or cinnamon and ginger. Use quatre-epices to add a more aromatic nuance to all meats, particularly game, or to add a Caribbean piquance to grilled or stewed meat.

Garam masala, traditionally used in Northern Indian cuisine, literally means "warm spice blend" because it is meant to heat the body. The blend is stirred into curries, pilafs and biryanis toward the end of cooking. Try substituting garam masala for cinnamon and nutmeg in oatmeal cookies. Dry-roast the whole spices in a hot pan over low heat before grinding them. Spices found in garam masala include cardamom, coriander, cumin, black pepper, cloves, cinnamon and nutmeg.

The word *curry* comes from the south Indian word kari, which means sauce. Curry is not a single spice but rather a spice blend with many variations. Spices found in curry may include coriander, cumin, red chili powder, turmeric, ginger, allspice, black pepper, cardamom, cinnamon, cloves, fennel seeds, fenugreek seeds, nutmeg or mace, saffron, asafetida, mustard seeds, nigella seeds, curry leaves, galangal, or sesame seeds. For something different, try adding a little curry powder to a fresh carrot soup. To maximize flavor, dry-roast the whole spices in a hot pan over low heat before grinding them.

Sometimes called *five-spice powder*, five-fragrance powder, five perfumes or five heavenly spices, this traditional Chinese blend of ground star anise, fennel seeds, Szechwan or white pepper, cassia or cinnamon, and cloves is used throughout southern China and Vietnam in stir-fries and in marinades for pork, beef, chicken or duck. It makes a wonderful addition to barbecued ribs or braised leeks.

Although there is no "classic" Latin blend, *chili powder*, composed of ground assorted chile peppers, cumin, Mexican oregano, fresh or ground onion, and garlic, is probably the most common. In Mexico, this powder is added to chili con carne dishes and all sorts of bean and meat chilis. A salt-free blend that adds lots of flavor, chili powder is also used to season fried tortilla chips and other snack chips.

Adobo seasoning, another Latin flavor, is composed of fresh thyme, oregano, cilantro, ground cumin, black pepper and garlic. Ingredients are placed in a blender and mixed with orange juice to make an adobo marinade. The ingredients mixed in their dried form make a spice rub commonly used in South American cooking. Adobo mix is also found on many of the Caribbean islands once occupied by the Spanish.

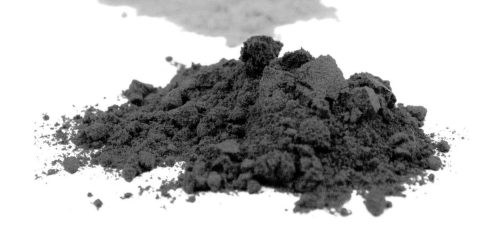

Ethnic Influences

Countries, regions, cities and even neighborhoods have traditional spice/herb combinations used for seasoning. Spice and herb shops, ethnic markets and catalogs offer single herbs and spices and blends. Some excellent sources for herbs and spices not typically available through food distributors are the Spice House at **www.thespicehouse.com**; McCormick Spices at **www.mccormick.com**; Penzeys Spice at **www.penzeys.com**; and Tones at **www.tones.com**.

Selected Spice Mixtures

Mixture	Country of Origin	Traditional Use	Form	Characteristic Spices
Bumbu	Indonesia	Used to flavor rendangs and gulais (spicy dishes served with sauce)	Dry spice mixture combined with coconut milk prior to use	Ginger, turmeric, chiles, cinnamon, cloves, coriander, black peppercorns, tamarind
Ras al Hanout	Morocco	All-purpose flavoring powder	Whole spices ground together	10 to 15 ingredients, usually including allspice, cloves, cumin, cardamom, chiles, ginger, peppercorns, mace, turmeric and caraway seeds
Berbere	Ethiopia	Cure for meats; added to condiments and stews	Ingredients mixed together then simmered prior to use	Chiles, cardamom, cumin, black pepper, fenugreek, allspice, ginger, cloves, coriander, ajowan seed, cinnamon
Harissa	Tunisia, Morocco, Algeria	All-purpose condiment, also used to flavor stews and sauces	Whole spices ground together then mixed with olive oil to moisten	Chiles, caraway, cumin, coriander, garlic
Baharat	Middle East (Lebanon, Syria, Gulf States, Saudi Arabia)	Widely used to flavor all types of dishes, particularly soups and stews	Whole spices ground together	Cloves, nutmeg, cinnamon, coriander, black pepper, paprika, cumin, cardamom, chiles
Curry Powder	Southern India	Used to flavor thin, soupy sauces	Fresh ground spices sautéed in oil at beginning of cooking process	Curry leaves, turmeric, chiles, coriander, black pepper and sometimes cumin, ginger, fenugreek, cinnamon, cloves, nutmeg, fennel seed, cardamom
Garam Masala	Northern India	Usually added at end of cooking to complete seasoning	Spices roasted whole then ground into a powder	Cinnamon, cardamom, cloves, cumin seeds, coriander, black peppercorns, nutmeg, mace
Panch Phoron (Indian Five-spice Mix)	Eastern India and Bengal	All-purpose flavoring for vegetable dishes	Sautéed in hot oil prior to cooking	Whole cumin seeds, fennel seeds, fenugreek, nigella, black mustard seeds
Gaeng Wan (Green Curry Paste)	Thailand	All-purpose flavoring, widely used in soups and sauces	Ingredients ground together in mortar and pestle to form a wet paste	Green chiles, lemongrass, ginger, coriander, cumin, white peppercorns, cilantro, green curry

Selected Spice Mixtures continued

Mixture	Country of Origin	Traditional Use	Form	Characteristic Spices
Massaman Paste	Thailand	All-purpose flavoring, widely used in soups and sauces	Ingredients ground together in mortar and pestle to form a wet paste	Chiles, coriander, cumin, cinnamon, cloves, star anise, cardamom, white peppercorns
Recado	Yucatan Peninsula of Mexico	Rubbed on food prior to cooking, also used as all-purpose flavoring for sauces and stews	Spices pounded to a paste in combination with vinegar, garlic and herbs	Achiote, cloves, black pepper, chiles, allspice, cinnamon, coriander, cumin, oregano
Chile Powder (pure ground chile peppers)	Mexico	All-purpose flavoring	Stems and seeds removed (if desired); dry toasted until fragrant then ground	Various chiles such as: • Ancho • Pasillo • Guajillo • Chiles de arbol
Chili Powder (blend of chile peppers and other spices)	Mexico	One of the most common spice blends in Mexican foods	Spices combined	Paprika, cumin, cayenne pepper, oregano, garlic power
Five-Spice Powder	China	Used as flavoring in a wide variety of Chinese dishes; frequently used in marinades	Whole spices ground into a raw powder	Anise, fennel seeds, cloves, cinnamon, peppercorns
Quatre Spices	France	Most often used in patês	Spices combined and then ground into a powder	Pepper, nutmeg, cloves, ginger, sometimes cinnamon
Pickling Spices	Europe	Used to add flavor to pickles and certain liquids	Raw whole spices	Mustard seeds, cloves, coriander seeds, mace, black peppercorns, allspice, ginger, chiles, cinnamon sticks, bay leaves
Cajun Blackening Spices	Louisiana	Used to coat fish prior to cooking	Ground raw spices	Mustard powder, cumin, paprika, cayenne pepper, black pepper, onion, garlic, thyme, oregano
Crab or Shrimp Boil	Chesapeake Bay	Add to water used for boiling crab or shrimp	Ground raw spices	Peppercorns, mustard seeds, coriander, salt, cloves, ginger, ground bay leaves
Mojo	Carribean South America	Marinade	Liquid with sour orange base	Garlic, oil, fresh herbs

Health Benefits Of Herbs And Spices

While herbs and spices have been used for thousands of years with purported benefits, research into the specific ways herbs and spices can improve health has increased significantly in the past few decades. Although research is in the beginning phase, certain compounds have been identified in herbs in spices that contribute to improved health.

In addition to the specific health-promoting compounds there are several other important nutrition benefits to consider with herbs and spices. Herbs and spices add unique flavors to foods that help increase palatability of meals while reducing added salt and sugar. As discussed in Chapter 6, Americans, to their detriment, consume too much sodium. Adding herbs and spices to vegetables makes them more appealing! It is no mystery why we don't like bland vegetables; add some fresh herbs or pungent spice and the vegetables become cravable. Herbs and spices have few calories, no fat and are low-sodium (unless they are processed into a salt – like garlic salt.)

Keep in mind, while herbs and spices have a very high concentration of antioxidants and other health-promoting compounds, they are consumed in small amounts. Vegetables and fruits are consumed in half-cup portions while herbs and spices are consumed in much smaller amounts. A specific herb or spice is not consumed every day, making nutrition contributions from each herb or spice very small.

Health Promoting Compounds in Herbs and Spices

Function	Health Benefit	Sources	
Antioxidants	Many compounds in herbs and spices fight oxidation and free radicals that can damage cell membranes. Oxidative damage and stress contributes to diseases including cancer, cardiovascular disease and Alzheimer's disease.	Cinnamon Calendula (Marigold) Cloves Garlic	Oregano Peppermint Thyme Turmeric
Anti-inflammatory agent	Chronic inflammation is thought to increase risk of cardiovascular disease and Alzheimer's disease.	Cumin Ginger Nutmeg Peppermint	Red pepper Rosemary Turmeric
Antimicrobial compounds	Traditionally used to keep meat safe from bacteria in warm climates. Role in maintaining healthy bacterial growth in the large intestine is being explored.	Basil Chiles Cinnamon Coriander Cumin	Garlic Ginger Nutmeg Oregano Rosemary
Anti-cancer	Certain compounds found in herbs and spices may help inhibit tumor growth, prevent cell mutation and influence enzymes that aid the liver in clearing potentially toxic substances.	Cayenne pepper Ginger Parsley Turmeric	
Blood sugar control	Keep blood sugar levels stable and enhance the effect of insulin in people who have insulin resistance or metabolic syndrome.	Cinnamon Fenugreek Ginseng	
Aid digestion	Fennel might aid in digestion by relaxing the colon.	Fennel	
Lift mood/relaxation	Some preliminary studies suggest that chamomile as tea might be helpful for generalized anxiety disorder. Studies on lavender for anxiety have shown mixed results.	Chamomile Lavender Saffron Sage Vanilla	

Health Promoting Compounds in Herbs and Spices *continued*

Function	Health Benefit	Sources
Reduce nausea and indigestion	There's some information from studies in people on the use of ginger for nausea. The natural oil in peppermint has anti-nausea effects when used in aromatherapy.	Ginger Mint Peppermint
Boost metabolism	The capsaicin in cayenne peppers may help boost metabolic rate. However, its effect is small and you may build up a tolerance.	Cayenne Chili peppers
Improve memory and brain function	There is promising evidence that sage extract can improve brain and memory function, especially in individuals with Alzheimer's disease.	Sage

Resources: National Center for Complementary and Integrative Health, **https://nccih.nih.gov/**; Office of Dietary Supplements, **https://ods.od.nih.gov/**; McCormick Science Institute, **http://www.mccormickscienceinstitute.com**; Healthline, **https://www.healthline.com/nutrition/10-healthy-herbs-and-spices**

The Issue of Salt

Regular **salt** is sodium chloride (NaCl). Some regular salts have added iodine and anti-caking agents. Sea salts and other natural salts have small amounts of additional minerals that may add color and other subtle flavors. Most sodium in the diet comes from salt added in food processing and preparation. Some comes from high-sodium ingredients like soy sauce. Relatively little comes from adding salt at the table. Successfully reducing the sodium content of foods requires a substantial change to fresher and less processed foods and ingredients. Currently, about three-quarters of the sodium in the American diet comes from processed foods, including snacks and fast foods.

As diners try to reduce their sodium consumption, culinary professionals are challenged to reduce salt and sodium-rich ingredients used during cooking. Knowing how much sodium is in a recipe requires calculation. Asian cuisines, such as Thai, Japanese and Chinese, tend to be high in sodium because they use salty fish and soy-based sauces and stocks liberally. Italian cuisine can be high in sodium when salted tomato products and cheese are used. Recipes with particularly high levels of sodium can be adjusted or portion size can be altered.

Salt's most obvious impact is on taste, but it also serves other functions in cooking such as increasing the water-binding capacity of proteins and increasing the juiciness of meat and poultry. Salt also helps stabilize batters and extends shelf life through its

antimicrobial effects. Small amounts of salt are added to many baked goods to balance and improve flavor. This should not be an issue as each portion served has very little added salt.

Sodium reduction in the American diet is long-standing concern. After nutrition labeling regulations mandated disclosure of sodium content, many food manufacturers began incrementally reducing the amount of sodium in prepared foods. The average American eats at least twice the amount of sodium recommended for a healthy diet. The *Dietary Guidelines* recommend that everyone gradually reduce sodium intake to less than 2300 milligrams per day (1 teaspoon of salt contains about 2,300 milligrams of sodium). This is a major challenge; currently, many menu items exceed the total daily recommendation. In June 2006, the American Medical Association called on the food and restaurant industries to cut salt levels by one-half during the next decade. But some scientists and the Salt Institute argue that individuals who are healthy and not salt-sensitive do not need to limit salt intake. [11]

As awareness of sodium's contribution to health risks increases, there will be more demand for food options with less sodium. Following repeated petitions from the Center for Science in the Public Interest and other advocacy groups, the Food and Drug Administration is considering removing salt from the list of foods it categorizes as "generally recognized as safe" (GRAS). [12]

Types of Salt

White, pink, grey or black – salt comes in many colors and forms and is found all over the world. Each variety has its own special characteristics.

Experiment with unique colors and flavors as garnishes for maximum visual and taste impact. (Remember to reduce the amount of salt in food as it is prepared.)

Type of Salt	Description
Table salt	Table salt is the most common kind of salt. It usually comes from salt mines and is refined with most minerals removed until it is pure sodium chloride. Most table salt is available either plain or iodized. It is mixed with a trace amount of an anti-caking agent such as calcium silicate to prevent clumping. Table salt is often preferred in baking for its fine-grained texture and accuracy of measure. One teaspoon of table salt contains 2,300 milligrams of sodium.
Iodized table salt	American salt manufacturers began iodizing salt in the 1920s after people in some parts of the country were found to be suffering from goiter, an enlargement of the thyroid gland caused by an easily preventable iodine deficiency. People require less than 225 micrograms of iodine a day. Iodized salt can be considered the first "functional food."
Coarse salt	Coarse salt is a larger grained sea salt crystal. It is less moisture sensitive so it resists caking. It is often used for salt crusts on meat or fish.
Kosher salt	Kosher salt is so named because it is used in the preparation of meat according to the requirements of Jewish dietary law. Its craggy crystals make it perfect for curing meat – a step in the koshering process. It contains fewer additives and has a more salty taste than ordinary table salt. Kosher salt generally comes in flakes rather than granules. The flakes dissolve easily and have a less pungent flavor than table salt. Many chefs enjoy using kosher salt because it tends to have a clean, natural flavor and sprinkles more evenly than other salts. This is the salt of choice for creating seasoning mixes. Diamond Crystal kosher salt has half the sodium of regular table salt. Because the crystals are hollow and lighter, 1 teaspoon has only 1,120 milligrams of sodium. Morton kosher salt crystals are not hollow and have the same amount of sodium per teaspoon as table salt.
Rock salt	Rock salt is composed of large, hard, chunky crystals. Rock salt is often used to regulate temperature when making ice cream in an ice cream maker. Sold in large crystals, rock salt has a grayish hue because it is unrefined. Rock salt makes a great bed for serving oysters and clams. It is not eaten.
Pickling salt	This salt is commonly used to brine pickles, sauerkraut, vegetables or turkey.
Sea salt	Sea salt is a broad term that generally refers to unrefined salt derived directly from an ocean or sea. It is harvested by channeling ocean water into large clay trays and allowing the sun and wind to evaporate the water naturally. Manufacturers of sea salt typically do not refine it as much as other kinds of salt, so it contains traces of other minerals including iron, magnesium, calcium, potassium, manganese, zinc and iodine that may impart color or flavor. Sea salt may be coarse or fine.
Smoked sea salt	Smoked sea salts are naturally smoked over wood fires. Smoked sea salts add a unique flavor to a wide range of dishes including roasts, chicken, salads and sandwiches.

Type of Salt *continued*	Description
Flake sea salt	Flake sea salt is a light crystal reminiscent of snowflakes. Seawater is evaporated using the natural processes of sun and wind, producing salt brine that is fed into an open evaporating pan. The brine is then slowly heated until delicate pyramid-shaped crystals appear.
Celtic salt	Celtic salt refers to naturally moist salts harvested from Atlantic seawater off the coast of Brittany, France. These salts, which are rich in trace minerals, are hand harvested in the traditional Celtic manner, using wooden rakes that allow no metal to touch the salt.
Fleur de sel	Fleur de sel (flower of salt) is an artisan sea salt composed of "young" crystals that form naturally on the surface of salt evaporation ponds. They are hand harvested under specific weather conditions by traditional paludiers (salt farmers). True fleur de sel comes from the Guérande region of France; different areas within Guérande produce salts with their own unique flavors and aroma profiles.
Grey salt	Grey salt is a moist unrefined sea salt usually found in the coastal areas of France. Its light grey, almost light purple, color comes from the clay found in the salt flats. The salt is collected by hand using traditional Celtic methods.
Grinder salt	Grinder salts are typically large dry crystals suitable for a salt mill or grinder. The white salt crystals are easy to grind and the lower moisture content allows the salt to flow through easily.
Hawaiian red alaea clay sea salt	Alaea sea salt is a traditional Hawaiian table salt used to season and preserve. A natural mineral called alaea (volcanic baked red clay) is added to enrich the salt with iron oxide. This mineral gives the salt its distinctive pink color. The clay imparts a subtle flavor that is said to be mellower than regular sea salt. Hawaiian sea salts have a nuance of sweetness that is rarely found in other salts.
Hawaiian black lava sea salt	Black lava Hawaiian sea salt is a unique combination of taste and mineral content. It can add drama and textural contrast when sprinkled over food. This salt is dried in high-tech solar evaporators and retains only 84% sodium chloride, the remainder being naturally occurring mineral elements.
Salt substitutes	Most salt substitutes are partially or entirely made from potassium chloride. They taste somewhat salty.
Light salt	A blend of salt substitute and salt that tries to capture the flavor of salt but with less sodium.

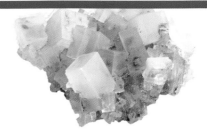

Reducing the Sodium Content of Food

Chefs can reduce sodium by optimizing the size and shape of salt flakes or granules. On a gram-for-gram basis, the sodium level is the same, but the flaky, less dense granules of some kosher salt, for example, mean less sodium per teaspoon – and less saltiness. A teaspoon of regular table salt (granular) has 2,300 milligrams of sodium; kosher salt has 1,120 milligrams per teaspoon (although variable by brand); and sea salt has about 1,870 milligrams per teaspoon. Tips for reducing sodium include:

- Read labels, become aware of sodium content and choose lower-sodium options as ingredients.

- Purchase ingredients, especially bases, that are labeled "low in sodium," "reduced-sodium" or "lower-sodium." Use reduced-sodium soy sauce routinely. Many Asian sauces are extremely high in sodium.

- Balance the sodium content of a favorite higher-sodium food with food choices naturally low in sodium, such as fresh fruits.

- Decrease salt in recipes whenever possible. In baked goods, leaving out the salt can affect quality and taste, but salt usually can be reduced by half.

- Make salad dressings and sauces with lower-sodium ingredients and with little added salt.

- Rinse canned beans before cooking to reduce sodium content by about 40%. Salt was added to preserve the beans' texture, but remains in the liquid.

- Salt provides flavor but no aroma. Use aromatic ingredients and assertive flavors to replace flavors lost when cutting down on salt.

Salt Substitutes

While most chefs will not use salt substitutes, there are situations – for example, cooking for people with severe salt restriction – in which using salt substitutes may be necessary. There are a number of salt substitutes available. The traditional salt substitute is a blend of potassium chloride and sodium chloride. Most people find these blends to have a bitter or metallic as well as salty flavor. Some substitutes use blends of potassium chloride, magnesium sulphate and the amino acid lysine hydrochloride. Other new salt products are blends of natural sea salts (both sodium and potassium chloride). Salt substitutes with potassium may not be a good choice for people with type 1 diabetes, kidney or heart problems who may need to limit potassium. Researchers in the United Kingdom are exploring the potential use of seaweed granules to replace salt in processed foods. Seaweed also adds minerals to the diet.

Another approach to salt reduction is to use flavor enhancers such as yeast extracts, yeast-based ingredients or monosodium glutamate (MSG), which activate taste receptors in the mouth and throat to amplify flavor and compensate for less salt as described earlier in this chapter.

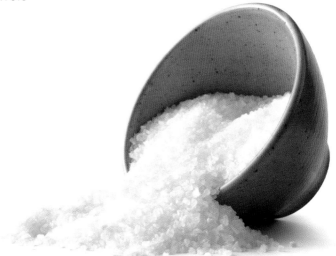

Opportunities for Chefs

Providing excellent flavor is a goal of all chefs. Chefs and culinary professionals are uniquely equipped to create healthy recipes that are full of flavor and appeal. Flavor involves the elements of taste, smell, texture, temperature, sight and sound. Herbs, spices, marinades, infusions, juicing and cooking methods can be used to enhance flavors in food. Traditionally, food preparers have relied on salt and sugar to add flavor to food. Today, we use other techniques and ingredients to optimize the flavors of foods.

Learning Activities

1. Using a selection of flavored jellybeans, close your eyes and select a bean. Pinch your nostrils closed and chew the jellybean. Can you identify the flavor? Unplug your nose. Can you identify the flavor?

2. Select several recipes (from a cookbook, magazine, website or cooking class). Identify ways to reduce the amount of salt in the recipes and ways to increase the flavor. Prepare recipes and compare the flavor of both versions.

3. Using a common spice (cinnamon, nutmeg, clove, etc.), gather various forms of the spice (ground, whole, toasted, etc.) and compare the smell and flavor of each form.

4. Compare the flavor of three preparations of an onion – raw, sweated and caramelized. Discuss the changes in flavor caused by cooking technique.

5. Conduct a tasting of sea salt, kosher salt, smoked salt and iodized table salt. Identify differences in grind, texture and flavor.

6. View "Reinventing Texture and Flavor," a lecture and demonstration given by Grant Achatz in 2010 at Harvard University School of Engineering, (www.youtube.com/watch?v=dYDe3RASpa0). Discuss in class.

For More Information

- McCormick Spices, www.mccormick.com
- Monell Chemical Senses Center, www.monell.org
- Page K, Dornenburg A. *The Flavor Bible: The Essential Guide to Culinary Creativity, Based on the Wisdom of America's Most Imaginative Chefs*. New York: Little, Brown and Company; 2008.
- Penzeys Spices, www.penzeys.com
- Salt Institute, www.saltinstitute.org
- The Spice House, www.thespicehouse.com
- Taste Science Laboratory, Cornell University, www.tastescience.com
- World of Flavors, Culinary Institute of America, www.worldofflavors.com

Chapter Ten

Healthful Cooking Techniques

Learning Objectives | *After completing this chapter, you should be able to:*

- Describe 15 healthful cooking methods or techniques
- Explain the nutritional advantages and disadvantages of various cooking methods
- Determine which healthful cooking method is best for specific foods
- List the factors that affect nutrient retention in food preparation
- Explain the process for developing and modifying recipes for healthful menus

Putting theory into practice is the purpose of this chapter. Using what you have learned about the essentials of nutrition and nutrition standards, it is time to focus on creating great tasting, eye-appealing, healthful dishes. This chapter describes the cooking techniques used to create such dishes. When plenty of positive choices are available on the menu, the service or waitstaff should be educated to promote these options based on their great flavors and unique ingredients.

Some people perceive healthful cooking as an unpleasant task requiring odd ingredients and unfamiliar techniques. In fact, many traditional cooking techniques from around the world can be used to prepare healthful food, sometimes with just a few modifications. The techniques described in this chapter work well with meat, poultry and fish as well as with vegetables, fruits, legumes and grains, and can help promote overall consumption of foods that are rich in protective nutrients. Proper serving temperature, portion size and attractive presentation also influence the perception of taste, quality and add pleasure to eating.

Cooking Techniques

There are four fundamental keys to healthful cooking:

1. Start with ingredients at their freshness and flavor peak.

2. Use a minimum amount of the type of fat necessary to provide excellent flavor and texture. Choose healthful fats when possible.

3. Use minimal amounts of added sugar and limit salt and other sodium sources.

4. Cook items at the right temperature and for the right amount of time, using sound cooking techniques.

From the Kitchen
Rakka
Chef/Owner
Café Rakka, Hendersonville TN

My style of cooking is a primitive desert-style, representative of the way we cook in my home country of Syria. The cornerstone of desert cooking is preventive lifestyle, and the best way to stay healthy is to utilize spices to create healthy and healing dishes. My personal approach is to show appreciation to nature's bounty by utilizing as many fresh herbs and spices as possible, blending and adapting them to each season to reach optimum health.

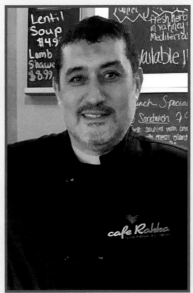

As for my diet, I eat a light breakfast of homemade cheese, olives, olive oil and fruit. Lunch is the main meal, where I'll typically eat whatever looks good on the menu that day, and for dinner I keep it light with a salad and lots of seasonal fruits. It's important to maintain a healthy relationship with food if you want a healthy life.

Café Rakka is a cozy, unassuming, 12-table cafe located in Hendersonville, a suburb of Nashville. It's a testament to Chef Rakka's unique passion and skill in the kitchen that this little Syrian café has landed on the map in a big way. His Lamb Korma, which was featured on Diners, Drive-Ins and Dives, simmers for three hours and includes upwards of a dozen spices, from cardamom to dried cherries to ajowan, an astringent spice reminiscent of thyme.

Rakka's mission is to bring Syrian cooking to the forefront of what he calls the modern tapestry of food and culture. Frustrated by the fast-food approach of most Middle-Eastern restaurants in the states, his approach is all about good old-fashioned practices: meats cooked low and slow, long-simmering sauces that require his full attention. He does it out of love—for his customers and his cuisine—but the byproduct is vibrant, delicious, wholesome food that is part meal, part tonic for the body and soul.

Café Rakka Lamb Korma

Serves: 10

Chef Rakka, Café Rakka
Chef/Owner Café Rakka

Chef Rakka uses the spices of his homeland, Syria, to infuse this rich creamy tomato lamb dish.

Coconut oil	4	ounces
Syrian black cardamom seeds	4	
Cardamom, ground	½	tablespoon
Cumin, ground	½	tablespoon
Coriander, ground	½	tablespoon
Garlic, crushed	4	cloves
Cinnamon	1	stick
Bay leaves	2	
Turmeric	1	tablespoon
Boneless leg of lamb, cubed	3	pounds
Lemon juice	2	tablespoons
Kosher salt	1	teaspoon
Saffron	½	tablespoon
Celery seeds	1	teaspoon
Ajowan	1	teaspoon
Tomato puree	16	ounces
Milk	1	cup
Yogurt	1	cup
Sour cream	¼	cup
Dried figs, quartered	4	each
Dried sweet cherries	1	ounce
Fresh cilantro	1	cup
Basmati rice, cooked	5	cups

1. To prepare the lamb: In a large saucepan put 2 ounces of coconut oil, 2 black cardamom seeds, ¼ tablespoon cardamom, ¼ tablespoon cumin, ¼ tablespoon coriander, 2 cloves of garlic, and ½ stick of cinnamon, 1 bay leaf and ½ tablespoon turmeric. Cook over medium heat to toast for about 2 to 3 minutes, then add the lamb, 1 tablespoon lemon juice and ½ teaspoon salt. Let it simmer for 20 to 25 minutes stirring occasionally. When meat is cooked add the saffron and turn off the heat.

2. To prepare the korma sauce: In medium saucepan add the remaining 2 ounces of coconut oil, and the remaining black cardamom seeds, cardamom, cumin, coriander, cinnamon, bay leaf and turmeric. Add the celery seeds and ajowan and toast for 2 to 3 minutes over medium heat. Stir in the remaining 2 cloves of garlic and the tomato puree, and mix well. Add the remaining 1 tablespoon of lemon juice and cook for 10 to 15 minutes over low heat. Stir in the milk, yogurt, sour cream and ½ teaspoon salt. Cover the pan and simmer for 45 minutes to 1 hour, stirring every 5 minutes, until the color turns bright orange. Add cherries and cook for 1 minute. Stir in the lamb, cook for 2 minutes, then turn off the heat.

3. Add a few cilantro leaves to the bottom of each serving bowl and ladle in the lamb korma. Garnish with more cilantro and enjoy it with basmati rice.

Per Serving

Calories	460		Cholesterol	80	mg
Fat	20	g	Sodium	370	mg
Saturated Fat	4	g	Carbohydrates	42	mg
Trans Fat	0	g	Dietary Fiber	2	mg
Sugar	8	g	Protein	29	g

Roasting and Baking

Roasting and *baking* are methods of cooking that cook food in dry heat in a controlled environment, usually an oven. Foods can be roasted or baked at low or high temperatures uncovered, which allows steam to escape. The term roasting typically applies to large pieces of meat, poultry, vegetables and fruits. Cooking on a rotisserie, with food turning mechanically, is also a form of roasting. Baking generally refers to seafood, starches, breads, cakes and pastries. The method of heat transfer in baking is generally the same as in roasting. There are exceptions – for example, pan-roasted salmon. This description has more to do with marketing than any real difference in cooking technique. Pan-roasted salmon just sounds better than baked salmon.

When vegetables and fruits are roasted, the heat caramelizes their natural sugars, making them sweet and soft on the inside but browned and crusty on the surface. Roasted fruits and vegetables are a flavorful way to incorporate more produce into menus and create unique flavors, color contrast and attractive plate presentations. Because they have little fat and salt, lots of protective nutrients, and relatively few calories, roasted fruits and vegetables are particularly good options for health-conscious diners and those with dietary restrictions.

When roasting poultry, it is preferable to keep the skin on to retain moisture and add flavor. The skin may be removed before serving or by the diner to reduce calorie and fat content. Most of the fat in poultry skin is unsaturated, so it makes little sense to remove the skin if other fats must be added.

Roasting on a rack allows rendering fats to drip from the food and air to circulate around the food. Generally, no additional fat is needed in preparation, but meat may be seared in a small amount of fat at the start of cooking to develop color and flavor. Tender, more expensive cuts of meat are usually used for roasting. Care should be taken to avoid overcooking roasted meats; use a thermometer to determine the degree of doneness.

Traditionally, fat drippings are used to make a roux for a pan gravy; however, after fat is removed, the pan can be deglazed and browned bits from the bottom of the pan used to make a delicious sauce with far less fat.

Fruits for Roasting or Baking

Apples	Oranges
Apricots	Peaches
Bananas	Pears
Figs	Pineapple
Grapefruit	Plucots
Mangos	Plums
Nectarines	

Beyond Potatoes and Onions: Great Vegetables for Roasting

Most roasted vegetables benefit from a light brushing of olive oil or a nut oil and the addition of herbs or seasoning before cooking. Go beyond roasted potatoes, sweet potatoes, onions, mushrooms, shallots and garlic with:

Acorn or other winter squashes	Fennel
	Leeks
Asparagus	Mushrooms including portobellos
Beets	
Bok choy	Parsnips
Broccoli	Radishes
Brussels sprouts	Scallions
Carrots	Sweet bell peppers
Cauliflower	Tomatoes
	Turnips

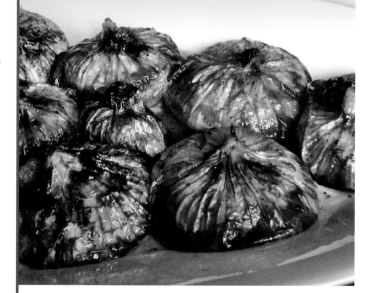

A fruit or vegetable salsa, a sauce using corn starch thickener or natural reduction can be lower-calorie, low-fat accompaniments.

Meat should have sufficient ***marbling*** (streaks of fat in lean meat) or it will become dry when roasted. Some meat must be basted during the cooking process with pan drippings or other liquids. When sauces or gravies are made from meat or poultry drippings, most of the fat should be removed and discarded before the deglazing liquid is added. Classically, lean pieces of meat and game were prepared for roasting by ***barding*** or larding – that is, adding fat either by wrapping or inserting pieces of fat with a special tool. Sometimes bacon is used for this purpose. You may want to consider braising as a healthier alternative for leaner or less tender cuts of meat or game.

Here are some suggestions for preparing healthful roasted foods:

- Trim most visible fat from meat prior to seasoning and cooking.
- Add more flavors to foods by using marinades or rubs prior to roasting.
- Use a range of herbs, spices and aromatics for seasoning.
- Roast on a rack to allow rendering fat to drip from the meat and poultry.
- Use fortified stocks, fruit concentrates or wine for flavoring sauces.
- Offer whole grain-based stuffings or dressings with roasts.
- Serve roasted meats with jus or jus lié.
- Serve main course items with a vegetable coulis, fruit-based sauce, salsa, chutney or relish.

Baking is the technique for most breads and desserts. The healthfulness of baked goods is more dependent on ingredient selection and portion size than on cooking techniques.

Crispy-Baked or Oven-Crisped

A crispy, fried-like texture can be achieved by topping food with a coating and then baking – for example, a crunchy topping on a baked chicken breast or fish fillet. The coating can be bread or panko crumbs, cornmeal, chopped nuts, cereal flakes, potatoes, or any starchy food with a small amount of added fat to help it adhere to the food surface. This cooking method was made popular by a product called Shake 'n Bake® and has recently been used by commercial kitchens in an effort to cut fat content and approximate a fried texture.

Seasoned potato sticks or strips can be crispy-baked with a resulting texture that is close to deep-fried French fries. Take care to describe cooking methods to patrons accurately and truthfully. Although the term "oven-fried" is sometimes used, it can create an expectation of texture and flavor that is seldom met. ***Deep-frying*** or ***pan-frying*** are cooking methods in which foods are cooked in hot fat; cooking foods in an oven with a crispy topping is clearly not frying.

The *Dietary Guidelines* tell Americans to eat fish or seafood at least twice a week, in 4-ounce portions, as a way of getting more heart-healthy fats. Thus, it is important to have some seafood on the menu that is not fried.

Broiling and Grilling

Broiling and grilling use very high heat to cook products quickly from the outside to the inside. Both methods involve dry heat with no additional moisture added during cooking.

Broiling uses radiant heat from an overhead source. Temperature is controlled by the intensity of the heat and how close the food is to the heat source. Typically, broiled foods are turned and broiled on both sides. Thicker cuts of meat, poultry and even seafood are often finished in the oven. A broiling variation for very tender foods, such as fish fillets, vegetables or fruits, is called ***au gratin***. Food is placed in a heatproof dish, covered with crumbs and broiled until a light crust forms. Although heat is applied only to the top surface, it is transferred through the heatproof dish so that the food is cooked thoroughly. This technique produces a crispy top similar to deep-fat-fried foods but without added fat.

Grilling uses a heat source located beneath the cooking surface. Kitchens use gas, electric, charcoal or wood-fired grills. Grilling is best for tender foods that cook relatively quickly and benefit from a smoky flavor. Preheating the grill, using a clean grill surface and turning the food in a controlled way create the distinctive crosshatch markings on grilled foods. Many grilled foods are marinated or brushed with oil and seasonings to add flavor. Use heart-healthy oils in marinades and for brushing and limit salt in rubs.

In addition to meats, poultry and seafood, consider grilled vegetables and fruits, which add color, flavor, texture and nutrient value to the meal. Grilled vegetables are also a welcome menu addition among health-conscious diners and vegetarians. Vegetables that are good roasted also may be grilled and used in hors d'oeuvres, appetizers, salads, entrées, sandwiches and accompaniments. Platters of grilled vegetables can be prepared in advance and served at room temperature as traditional antipastos. Romaine lettuce can be grilled for upscale Caesar salads. Flatbreads, such as pizza, and some fruits, such as pineapple, are also excellent for grilling.

Grilling is also a term used when cooking on a **griddle**, a solid flat plate of metal with a gas or electric heat source. Using a griddle, however, does not impart the flavor of foods grilled over fire. Griddles are often used for pancakes, eggs, flatbreads and sandwiches. When using a griddle, some fat may be needed – such as a vegetable oil spray or light brushing of oil – to keep foods from sticking. Heat is usually 350° F. Some griddles have an upper and lower plate to press grilled sandwiches such as paninis or Cuban sandwiches. Other griddles have raised grooves on their surface to simulate the crosshatching of grilling.

Barbecuing is a roasting or grilling method that requires a wood fire made from charcoal, various hardwoods, teas and/or herbs. Traditional barbecue is done in a smoke-filled chamber or in pits. The flavor of the finished product depends on the type of wood or plant used. A barbecue with a cover, sometimes called a kettle, can be used to smoke food and contain the heat. Meats can be enhanced by using a variety of seasonings as rubs applied prior to barbecuing.

The advantages of broiling or grilling include:

- When food is cooked on a grill, rendered fats drip away from it. Thus, after broiling or grilling, meat and poultry have less fat content than before cooking, which is important to estimate or deduct when calculating nutrient content.

- Broiled or grilled food can be cooked quickly to order.

- Foods receive flavor from high-heat searing, caramelizing and the distinctive flavors of various woods used in the grill.

- Barbecued foods and foods cooked with aromatic woods have distinctive and enticing aromas that are appealing to many diners.

Some limitations of broiling and grilling include:

- Both techniques require relatively tender cuts of meat, fish and poultry that usually are more expensive than less tender cuts.

- Dense vegetables, such as potatoes, other root vegetables and hard squashes sometimes require precooking.

- Grilled foods do not usually hold well in the prolonged heat of a steam table or for extended food service; however, food can be marked by grilling and finished in the oven as needed.

Here are some suggestions for preparing healthful broiled and grilled foods:

- Marinate or season the product prior to grilling.

- Low-fat marinades add flavor. Use herbs, rubs or spices for seasoning.

- Oil the grill to prevent food from sticking. Most of the oil will burn off, so there should be no concern about that added fat.

- Apply sauces with sugar, such as barbecue sauce, toward the end of the cooking process to prevent burning or excessive charring.

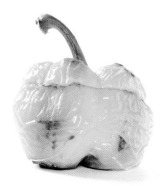

Smoke-Roasting or Pan-Smoking

Smoke-roasting or pan-smoking, also called hot-smoking, is done in a closed container using wood chips and, if desired, aromatics, herbs or tea to make smoke. This technique is best for small, tender, quick-cooking items such as poultry pieces, tender meats, fish, shellfish, game, lean sausages and some vegetables. It adds flavor without adding fat, salt or calories. Foods intended for smoke-roasting are often cured or brined for flavor. This step can easily be skipped to avoid high-sodium content. It is important, however, to season well with other herbs and spices.

Smoke-roasting is an excellent cooking technique for vegetables such as corn on the cob, peppers or tomatoes. It imparts a smoky "meaty" flavor. If left in the smoke too long, however, food may develop a strong, bitter and unpleasant flavor.

Here are some suggestions for preparing healthful smoke-roasted foods:

- Use various woods or aromatics for unique flavors.
- If the food is large or dense, it may be finished in the oven.

The Grilling Question

Grilling and broiling are excellent cooking techniques and many people love the resulting flavors. Chefs should be aware, however, that dietary advice for the prevention of cancer suggests limiting char-grilled foods.

Substances in the muscle protein of red meat, poultry or seafood react under high heat to form compounds called *heterocyclic amines (HCAs)* that can damage genes, thus triggering development of cancer.

Consumption of HCAs is linked most clearly to cancers of the colon and stomach. One study found that people who eat the most barbecued red meat (beef, pork and lamb) almost double their risk of colon polyps, compared to those who do not eat these foods. The more meat is cooked past ideal temperature, especially charred surfaces, the more HCAs will form. A higher consumption of well-done meat is linked with two to five times more colon cancer and two to three times more breast cancer. Risk of cancers of the stomach, pancreas and prostate may also increase.

To reduce HCA formation when grilling, turn the gas down or wait for charcoal to become low-burning embers. Raise the grilling surface from the heat source to reducing charring and flip meat often. Also consider cooking meat at lower temperatures, such as roasting or stewing. Pan-frying also should be done at a lower temperature. Research shows that frying meat at a high temperature, which saves only 2 minutes of cooking time, produces three times the HCA content of meat cooked at medium temperatures. In addition, marinating can decrease HCA formation by up to 96%, although studies are still underway to determine which ingredients help the most.

Vegetables and fruits are the best choice for grilling because they do not have protein so they don't form HCAs while they supply a range of cancer-fighting nutrients. In addition, the phytochemicals in vegetables stimulate enzymes that can convert HCAs to an inactive, stable form that is easily eliminated from the body.

Four factors influence HCA formation:

1. **Type of food**. HCAs are found in cooked muscle meats.
2. **Temperature**. Temperature is the most important factor in the formation of HCAs.
3. **Cooking method**. Frying, broiling and barbecuing produce the largest amounts of HCAs because these cooking methods require very high temperatures. Roasting and baking require lower temperatures, so they result in formation of lower HCA levels. Gravy made from meat drippings, however, does contain substantial amounts of HCAs. Stewing, boiling or poaching are done at or below 212° F; cooking at this low temperature creates negligible amounts of HCAs.
4. **Time**. Foods cooked a long time ("well-done" instead of "medium") form slightly higher HCA levels.

To avoid a different class of cancer-causing compounds called polycyclic aromatic hydrocarbons (PAHs), grill leaner meat cuts that will drip less and cause fewer flare-ups and smoke. PAHs form in smoke and are deposited on the outside of meat.

Source: American Institute for Cancer Research, **www.aicr.org/site/New s2?page=NewsArticle&id=8484&news_iv_ctrl=0&abbr=pr_hf_**

Sautéing, Searing, Stir-Frying, Pan-Frying and Deep-Frying

Generally, the term **frying** means cooking foods in hot fat or oil. In all forms of frying, choose as heart-healthy a fat as possible. Fry foods at temperatures that will cause the least amount of fat absorption.

Sautéing

A traditional **sauté** is a dry-heat method using some fat and medium-to-high heat. Sautéing is done in a shallow pan, turning or tossing the food to cook the outside surface evenly without overcooking the inside. Sautéing is a technique generally used with delicate foods that cook quickly – scallops, shrimp, tender strips or medallions of meat, poultry, fish fillets, and tender vegetables. In many recipes, onions are sautéed to a light golden color to bring out the natural sweetness and to create and impart flavor to a dish.

Traditionally, sautéed meats are served with a pan sauce with shallots, garlic, pepper, herbs and other seasonings. In the case of seafood, butter is often added and browned and served over the finished product. Omitting this last step will reduce the fat and caloric content of a sautéed dish.

In dry **sautéing**, no added fat is used. High heat is necessary to sear food and there must be enough space in the pan for proper browning without steaming. Nuts, grains and seeds may also be dry sautéed (toasted) to bring out their natural flavors and intensify aromas. Foods, such as onions, receive flavor from caramelizing. For some foods, such as mushrooms, water is released and the natural flavors of the vegetable intensify. Although dry sautéing is an excellent technique for serving health-conscious diners, it does have some disadvantages. Dry sautéing requires tender, often more expensive cuts of meat, poultry or fish. It works best when a food has some internal fat to help with browning.

Dense vegetables, such as carrots and potatoes, usually need to be precooked before sautéing. Generally, sautéed foods are prepared or finished when the order arrives in the kitchen, thus lowering nutrient loss from holding. Sautéed foods do not hold well on the steam table.

Safety of Nonstick Cookware

Nonstick cookware has been used for years to reduce the added fat needed in cooking. The safety of this cookware continues to be examined with no clear answer. At issue is the use of **perfluorocarbon acid** (PFOA). PFOA is used in manufacturing fluoropolymers, which impart fire resistance and oil, stain, grease and water repellency. Fluropolymers are used to make most nonstick surfaces on cookware and to waterproof breathable membranes for clothing.

PFOA has been shown to cause cancer, low birth weight and a suppressed immune system in laboratory animals exposed to high doses. Studies have shown the chemical to be present at low levels in the bloodstream of nine out of 10 Americans. And although the effects of PFOA at lower doses in humans are disputed, there does seem to be a link between PFOA and raised levels of cholesterol.

Manufacturers claim that PFOA does not leach into food cooked in nonstick pans made with perfluorocarbon acid. Although indicating that the science is still coming in, the Environmental Protection Agency launched a global stewardship program in 2006 that asked companies to reduce the presence of PFOA in products by 95% by no later than 2010 and to work toward eliminating sources of exposure no later than 2015. Many newer non-stick pans are not made with PFOA.

Until science has determined the complete safety of nonstick cookware, follow these guidelines:

- Never leave nonstick pans unattended on an open flame or other heat source.
- While cooking, don't let temperatures get hotter than 450° F. It is best to cook at low-to-medium heat.
- Don't use metal utensils that can scratch the surface of nonstick cookware.
- Wash nonstick cookware by hand using non-abrasive cleaners and sponges (do not use steel wool).
- Do not put nonstick cookware in a dishwasher.
- Don't stack pieces of nonstick cookware on top of each other to avoid scratched surfaces.

Searing, a variation of sautéing, calls for browning foods on all sides in a very hot pan over medium high to high heat to develop a brown and flavorful crust. A little oil may be used in the pan to prevent sticking. Food is sometimes served seared, such as thinly sliced seared tuna or very rare beef. Often searing is followed by braising or stewing, as in lamb shanks, osso bucco, short ribs and beef stew.

Stir-frying, another variation of sautéing, is traditionally found throughout Asia. Stir-frying is done in a wok or large pan with sloping sides and involves constantly turning food as it cooks. Cut vegetables and boneless meats and shellfish are often stir-fried. Foods are added to the stir-fry in sequence of longest to shortest cooking time so that at service, all ingredients are completely but gently cooked. Take care when seasoning stir-fries. The soy sauce, fish sauce and other Asian condiments included in many stir-fry recipes are typically very high in sodium. Reduced-sodium varieties are available and preferable.

Here are some suggestions for preparing healthful sautéed foods:

- In mixed dishes, use more vegetables and less protein. This is a great way to boost the volume of vegetables and moderate the protein portion.
- Use a well-seasoned or nonstick pan so that little or no additional fat is needed.
- Use herbs, spices and aromatics for seasoning.
- Use low-fat liquids to deglaze the pan and make the sauce.
- Use arrowroot or cornstarch to thicken the sauce if appropriate.
- Limit amounts of high-fat ingredients (butter, cream or cheese) to enrich and finish the sauce, or use only if necessary.
- Limit condiments and sauces high in salt or sugar.
- Serve sautéed foods with light, flavorful sauces made from vegetables or fruits.

Pan-Frying and Deep-Frying

Generally, pan-frying, and especially deep-frying, are not healthful techniques because frying in fats and oils usually creates a product that has a considerable amount of added fat. Eating fried foods frequently is likely to increase calories and weight. On healthful menus, fried foods are limited, portions of fried foods are modest and while fried foods can be requested as side dishes, they should not be routinely served as accompaniments to main course items. In fact many food service kitchens (especially in schools and healthcare facilities) no longer include fryers.

To **pan-fry** means to cook in a moderate amount of fat, typically a vegetable oil. To **deep-fry** means to cook a food submerged in hot fat. While frying may not seem to be compatible with healthful cooking, it can be used prudently. Modest amounts of fried foods can be used to add visual appeal, crunchy texture and unique flavors – for example, crispy fried leeks used as a garnish on a poached fish or a fried sage leaf on top of butternut squash soup. When fried foods are incorporated in healthful cooking, they should be front and center – used for visual and flavor impact in the first bites.

Limiting the fat in fried foods depends on cooking technique. Less fat is absorbed if no batter or breading is used. After a food has been fried, it should be removed from the oil and drained on an absorbent surface or rack. Most foods are fried at 350° F to 375° F. The fat should be hot enough to sizzle when food is added but not hot enough to smoke. Frying at too low a temperature usually causes excessive greasiness and contributes to excessive fat absorption in fried foods. When foods are pan-fried or deep-fried, care should be taken to choose oils that are mono- or polyunsaturated and trans-fat free.

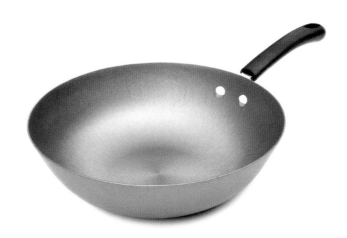

Microwave Cooking

Microwave ovens can cook some foods, but their main use is to reheat quickly. Foods like soups, stews, many sauces and grain dishes can be prepared in advance, divided into small batches and reheated before serving. Sometimes microwaving can also be used to precook root vegetables before finishing by grilling. Microwaving reduces the need to keep large batches of food hot through service, which can result in nutrient loss, reduced food quality and waste.

Poaching, Simmering, Boiling, Sous Vide and Blanching

Poaching, simmering, boiling and blanching are methods of gently cooking food in a liquid. Poached, simmered and boiled food can take flavor from the liquid used. Flavorful liquids include stock, broth, wine, vegetable or fruit juices or spiced teas often with aromatics added.

To **poach** means to cook in a small amount of liquid that is hot but not bubbling, about 140° F to 180° F. Often, the poached food (especially fruit) is cooled in the liquid to absorb its flavors. If the poaching liquid is flavorful, it is sometimes reduced to make a sauce that can be thickened with arrowroot or cornstarch. Poaching is a good technique for tender, delicate fish fillets, chicken breasts, eggs, some meats and fruits. Some classic recipes even poach filet mignon.

To **simmer** means to cook in a liquid that is bubbling gently, at a temperature no higher than 185° F to 205° F. Simmering may also be used to reduce the volume of a liquid, such as when making a tomato sauce thicker or reducing a wine or fruit sauce. Because simmering is done at a higher heat than poaching, it has a tenderizing and rehydrating effect. It is a good technique for cooking dense vegetables, grains, legumes, poultry, meat and dried fruits.

To **boil** means to cook in a rapidly bubbling liquid, often water or stock, at about 212° F. Boiling is typically used for certain vegetables and starches. Boiling toughens the proteins in meats, fish, poultry and eggs and breaks up delicate foods.

Sous vide (the French term for "under vacuum") or reduced-oxygen packaging (ROP) is a method of cooking in vacuum-sealed plastic pouches at precise temperatures. The result is a final product with superior texture and concentrated flavors. Sous vide is being used to serve food to large numbers of people at hotels and casinos, on airplanes and cruise ships and in the military. It is also a favorite of many top-tier chefs, who say the technique can be used to create unique, individual dishes for their discriminating clientele. It is an effective way to consistently turn out the same quality dish day after day and saves a great deal of time. A large quantity of sauce, for example, can be prepared and packaged in single portions for use as needed.

The sous vide plastic-film packaging prevents the loss of moisture and flavors. Consequently, flavors are concentrated and fewer spices and less salt is required, lowering the overall sodium content of sous vide foods. Seasoning can be a little tricky when cooking sous vide. While many herbs and spices act as expected, others are amplified and can easily overpower a dish. Additionally, aromatics (such as carrots, onions, celery, bell peppers, etc.) will not soften or flavor the dish as they do in conventional cooking because the temperature is too low to soften the starches and cell walls.

Sous vide is a very healthful method of cooking. Little or no fat is needed in the preparation and nutrients are preserved. Essential minerals are typically leached into cooking water, reducing the mineral content of foods processed by traditional means. The pouch eliminates mineral loss, preserving the mineral content of fresh foods. All the flavor and most of the nutrients are retained.

The drawback is that the sous vide process cannot produce a browning of surfaces or crispy texture. In addition, cooking produces no food aroma. Food safety, however, is probably the biggest concern with sous vide cooking. The hermetically sealed plastic bags form oxygen barriers that slow the growth of **aerobic bacteria**, delaying spoilage. While this certainly can be a benefit, the downside is that anaerobic bacteria may thrive under the right conditions. Unfortunately, the most deadly food-borne illness is **botulism**, caused by *Clostridium botulinum*, an anaerobic bacteria. Because of this, foods must be of the highest quality and handled within strictly maintained temperature ranges according to Hazard Analysis Critical Control Point (HACCP) procedures. The Food and Drug Administration's 2009 Food Code sets out strict procedures, including chilling the bagged products to 34° F and storing them for no more than 30 days to eliminate the possibility of listeria or botulism poisoning. [1]

Blanching is a two-step process. First, the food is completely submerged in boiling water for a short time. Then it is removed and plunged into ice water. The quick chill stops the cooking process and sets the color, especially bright oranges and greens. Since vegetables with green, orange, deep yellow and red pigments are particularly rich in vitamins, minerals and phytochemicals, every effort should be made to serve as many of them as possible to maximize the healthfulness of menu offerings.

Crudités platters with blanched rather than raw carrots, broccoli, green beans, asparagus, cauliflower, sugar snap peas, etc., are more attractive, colorful and taste better. Blanching also increases the bioavailability of some vitamins.

Blanching can also be used to:

- Speed the peeling process (for tomatoes, peaches, etc.).
- Soften herbs.
- Remove excessive saltiness.
- Reduce strong flavors from meats and game.
- Precook vegetables prior to stir-frying or grilling.

The amount of nutrients lost during poaching, simmering, boiling and blanching depends on the heat stability of the nutrients present and the length of cooking time. Some vitamins, but not all, are destroyed by heat, especially when there is a long cooking time. In some cases, nutrients from vegetables leach into the cooking liquid. If the liquid is used in a soup or reduced sauce, those nutrients are consumed. Often, however, the cooking liquid is discarded. It is wise to save the cooking liquid for use in soups and sauces. For many vegetables, cooking softens the fibers and makes the nutrients more available. Cooked carrots, for example, are more nutrient rich than raw carrots.

In doing nutrient calculations, it is important to enter the values of vegetables in the state they are eaten, rather than how they are listed on the ingredient list. The same vegetable, raw or cooked, has different nutrient levels.

Here are some suggestions for preparing healthful poached, simmered, boiled and blanched foods:

- Use flavorful cooking liquids, such as juices, wines and stocks.
- Trim surplus fat from food before cooking.
- Use cooking liquid for sauces or retain for use in soup when possible.
- Cook food only as long as necessary.
- Maintain proper cooking temperatures.

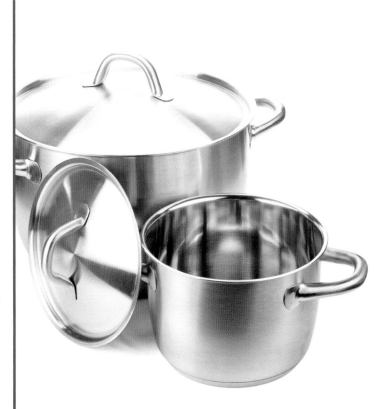

Poached Chicken Breast with Root Vegetables

Yield: 10 servings

Orange zest and ginger create a flavorful poaching liquid and enhance this appetizing dish. Lightly searing the chicken breast before poaching adds to both flavor and appearance. This main course is beautiful in its simplicity and perfect for most guests with special dietary needs or restrictions.

Broth:

Chicken broth, defatted, high-quality	1 ½	quarts
Red onion, chopped	¾	cup
Garlic, minced	2	cloves
Orange, peel of	1	each
Ginger, fresh, peeled, chopped	1	tablespoon
Bay leaf	1	each

Chicken:

Chicken breasts, fat trimmed, with wing bone and skin	10	5 ounces each
Salt	½	teaspoon
Black pepper, freshly ground	½	teaspoon
Olive oil	2	tablespoons

Vegetables

Carrots, baby	30	each
Fingerling potatoes	20	each
Pearl onions, peeled, fresh or frozen	2	cups
Asparagus, top half only	40	baby
	20	medium
Orange zest, julienne	2	tablespoons

Garnish:

Garlic cloves, peeled, roasted	20	each
Chives, cut or parsley, chopped	1	tablespoon

1. In a large pot, combine broth ingredients and bring to a boil. Reduce heat and simmer 15 minutes. Adjust seasonings as needed.

2. Season chicken with salt and pepper. Heat fry pan with olive oil and sear chicken breast on both sides until lightly browned but not cooked through.

3. Add chicken pieces to seasoned broth. Add the carrots, potatoes and pearl onions. Cover and simmer 20 minutes until chicken and vegetables are cooked.

4. Add orange zest and asparagus tips. Cook 5 minutes more. Remove bay leaf.

5. To serve, put 1 chicken breast in each flat bowl, top each with potatoes, carrots, pearl onions and asparagus. Add ½ cup broth to each bowl. Top with 2 roasted garlic cloves and cut herbs.

Per Serving

Calories	310	Cholesterol	75	mg
Fat	8 g	Sodium	250	mg
Saturated Fat	2 g	Carbohydrates	28	mg
Trans Fat	0 g	Dietary Fiber	3	mg
Sugar	4 g	Protein	30	g

Adapted from Chicken Breast in Herb Broth with Root Vegetables and Roasted Garlic. Gielisse V, Kimbrough M, Gielisee K. *In Good Taste: A Contemporary Approach to Cooking*. Upper Saddle River, NJ: Prentice Hall; 1999.

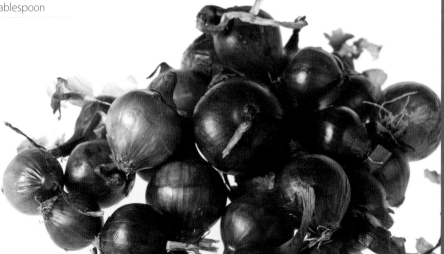

Steaming

Steaming cooks foods by surrounding them with a vapor bath. Many kitchens have pressure steamers that create steam under pressure to cook foods quickly while preserving nutrient value. Pressure steamers are typically used for vegetables, especially in large volume.

Steaming is a very quick cooking method that retains a maximum of nutrients. Although used mostly for vegetables, steaming can also be used for seafood and shellfish, chicken breasts, doughs, some grains and other foods. Steaming helps food retain its shape, color, flavor and texture better than boiling, simmering or even poaching. Foods must be carefully placed within the steamer so they cook evenly. Sometimes foods for steaming are encased in a wrap such as seaweed, cornhusks, banana leaves, leek strips or cabbage leaves. Steamed foods can easily be overcooked.

In ***pan-steaming***, foods are placed in a closed vessel, above – but not touching – the liquid. The heat must be high enough for the liquid to boil and create steam to cook the food. Ingredients placed in the liquid can infuse delicious flavors and aromas into steamed food. Mussels and clams are often steamed with aromatics, such as lemon zest, and the pan liquids are served as the sauce. The flavored liquid used to pan-steam vegetables may be reduced to make a sauce or glaze. Chinese cooking techniques include steaming many foods over water or stock, including filled buns, pot stickers and seafood in stacked bamboo baskets.

En papillote is a variation of steaming in which the main item, often fish and accompanying ingredients such as vegetables and herbs, are encased in parchment paper and cooked in a hot oven. The natural juices of the fish and vegetables create their own sauce. When the packet is opened for the diner, aromatic steam is released.

Braising and Stewing

Braising is a method of cooking that involves both dry and moist heat. It is an ideal way to prepare less tender cuts of meat and sturdy root vegetables. Braised meat is generally seasoned and seared in a large roasting pan and then covered and simmered slowly in the oven in liquid with mirepoix and aromatics. ***Stewing*** is similar to braising but the main item is cut into bite-sized pieces. Legumes, poultry and non-root vegetables can also be braised or stewed.

The amount of liquid used should cover the product by one-third to two-thirds, depending on how much sauce is desired. The long cooking process tenderizes the meat and produces a concentrated flavorful liquid. The addition of tomato products adds flavor and tenderizes meat. Vegetables are added partway through the process to avoid overcooking them. The liquid is strained and seasoned and the meat and vegetables are returned to the liquid to cool. Braises and stews are best prepared a day ahead and refrigerated so the cooking liquid can be absorbed into the product and the fat can rise to the top to be easily removed before reheating the dish to serve.

The long cooking times of braised and stewed dishes allow the development of wonderful flavors. Because the liquid is consumed as part of the dish, nutrients that are not destroyed by heat are retained and consumed.

When wine or an alcohol-containing liquid is added to food during cooking, some of the alcohol is "burned off." In fact, in a long, slow braise, such as Beef Bourguignon, most of the alcohol has been released in the steam after two hours of cooking. Although long cooking times and very high heats cause alcohol loss, the alcohol flavor remains in the food. Virtually all the added alcohol remains, however, when food is uncooked or cooked only briefly.

Because some individuals choose not to consume alcohol for various reasons, any food with alcohol as an ingredient should be described in a way that mentions the source of the alcohol. Recipes with alcohol-containing ingredients need to be calculated carefully, and the calories must be adjusted for the amount of retained alcohol. Refer to Chapter 6 for information regarding the amount of alcohol retained during the cooking process.

Here are some suggestions for preparing healthful braised and stewed foods:

- Use lean meats or poultry.
- Trim excess fat before stewing.
- Where suitable, marinate food to tenderize and add flavor.
- Use little or no fat for searing.
- Skim the sauce to remove extra fat.

Sauces

Sauces have always added interest, flavor and moistness to menu items, but it is no longer mandatory that sauces be roux- and cream-based, calorie- and fat-laden mixtures. Sauces have evolved into flavorful, colorful and nutritious additions to many meals. Traditional grand or leading sauces – béchamel, veloute, brown, tomato, and hollandaise – are making room for lower-fat and calorie-reduced coulis, salsas, infusions and natural reductions.

A flavorful poultry, meat, fish or vegetable stock can be the foundation of many good sauces and adds few calories and little fat. Ideally, stocks should be made on-site and without added salt. If this is not possible, look for good quality, reduced-sodium stocks. Salt, if needed, can be added when preparing the sauce.

A **reduction** is often used with sautéed items. The sauté pan is deglazed with a liquid – often stock, juice or wine – to capture the flavorful bits left on the bottom of the pan. Other flavoring agents are added and the sauce is reduced by simmering to the desired consistency. Sometimes a thickening agent, such as arrowroot or cornstarch, is used. Garnishes, such as bruinoise of vegetables or juniper berries, can be added. Reductions can add flavor and moisture with minimal calories or added fat. Because of the intensified flavor of a reduction, little added salt is necessary.

In addition to adding color and flavor to any dish, salsa adds healthful fruits or vegetables. The traditional *salsa* is a Mexican, tomato-based mixture used for dipping chips. Today's chefs, however, are creating salsas using a wide variety of fruits and vegetables. Examples include mango and red pepper salsa, watermelon and red onion salsa, pineapple and green pepper salsa and strawberry and mint salsa.

Pestos can be a healthy way to add flavor to dishes, assuming they're moderate in fat. Italian for "pounded," **pesto** is traditionally an uncooked sauce of fresh basil, garlic, pine nuts, olive oil and Parmesan cheese. Today, however there are a myriad of pestos made from other ingredients, including greens such as parsley, kale and arugula. When the oil, nuts and cheese are minimized, pesto can be a healthy way to boost flavor, as a little goes a long way. Along the lines of pesto, chimmichurri is a thick herb sauce common in Argentina and South America. It's a mélange of olive oil, vinegar, and finely chopped herbs, onion and garlic. It frequently accompanies grilled meats.

Coulis are fruit- or vegetable-based purees. Like salsas, they add color and flavor to a dish as well as fruit and vegetables. Typically, coulis have little added fat and are generally low in calories. Examples of popular coulis are carrot, fresh pea, asparagus, roasted red pepper coulis, raspberry or mango coulis and applesauce (although it is not strained as other coulis sometimes are). Placing a meat serving atop a pool of colorful vegetable coulis can be an attractive and healthful presentation.

Rich cream-based and roux-thickened sauces can be modified to be more healthful. Start with a full-flavored stock. For cream, substitute lower-fat dairy products such as evaporated skim milk, which has better body and a more cream-like flavor than skim milk. Buttermilk, which ironically has no fat and no butter, is another substitute suitable if its acidic flavor is appropriate. Yogurt and reduced-fat cream cheese also work well in some sauce recipes. For thickening, try starches such as arrowroot or cornstarch.

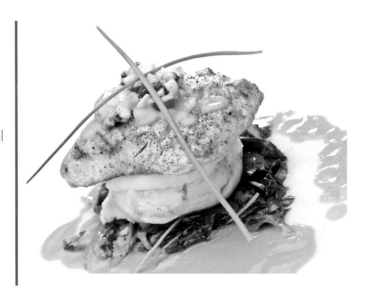

Nutrient Retention

Nutrients – especially vitamins, minerals and phytochemicals – are found in a wide variety of food products, from meat, fish, poultry and dairy to fruits, vegetables and whole grains. The nutrient content of food can vary and is affected by how the food is handled and processed. Factors such as soil quality, degree of maturity at harvest, length of transportation time, storage time and exposure to the elements – heat, oxygen (air), light, extremes in pH (acidity or alkalinity) and moisture – all affect nutrient content.

The range of nutrient loss will vary among different produce. One study showed that vitamin C loss in cut fruits stored for six days can range from 5% (for cut watermelon) to 25% (for cut cantaloupe). Carotenoid loss ranged from none in kiwifruit to 25% loss in pineapples. This same research concluded that cut and whole fruits deteriorate nutritionally at about the same rate in refrigerated temperatures. [2]

What Is Fresh?

Keep in mind that "fresh" is not always truly fresh. Fresh-picked produce and the same produce after a week or more of storage and distribution can have differing amounts of nutrients. Buying local produce from known sources will help ensure freshness. The nutrient value of frozen produce will usually be comparable to (or better than) fresh produce. Generally, produce is frozen within hours of being picked, and freezing slows down nutrient loss. Drying fruits and vegetables will decrease vitamins A and C and folate. Drying fruits will also concentrate calories and sugar. Fruits commercially dried on iron racks will absorb some iron, which is why raisins are higher in iron than grapes and dried plums (prunes) are higher in iron than fresh plums.

Often, the same procedures used to maintain food quality will also protect nutrients. For example, refrigerating most produce will maintain quality and preserve vitamins; likewise, cooking vegetables properly will maintain both quality and nutrients. Vitamins and, to a certain extent, minerals will leach into the water when cut vegetables and fruits are washed or cooked. Removing the peel will expose even more of the vegetable's flesh (and will remove fiber as well). In cases such as peeled tomatoes, asparagus and potatoes, however, maintaining sophisticated culinary standards often overrides maximizing nutrient retention.

To minimize nutrient loss, wash food just before cutting. Minerals are quite stable and are unaffected by high temperatures. To preserve vitamins, however, avoid high heat and use the shortest appropriate cooking times. Steam or microwave vegetables instead of boiling them. Reserve nutrient-rich cooking liquids for use in preparing soups and stocks, to braise or poach meats, poultry and fish, and to cook starches. [3]

Cooking Methods

To cook most vegetables, steam them over rapidly boiling water for a short time until just done. Remove and serve or, if not served immediately, stop the cooking process by plunging the vegetables into ice water and then draining them quickly and thoroughly. Cover and refrigerate until ready to reheat and serve. If steaming is not practical, blanch vegetables for a short period in rapidly boiling water. Follow the same ice-water process for maximum nutrient retention. Avoid adding acid during cooking or holding as acid will destroy the color of vegetables. An old-fashioned trick for maintaining the color of vegetables is to add baking soda (alkaline) to the cooking water; however, this addition will change the texture of the vegetable and rob it of nutrients. When possible, cook vegetables from the raw state and serve them immediately.

Using the microwave to reheat starches and soups is an ideal way to decrease cooking time and retain quality and nutrients. To maximize the nutrient value of soups, avoid holding them in a steam table. Some restaurants prepare the soup; cool it immediately; portion it into cups or bowls; reheat portions in the microwave and garnish immediately before serving. A more common practice is to cook and chill soup and then reheat in batches on the stovetop.

Starches, such as rice, pasta and potato, held on a steam table will overcook and dry out, thus increasing nutrient loss. When precooking any starch, make sure that it is cooled and stored properly and reheated in a microwave or oven.

Proper storage is crucial to maintaining the quality of a food product and its nutritional value. Know your inventory needs and label chilled, stored food with preparation date. Overstocking anything may lead to serving poor quality products with deteriorated nutrient content. It is important to follow "the first in, first out" (FIFO) procedure in order to rotate all inventory but particularly fresh produce, fish, meats, poultry and dairy products. Allocate time and staff to make sure this procedure is followed to maintain quality while reducing spoilage and holding down food costs.

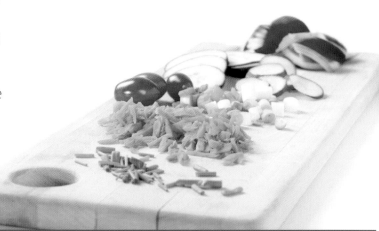

Cooking Vegetables to Retain Nutrients

1. **Cook vegetables in the smallest amount of liquid possible.**

   Vegetables have some vitamins that dissolve in water and are lost when the cooking liquid is discarded. Water-soluble vitamins include C and the B vitamins riboflavin, thiamin and niacin. Liquids in which vegetables are cooked can be added to soups and stocks to boost flavor and nutrient content. Commercial steamers are excellent for cooking large quantities of vegetables while retaining maximum nutrients.

2. **Cook vegetables for the shortest amount of time to desired tenderness.**

   Vegetables contain vitamins that are destroyed by heat. Prolonged cooking can reduce vitamin and phtyochemical levels. Use a commercial steamer or a microwave oven, if possible.

3. **For vegetables with skin, scrub well and cook with the skin on whenever possible. If the skin must be removed, peel the vegetable as thinly as possible.**

   Vegetables such as potatoes, carrots, parsnips and turnips have a valuable layer of nutrients right under the skin. Peeling will remove these nutrients as well as fiber. Fiber is also removed when a tomato or staik of asparagus is peeled. Removing the seeds of tomatoes or cucumbers also reduces fiber.

4. **When cutting vegetables, use a sharp blade and cut pieces as large as possible to suit the recipe. Pieces should be uniform to allow for even cooking. Large pieces help preserve the nutrient content of the vegetable. This guideline contradicts the "green advice" that smaller cuts reduce cooking time. In practice, choose the cut that makes the most sense for the dish you are preparing.**

   A sharp cutting blade will make a clean cut without bruising the vegetable. Bruising causes a rapid loss of vitamin C in green, leafy vegetables such as cabbage.

5. **Cook vegetables just before service.**

   Holding vegetables after cooking causes some nutrient loss and diminishes quality, particularly texture. Vegetables may be precooked, chilled and reheated at service. Batch cooking, preparing vegetables in small quantities as needed, is recommended for maximum nutrition and quality.

Effects of Processing on Nutrients in Foods

Nutrient	Popular Food Source	Effect of Processing
Fat	Vegetable oils, butter, lard	• Oxidation and spoilage accelerated by light
Protein	Meat, fish, poultry	• Structure altered by heat and acids
Vitamin C	Citrus fruit, tomatoes, strawberries, peppers, broccoli and greens	• The least stable of all vitamins • Decreases during storage, drying, heating, oxidation, chopping
Thiamin (B₁)	Pork, organ meats, whole grains, enriched grains and cereals	• Sensitive to light in alkaline and neutral condition • Moderately heat stable under neutral conditions • Sensitive to heat under alkaline conditions
Riboflavin (B₂)	Milk, liver, eggs, cereal/grains, dark leafy greens	• Sensitive to light in alkaline and neutral conditions • Moderately heat stable under neutral conditions • Sensitive to heat under alkaline conditions
Vitamin B₆	Whole grains, vegetables, meat and fish	• Heat stable • Pyridoxal (a form of vitamin B₆) changes when heated
Niacin	Lean meats, whole grains, eggs and legumes	• Stable to heat and light • Leaches into cooking water
Folate	Beef liver, pinto beans, asparagus, lentils, avocado, enriched cereal, leafy green vegetables	• Decreases with storage or prolonged heating • Lost in cooking water
Vitamin B₁₂	Beef, pork, cheese, tuna, fish	• Destroyed by light and high acidity
Vitamin A	Dark leafy greens, yellow and orange vegetables, cantaloupe, milk and eggs	• Easily destroyed by heat • Easily oxidized (exposure to air)
Vitamin D	Fortified milk	• Destroyed when exposed to heat and light
Vitamin E	Vegetable oils, whole grains, cereals, leafy vegetables, nuts and beans	• Oxidizes readily
Vitamin K	Leafy vegetables, vegetable oils, wheat bran	• Destroyed by acids and light
Minerals	Many foods	• Generally stable but leaches into water or other cooking liquid

Source: Adapted from: Morris A, Barnett A, Burrows O. *Effect of processing on nutrient content of foods*. Cajanus: The Caribbean Food & Nutrition Institute Quarterly. 2004. 37(3). **www.paho.org/English/CFNI/cfni-caj37No304-art-3.pdf**

Healthful Recipe Development

Understanding the *Dietary Guidelines for Americans*, applying what you know about nutrition, selecting appropriate cooking methods and adding a generous portion of your own creativity will result in recipes that delight and meet the nutritional needs of your customers. When creating healthful recipes, think about the ingredients and components, flavoring agents and seasonings, garnishes and accompaniments, and cooking methods.

- **Ingredients:** Start with healthful ingredients – lean meats, fish and seafood, legumes, whole grains, and plenty of fruits and vegetables. Can you use a whole grain as a crust on the protein item? How about using fruit for the base of a sauce?

- **Flavoring agents and seasonings:** Look for ingredients that add lots of flavor but little fat or sodium. If you are creating an ethnic-inspired dish, look to the flavoring agents commonly found in that region.

- **Garnishes:** Almost as important as the center-of-the plate item, garnishes should complement the dish and blend with the flavors. Remember to ask yourself, "Does it make sense?" An orange slice adds color to a dish, but does it make sense with the food? Toasted or black sesame seeds atop an appropriate dish add texture, nutrients and a dash of fiber, as well as visual interest. Thoughtful garnishes add flavor and nutrients, such as vitamins, minerals and phytochemicals.

- **Accompaniments:** Look beyond "vegetable-of-the-day." Vegetable and starch accompaniments should complement the dish and are an opportunity to add healthful ingredients. Sauces should be low in fat and full of flavor. If a rich sauce is optimal, use it sparingly. Explore ways to use legumes, fruits and vegetables (whole and juices) in sauce preparation.

- **Portions:** Serve reasonable portions. Certainly the serving size should look gracious but using smaller glasses, plates and bowls, or ones with interesting shapes and textures can make a smaller portion very appealing. Arranging food attractively also helps. If guests are taking excess food home, re-think how much you are serving. A portion should be appropriate for one meal - not two or more.

- **Cooking methods:** Selecting the appropriate cooking method is as important as choosing the right ingredients. For example, deep-frying or pan-frying tilapia can undo the best healthful intentions. Select cooking methods that add flavor while minimizing added fat, salt and calories. Identify challenging areas and consider alternatives. For example, with fried fish the challenge might be added fat from frying. In this case, consider baking the fish using a panko crumb crust to create the crunchy texture. An understanding of how ingredients function is important when thinking about substitutions: Is the sugar part of the structure of a dessert, or is it just adding sweetness?

Modifying favorite recipes to create more healthful alternatives can be a challenge when you know customers will inevitably compare the two versions. "This low-fat crème brulée is almost as good as … " is not a compliment. If a particular favorite food does not lend itself to modification, and a substitute with a good nutritional profile is not a reasonable option, instead serve a smaller size portion of "the real thing." Balance an indulgence with several healthful choices at the same meal. Make as many of the foods you serve as healthful as you can, but keep in mind that even the most nutritious food will not be enjoyed unless it tastes delicious.

casebycase | The 'Family' Dining Table

At the University of New Hampshire (UNH), Todd Sweet, CEC, CCA, assistant director of culinary, and Rochelle L'Italien, MS, RDN, LD, culinary registered dietitian, have made student dining a leading-edge example of fresh, healthy, local, sustainable, and culturally and medically sensitive food service. Students who prefer vegan, halal, pork-free, non-GMO, or gluten-free foods have a array of choices.

Todd, a Culinary Institute of America (CIA) graduate, came to UNH hospitality services in 2010, joining Rochelle, a 27-year veteran. With almost 900 employees and a $40 million operating budget, UNH kitchens spend $200,000 on food weekly and serve 15,000 meals a day. "We are self-operated, so we can be creative and flexible," says Todd. "Our three dining rooms, which are open until at least 9:00 pm daily, are like big family dining tables, and chefs from our three dining halls are available for individual appointments to review student and parent concerns and special needs."

UNH focuses on "plant-forward" healthy menu items but doesn't always market them aggressively. Some customers believe such foods are poor substitutes for the "real thing." "Our menus are promoted for what they are," Rochelle explains, "and that's 'flavor-forward' and transparent."

In 2014, UNC joined the Menus of Change (MOC) initiative, created by the CIA and Harvard School of Public Health, and the Partnership for a Healthier

America's (PHA) Healthier Campus Initiative, which was inspired by the former first lady Michelle Obama's Let's Move! program.

Menus of Change charges universities with advancing healthier, more sustainable life-long food choices among students, some of whom will soon be parents and adult decision makers. UNH follows MOC's guidelines for menu planning and product sourcing and has adopted the initiative's 24 Principles of Healthy Sustainable Menus. "One of the MOC recommendations that we have enthusiastically embraced," notes Todd, "is to feature cuisines from other cultures that naturally reflect MOC recommendations. We use the same ingredients and cooking processes to give our items an authentic flavor profile."

PHA's Healthier Campus Initiative urges colleges and universities to adopt guidelines around nutrition, physical activity and programming.

UNH Dining Services chose 10 PHA food and nutrition areas for assessment and verification, including wellness meal combos that adhere to specific food group and nutrient profile criteria. With Rochelle's guidance, university dietetic interns created a variety of wellness meals that use items regularly available in the dining halls.

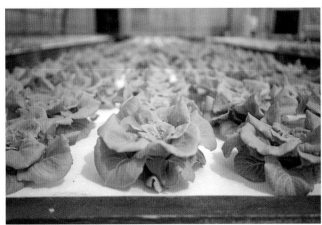

Photo Credit: University of New Hampshire

Researchers at UNH recently grew aquaponic Boston butterhead lettuce in 35 days from seed to harvest and hit the magical 150g head weight using only nutrients from fish. Hospitality Services is now purchasing approximately 800–1000 heads of fresh Boston butterhead lettuce per week, which is used in the dining halls. Guests look forward to enjoying the lettuce in salads and menu offerings like Southwest lettuce wraps.

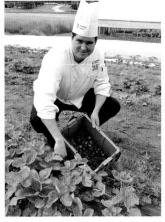

Photo Credit: University of New Hampshire

Assistant Director of Culinary
Todd Sweet

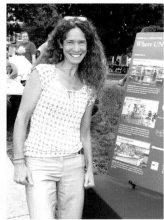

Photo Credit: University of New Hampshire

Registered dietitian nutritionist
Rochelle L'Italien MS, RDN, LD

Opportunities for Chefs

At the center of nutritional cooking is properly executing healthful cooking techniques. As this chapter demonstrates, these techniques are not a great deal different from traditional cooking techniques – but require attention, a level of skill and precision. From sautéing to poaching, most every technique can be used or adapted in preparing healthier foods. A culinary professional is always mindful of retaining the nutrients in foods prepared and served. Providing more healthful options, without a nutrition "hard-sell" shows that you care about your customers' healthy and will encourage repeat patronage.

Learning Activities

1. Select a food item and prepare it using three healthful cooking techniques. For example, slice an onion and steam it, sauté one until it is caramelized and roast one. Compare color, texture and taste.

2. Using the U.S. Department of Agriculture's Nutrient Data Library (**www.nal.usda.gov/ fnic/ foodcomp/search**), select a meat item and compare the calories and fat of three different preparation methods. For example, chicken breast – roasted, fried, poached or stewed, baked, etc.

3. Using the recipe index of a quality consumer food magazine, choose 10 recipes from the appetizer, main dish, vegetable, side dish or pasta/rice categories. Go to those recipes and identify which incorporate healthful cooking techniques and list techniques used. How could the others be modified to incorporate healthful cooking techniques?

For More Information

- The Culinary Institute of America. *The Professional Chef*, 9th ed. New York: John Wiley & Sons, Inc.; 2011.

- The Culinary Institute of America. *The Professional Chef's Techniques of Healthy Cooking,* 4th ed. New York: John Wiley & Sons, Inc.; 2013.

- Gielisse V, DeSantis R. *Modern Batch Cookery*. New York: John Wiley & Sons, Inc.; 2011.

- Gisslen W. *Professional Cooking*, 9th ed. Hoboken, NJ: Wiley; 2018.

- Gisslen W. *Professional Baking*, 7th ed. Hoboken, NJ: John Wiley & Sons; 2016.

- Labensky S, Hause AM, Martel PA. *On Cooking: A Textbook of Culinary Fundamentals*, 6th ed. Boston, MA; Pearson; 2018.

- Lopez-Alt JK. *The Food Lab: Better Home Cooking Through Science*. New York, NY: W.W. Norton & Company, Inc.; 2015.

- Molt M. *Food for Fifty*, 14th ed. Boston, MA: Pearson; 2017.

- Murphy EW, Criner PE, Gray BC. Comparison of methods for determining retentions of nutrients in cooked foods. (0.4 Mb). J Ag Food Chem. 1975;23:1153.

- Myhrvol N, Young C, Billet M. *Modernist Cuisine: The Art and Science of Cooking*. Bellevue, WA: The Cooking Lab; 2011.

- U.S. Department of Agriculture. Table of Nutrient Retention Factors, Release 6. 2007. **https:// www.ars.usda.gov/SP2UserFiles/Place/ 80400525/Data/retn/retn06.pdf**

Chapter Eleven

Communicating Nutrition Messages

Learning Objectives | *After completing this chapter, you should be able to:*

- Discuss effective ways to communicate and promote a healthful foods program to guests
- Explain the U.S. Food and Drug Administration's definition of "healthy"
- Identify the various ways of flagging healthful items on your menu
- Explain the national menu labeling program
- Describe the process for calculating nutrient data
- Develop a staff training program for communicating your nutrition message
- Discuss the value of cause-related marketing

Bottom line: What's the point of preparing healthful, great-tasting food, if no one is going to eat it? Because "healthy" can mean different things to different people, it's important to understand how to promote healthful menu items. In the past, these foods met with customer resistance because they didn't look as appealing or taste as good as "regular" menu items. Many customers are still stuck in this old mindset. Consequently, while they say they want healthful food options, they order everything else. Interesting high-quality, healthful food can change this behavior pattern. Patrons who know your food is both delicious and nutritious are likely to become regulars.

The menu is the most common tool for communicating nutrition to your guests and customers. Newsletters, websites, blogs, social media and media stories also shape messages to your guests. Increasingly, chefs are using their status and influence to communicate nutrition and health messages. Service staff are also important tellers of your nutrition story and should be properly trained to communicate your message.

Healthy: What's in a Word?

In everyday conversation, most people use the terms "healthy" and "healthful" to describe certain foods and menus. The U.S. Food and Drug Administration (FDA), however, takes these terms very seriously. FDA considers them "implied claims" and sets guidelines for their use on food labels. These guidelines also apply to restaurant menus.

The term "healthy" and related terms ("health," "healthful," "healthfully," "healthfulness," "healthier," "healthiest," "healthily" and "healthiness") may be used if the food meets the following requirements:

- An individual food or main dish must contain no more than 3 grams of fat per standard serving. For seafood, meat and game, the guideline is less than 5 grams of total fat and less than 2 grams of saturated fat per 100-gram portion. Note that 100-gram portions are smaller than what most restaurants serve, so the amount of fat and saturated fat must be calibrated to the portion served. This guidance has been modified to include an individual food or main dish that has mostly mono and polyunsaturated fats. Foods that use the term "healthy" that are not low in fat should consist predominantly of mono and polyunsaturated fats, that is, the sum of monounsaturated fats and polyunsaturated fats must be greater than the total saturated fat content. This modification of the guidance allows for nuts and nut products to be labeled "healthy."

- An individual food must have less than 480 milligrams of sodium per standard serving size (referred to as RACC or reference amount customarily consumed per eating occasion, the amount used on food labels) or 50 milligrams if the RACC is 30 grams or less. Meals or main dishes may have up to 600 milligrams per serving.

- Seafood, meat, game and main dishes or meals must have 90 milligrams or less of cholesterol.

- An individual food must contain at least 10% of the Daily Value per standard reference serving size of one or more beneficial nutrients – vitamins A or C, calcium, iron, protein or fiber. Main dish products must have at least 10% of the Daily Value of two nutrients; meals must contain at least 10% of the Daily Value for three beneficial nutrients. Because vitamin D and potassium are now nutrients of public health concern, a food can now bear a "healthy" claim even if it does not contain 10% of the DV per RACC of vitamin, A, Vitamin C, calcium, iron, protein, or fiber if it contains at least 10% of the DV per RACC for potassium or vitamin D.

- All raw fruits and vegetables and frozen or canned single-ingredient fruits and vegetables are considered "healthy."

- Enriched cereal or grain products that conform to standards of identity are considered "healthy."

Source: U.S. Food and Drug Administration. Guidance for Industry: A Food Labeling Guide, **www.fda.gov/Food/GuidanceComplianceRegulatoryInformation/GuidanceDocuments/ FoodLabelingNutrition/ FoodLabelingGuide/ucm064916.htm**

Nutrition on the Menu

There are several schools of thought – and even some controversy – concerning the best way to identify healthful items on menus. One approach uses symbols or icons to designate items as healthier alternatives. Clear and concise, symbols eliminate guesswork and help guests make their selections without a lot of server assistance.

Designing a separate menu or menu section is another approach. The obvious benefit for the guest is that healthier alternatives are easy to identify. Research is needed to determine if people are more likely to order healthier items if they are integrated in the main menu or presented separately.

A third approach – offering but not highlighting healthful alternatives – is based on the concept that special labeling sends a negative message and may lead guests to wonder, "If these items are healthy, does that mean the rest of the menu is unhealthy?" A more positive approach is to let menu items speak for themselves and rely on a combination of guests' knowledge and personal interest in healthful selections and servers' ability to promote the items appropriately.

A fourth approach is to position a restaurant as a provider of healthful foods, serving only foods that are under a specific calorie levels, using only heart-healthy fats and focusing on nutrient-rich ingredients. While some consider this a limited market, chains and restaurants such as Seasons 52, Rouge Tomate and others have loyal clientele.

Yet another approach is to offer **small plates** or reduced portions of entrées, salads or desserts. Pricing can be a problem with this approach. A guest may expect a 4-ounce portion of a protein entrée to be priced at half the price of an 8-ounce portion when typically, the half portion is priced at about 75% of the larger portion. Overhead, dishwashing, service, utensils and labor are cost factors independent of the difference in portion size. For many patrons, a better choice might be sharing one entrée, ordering two appetizers and no entrée, ordering a salad or soup and an appetizer as an entrée, or splitting desserts. Many people think

that sharing limits portions and calories. This approach works only if less total food is ordered. Two people sharing two entrées or two desserts does not cut calories; it just redistributes them.

Menu Labeling and the Healthcare Reform Act

The Patient Protection and Affordable Care Act, commonly known as the Healthcare Reform Act, was signed into law in March 2010 and went into effect in May 2018. One section of the bill – Section 4205 – requires restaurants with 20 or more locations nationally to add calorie counts to menus, menu boards and drive-thru menu boards for standard menu items. It also requires those restaurants to make additional nutrition data available to guests upon request. [1] This mandate provides a single, consistent national standard for nutrition disclosure in restaurants that helps consumers make choices that are best for themselves and their families. The federal standard provides uniform nutrition-labeling requirements that multi-state restaurants can implement nationwide. Before the law, restaurant operators had to comply with a patchwork of state and local menu labeling regulations. The differing requirements made it difficult for restaurants to comply and for consumers to understand.

Restaurants and similar retail food establishments that are covered under the new federal rules are no longer subject to state or local menu labeling laws, except to the extent they are identical to the federal requirements. Smaller chain and individual retail food establishments are not subject to the new federal law; however, they may still be subject to all state and local nutrition-labeling laws and associated regulations. If these restaurants and similar retail food establishments voluntarily register with the Food and Drug Administration (FDA), they will no longer be subject to state or local nutrition-labeling requirements.

The law also requires those restaurants to make available additional written nutrition data about **standard menu items** upon request. The term standard is used to designate items that generally appear on the menu and are usually available. Daily specials or menu items being introduced are not required to have full information.

The nutrition disclosure requirements also apply to restaurants that are part of a chain that operates 20 or more locations under the same trade name, regardless of the ownership type of the locations, which offer "substantially the same menu items" for sale. The law also applies to retail food establishments that are similar to foodservice operations. It doesn't define those establishments. Based on the way the FDA has interpreted other parts of the Food, Drug and Cosmetic Act, it likely means that the new restaurant labeling requirements apply to any establishment owned by a company with 20 or more locations under the same trade name where food is served for immediate consumption. For example, this category could include foodservice facilities in hospitals or schools, food at convenience stores served for immediate consumption, and food served from mobile carts. The law also applies to vending machines owned by companies that operate 20 or more machines.

Covered restaurants are required to provide the following information for standard menu items:

- Number of calories per standard menu item. The calorie count per serving must appear next to the menu item name. This count is based on actual serving size of a single portion, not on a predetermined amount or RACC (reference amount customarily consumed). FDA will provide more details on how restaurants must display this information.

- A prominent, clear and conspicuous statement about the availability of additional nutrition information. Additional information includes values for:

  - Calories
  - Calories from total fat
  - Saturated fat
  - Cholesterol
  - Sodium
  - Carbohydrates
  - Sugars
  - Dietary fiber
  - Protein

- A succinct statement concerning suggested daily caloric intake posted prominently on the menu to help guests understand calories in the context of a daily diet. FDA specifies the language for this statement in its regulations.

Congress recognizes that there is variation in preparing restaurant meals. A main course salad, for example, might not have the same amount of vegetables, croutons or exactly the same amount of dressing each time it's prepared. As a result, the new law doesn't require an exact count for prescribed nutrient levels. It does, however, require that restaurants show they have a reasonable basis for the nutrition data they present. Restaurants must demonstrate that they have used reasonable means to derive their information, such as nutrient databases, cookbooks, laboratory analysis and other reasonable means described in FDA regulations and related guidance.

The law directs the FDA to look at all the factors that could cause variations in restaurant nutrition content. Some factors the FDA must consider in determining restaurant compliance include:

- Reasonable variation in serving size and formulation of menu items
- Standardization of recipes and preparation methods
- Inadvertent human error
- Employee training
- Ingredient variations

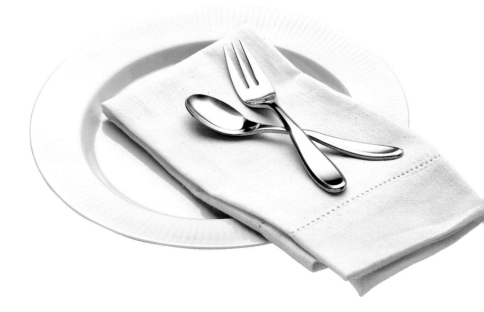

Benefits and Obstacles of Menu Labeling

A majority of consumers express a strong interest in having nutrition information, particularly calorie information, on restaurant menus or otherwise near the point of purchase. Only 10 percent of Americans oppose menu labeling requirements. [2]

Some of the benefits of menu labeling include:

- Increased consumer education. Theoretically, consumers will use calorie counts to make informed food choices.

- Reformulation of products. As foodservice operators look at menu balance from a nutrition viewpoint, they may choose to create a broader spectrum of food choices. Questions to ask include:
  - What menu items will I keep?
  - What items will I remove?
  - What items will I change?
  - How will I change these items?
  - What items will I add?
  - What commonly used ingredients will I substitute for currently used products?

- Right-sized portions. As calorie amounts are revealed, portion distortion will become more obvious, which may lead to a reduction in portion size, lowered food costs and more healthful options.

Some of the potential obstacles of menu labeling include:

- Restaurants and cafeterias that do not routinely use standardized recipes may unintentionally provide inaccurate information.

- Cooks will require more training to ensure they consistently measure ingredients and use standardized recipes.

- Labeling may limit flexibility in changing the menu.

- Providing nutrition information can be costly.

- Providing nutrition information might lead to reduced demand for profitable menu items.

- Customers may not return to a restaurant that has many menu items that they perceive as having too many calories.

- Training employees to respond to questions about menu labeling will take time and may be difficult.

Does Calorie Knowledge Lead to Calorie Control?

In a 2013 synthesis of existing menu research titled *Impact of Menu Labeling on Consumer Behavior: A 2008–2012 Update* Healthy Eating Research, A Robert Wood Johnson Foundation program, reported:

- Most customers and the majority of the general public want restaurants and cafeterias to have menu labeling.

- Customers rarely seek out nutrition information from sources not available at the point of purchase (e.g., websites, brochures), but they do see menu labels at the point of purchase and those labels increase their awareness of nutritional information.

- Evidence from surveys and simulation studies suggests menu labeling reduces calories purchased or consumed, but evidence from real-world cafeteria and restaurant studies regarding calories purchased or menu items selected is mixed.

- The impact of menu labeling is not uniform. It may have a greater effect on women than men, on higher calorie items, and among certain types of restaurant chains.

- The optimal format for providing nutritional information on menus is not known, but providing calories, use of "healthy choice" symbols, displaying total caloric intake needs, and presenting items in order of caloric content might have some effects on reducing calories purchased.

- Emerging evidence suggests that menu labeling does not impact revenue and could have positive effects on the reformulation of menu items and other aspects of the environment (e.g., promotion and signage).

- Menu labeling may result in lower total daily caloric intake by influencing customers' food choices apart from those made in the restaurant or cafeteria with labeling, but more definitive evaluation of this is warranted.

Source: Healthy Eating Research. Impact of Menu Labeling on Consumer Behavior: A 2008-2012 Update. Research Review. June 2013. Available at **healthyeatingresearch.org/wp-content/uploads/2013/12/HER-RR-Menu-Labeling-FINAL-6-2013.pdf**. Accessed April 10, 2018.

Menu Descriptions

What compels a diner to order a particular menu item? Personal food preferences, health concerns, economics, peer pressure and taste generally dictate what people order at a restaurant. How a menu item is described gives diners the information they need to make a selection. Menu descriptions can also provide clues about the healthfulness of an item.

- **What is it?** Healthful key ingredients – for example, scallops, salmon, greens, whole grains, legumes or organic fruit – are a guest's first indication that the menu item may be among the restaurant's healthier choices.

- **How is it prepared?** Poaching, steaming, grilling, roasting and infusing are generally low-fat, high-flavor cooking methods. Indicating preparation method can suggest the healthfulness of the dish. Fried foods, on the other hand, are not considered healthful unless the fried item is used in small amounts as a garnish, such as fried sage atop a pasta with sundried or chopped fresh tomatoes and herbs. Adjectives like "crispy" or "crunchy" generally suggest a food is fried. "Creamy" suggests use of cream or a high-fat product.

- **What are the food's special qualities?** Foods that are free range, organic, grass fed and/or locally grown indicate that ingredients have been carefully selected for nutrition and taste and are "green" – that is, grown in ways that are good for the environment. More and more restaurants are featuring the source names of the farm, ranch, cheesemaker or grower.

- **What are the ingredients?** Words like "creamed," "buttered," "larded" and "glazed" are indications that a menu item may be higher in fat or sugar. "Fruit coulis," "vegetable puree," "beans" and "whole grains" are telling patrons that the menu item is probably healthier.

- **What is the serving size?** Words like "abundant," "family style," "bountiful," "generous," "big," "giant" and "heaping" suggest super-sized portions. "Small," "4-ounces" and "garnished with" indicate modest portion sizes. Inviting customers to share an appetizer, salad, pasta, side dish or dessert encourages sales and moderate eating. The trend to small plates, half-portions and bite-sized desserts helps patrons enjoy a wide variety of foods without excess.

Sharing Your Story

Newsletters, websites, blogs, social media and media articles are viable avenues to share your story and promote your foodservice operation. These are excellent places to expand your nutrition message and garner customer support. Some ideas for sharing your story include:

- Post pictures of your restaurant garden and share how you are using more vegetables on the menu.

- Include short biographies or photos of the farmers or growers and producers you patronize on your website.

- Have you recently improved your health? Maybe you have lost weight? Share your success with your guests and let them know that you can help them, too.

- Share your healthful recipes in your newsletter or website to highlight your expertise.

- Showcase your most healthful recipes when teaching classes, hosting events, contributing products to charity events or doing demonstrations.

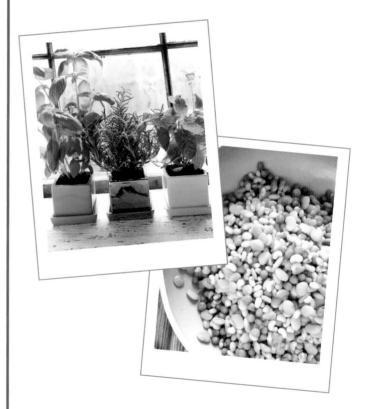

Garnering Recognition for Healthful Foods

- Give cooking demonstrations or classes for the community. Choose items that feature healthful ingredients and cooking techniques.
- Market the restaurant through cooking competitions, food tastings and media interviews that promote healthy dining.
- Offer getaway weekends with cooking demonstrations, nutrition seminars, exercise workshops and other lifestyle enhancers.
- Tie into hotels or fitness centers with a juice and smoothie bar, healthy snack items, body-fat testing and a menu for the hotel/fitness center restaurant.
- Become the restaurant of choice or caterer of events sponsored by health-related organizations (American Heart Association, American Diabetes Association, etc.) or organizations of health professionals such as district dietetic associations.
- Work with hotels that host conferences to provide special food and/or nutrition seminars for programs or lifestyle-enhancement seminars such as healthful entertaining, how to survive business lunches, staying fit on the road and eating to increase productivity.
- Be sure your establishment is included in listings of healthful restaurants in your community.
- When being quoted or when providing recipes to the media, use your most interesting and popular healthful recipes.

Community and Professional Involvement

Building a reputation for doing the right thing can be the best marketing plan. Many chefs and foodservice professionals are realizing they have a responsibility to use their influence to foster change. Celebrity chefs are leading campaigns to improve school meals, lose weight, increase produce consumption, protect the environment and be more physically active. How can you become part of this movement? Consider:

- Working in the kitchens of a local school district
- Supporting and promoting local farmers and growers
- Supporting community food pantries and hunger organizations
- Donating left-over food to homeless shelters and hunger organizations or volunteering to provide or cook meals
- Teaching a series of cooking classes at the local Boys and Girls Club
- Inviting students to dine in your restaurant
- Teaching parents or guardians how to prepare easy and healthful meals
- Conducting demonstrations at your local farmers' market
- Pushing your local, state and federal legislators to support more healthful food choices at schools and community feeding sites
- Donating or providing healthful food at community events

Cause-related marketing allows you to help non-profit organizations within your community and reap the rewards from the publicity surrounding charitable events.

- Establish a connection with a community-service organization to galvanize positive public perception about your business. Find charitable organizations through your customers, employees or vendors. Pick a cause that employees are excited about so they will continue to participate in your community-service project. Spark employee activism by exchanging an afternoon or evening off for donating a certain number of hours to charity events.
- Be sure the charity or event acknowledges your restaurant to let the community learn of your efforts.
- Maximize publicity by printing T-shirts with your restaurant's logo for employees to wear while they perform volunteer service.
- Distribute bumper stickers urging the public to support your chosen organization. The stickers should include your establishment's name and logo.
- Post a bulletin board in your restaurant where customers can see photos of your staff's volunteer activities. Display flyers urging patrons to sign up as well.
- Include your charitable activities in your restaurant's newsletter and website.

- Have staff wear buttons promoting your charitable organization or event so customers will inquire about it.

- Work with a publicist to increase business. Highlight that your operation has added menu items to meet the needs of health-conscious diners in your publicity and public relations efforts.

Non-Commercial Foodservice

Many innovations that are focused on quality foods are happening in the healthcare arena. Culinary teams led by certified and/or culinary-trained chefs are partnering with registered dietitians to create nourishing quality meals. The traditional trayline is being replaced by the room service model in which patients are able to have more control over what and when they can eat a meal. Patients can order what they feel like eating when they are ready to eat rather than at set mealtimes. As hospitals and other healthcare operations try to differentiate themselves from the competition, they often look to value-added services. The food served is certainly an area for differentiation, and good food is always appreciated. The days of strict diets have been replaced with a more liberal approach to the menu in hospitals and in healthcare and senior-living facilities.

---

casebycase | Marketing Healthful Menus: Five Ways to Use Social Media

With the rise of social media, it's easier than ever to promote your establishment – even with a limited marketing budget, according to food blogger and public relations executive *Janet Helm, MS, RDN*, who is the chief food and nutrition strategist for Weber Shandwick, one of the world's leading public relations firms.

"Social media is all about storytelling and visuals, which makes it an ideal platform for food," Helm explains. "It's about building a community, starting conversations and providing engaging content that people want to read and share. All of that can translate to more customers for you."

When you have a good story to tell about a healthful menu, that's even better. "Food and health are two of the major topics that people search for online," Helm says. "So you have a tremendous amount to gain if you build an online presence." Here are five steps to get you started.

Start with Instagram. This visual platform has emerged as a dominant marketing channel for food. Create your own profile for sharing photos of menu items, and be sure you're using popular hashtags to be more discoverable, such as #instafood, #healthyfood and #plantbased. Be sure your plating and presentation are Instagram-worthy, and encourage diners to share their experiences on Instagram, including Instagram Stories.

Create a Facebook page. Set up a business page to curate your story. Post photos of your healthful menu items, promote specials and share behind-the-scenes video of your team. Encourage followers to "check in" when they visit and post photos of their experience. Engage with your followers and respond to comments.

Connect on Twitter. Many of the country's top chefs have developed large followings on Twitter. Set up your own profile and start tweeting. It's a great way to create a personality for your establishment, network with other professionals, and be discovered by customers. You can use Twitter to post pictures and to enter conversations about food and nutrition that give you a chance to talk about your healthful offerings.

Engage with food influencers. Invite local food bloggers to visit your establishment and post about their experiences. Host a mini-event for registered dietitians to dine and encourage media interviews and blog posts about their "top picks" from the menu.

Combine your online activities with offline publicity. Offer to do a cooking segment for a local TV station and use it as an opportunity to showcase new healthful menu items and to provide recipes for viewers to make at home. Bring food to radio personalities and ask them to talk about special items and promotions. Be a resource to the food editor of your local newspaper.

Students and people of all ages in residential facilities appreciate the strides foodservice directors are making to serve food that is both healthful and delicious. Many food establishments are adding salad bars, baked potato bars, soup and sandwich lines, vegetarian and stir-fry entrées, homemade whole-grain breads, low-fat entrées and dairy products, light salad dressings, and grilled and petite meat portions. Many facilities are planting gardens or featuring produce from local sources. Display cooking – moving the final stages of preparation to the front of the house – has become popular in colleges and hospitals.

New food options can be promoted in newsletters to students, parents or residents, on websites, on bulletin boards and posters, on table tents in the cafeteria, and in presentations to classes or group meetings. Let the dietary department of your local hospital and dietitians who do counseling in your community know that your operation is serving more heart-healthy or moderate-calorie options so that they may suggest your restaurant. Of course, instruct the cooking and serving staff, residents and teachers on nutrition benefits and reasons for change first. Caring about customers' health and well-being, as well as your own and your staff's, can increase sales and create the dividend of better health for all.

From the Kitchen
Samantha Cowens-Gasbarro
Executive Chef
HealthySchoolRecipes.com

I believe that food is medicine for your body. Eating well keeps your body functioning and healthy so life can be spent living and not at the doctors. There's a lot of focus on food as the cause of disease, but food can also be the cure. There's also a misconception that you have to sacrifice flavor and taste if you want to prioritize healthy eating. Once you begin omitting processed foods, and eating real, whole foods, your taste buds actually become more sensitive, allowing you to fully appreciate the inherent natural flavor of food.

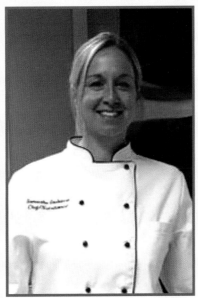

Personally, I mostly stick to a plant-based diet. I love vegetables, and there are so many delicious ways to prepare them. I often feel people don't like vegetables because they have not had them prepared well. I cook a lot at home and put a priority on healthy, balanced meals.

Substitutions are often useful, such as using yogurt in place of butter and cream. But even more important is enhancing each dish with full-flavor ingredients and spices. Favorites include sesame oil, ginger, citrus, and smoked sea salt. Salt is so important to enhance flavor in cooking. It is just that our food system has it all wrong by using it has a preservative in processed foods. Healthy food can be delicious; it is all about highlighting the best feature of any given food (vegetable,

protein, grain, etc.) in the appropriate way to bring out the best flavor. In other words, using food to complement food.

Samantha Cowens-Gasborro began her cooking career as a personal chef for professional athletes. It wasn't long before she noticed the effect a specific diet could have on athletic performance. Around the same time, she began teaching kids to cook and saw that if kids made the food, even the pickiest eaters were more likely to eat it. Since then she has made it her personal mission to inspire young eaters to get in the kitchen, showing them that food can be fun and delicious, not scary. She is determined to help create a generation of healthy eaters by giving them delicious and healthy food and teaching them how to prepare it.

In her position working in school foodservice, she serves around 2200 kids a day for lunch and 1500 for breakfast. The meals she prepares are from scratch with a focus on being delicious as well as nutritious, and because of this, even the pickiest eaters enjoy what's on the menu. In teaching nutrition education to kids, her philosophy is simple: if kids cook it, they are way more likely to eat it. She credits this approach as the secret behind getting kids to eat, say, quinoa and enjoy it. It's all about letting them participate and cook.

Roasted Butternut Squash Quinoa Salad
Serves: 10 ½ cup servings

Samantha Cowens-Gasbarro
Executive Chef,
HealthySchoolRecipes.com

Butternut squash, peeled, seeded, and chopped into ½-inch cubes	1	each
Olive oil	2	tablespoons
Salt	½	teaspoon
Black pepper, freshly ground	½	teaspoon
Quinoa	2	cups
Water	3	cups
Salt	¼	teaspoon
Dried cranberries	½	cup
Scallions, minced	2	each
Sunflower seeds, roasted	½	cup

Dressing:

Orange (zest and juice)	1	large
Olive oil	¼	cup
Honey	1	tablespoon
Salt	¼	teaspoon
Black pepper		to taste

1. Heat the oven to 425 °F. Place cubed butternut squash in a large bowl and toss with olive oil, salt and pepper until squash is well coated. Place seasoned squash on a parchment lined sheet pan and roast the squash for 30 minutes, turning once, until tender.

2. While the butternut squash is roasting, cook the quinoa. Add quinoa, water, and salt to a medium saucepan and bring to a boil over medium heat. Boil for 5 minutes. Turn the heat to low, cover and simmer for about 15 minutes, or until water is absorbed. Remove from heat and let stand for 15 minutes. Then fluff with a fork. Let quinoa cool to room temperature.

3. In a large bowl, combine quinoa, butternut squash, dried cranberries, scallions and sunflower seeds.

4. In a small bowl, whisk together the zest of the orange and the juice of the orange, olive oil, and honey. Season with salt and pepper, to taste. Drizzle over quinoa salad. Toss until ingredients are well dressed.

Per Serving

Calories	310	Cholesterol	0	mg
Fat	14 g	Sodium	350	mg
Saturated Fat	7 g	Carbohydrates	42	mg
Trans Fat	0 g	Dietary Fiber	5	mg
Sugar	16 g	Protein	7	g

Turkey Meatloaf
Yield: 51 ounces
Serves: 12 slices, 4 ounces each

Chef Ann Cooper
Director of Foodservice, Boulder Valley
School District, Boulder, Colorado

This delicious, mild-flavored meatloaf can be adapted for many audiences. It can be used in schools, long-term care or family-style restaurants. Chilled and thinly sliced, the loaf makes delicious meatloaf sandwiches with whole grain breads, lettuce and tomato. The mixture can also make mini meatloaves in cupcake pans.

Onion, small dice	4	ounces
Garlic, minced	1	teaspoon
Carrots, shredded	2	ounces
Canola oil	1	tablespoon
Turkey, ground	3	pounds
Parsley, chopped	1	tablespoon
Japanese (Panko) bread crumbs	½	cup
Eggs	3	
Kosher salt	1	teaspoon
Black pepper, freshly ground	¼	teaspoon
Ketchup	3	tablespoons

1. Preheat oven to 350° F. Prepare a 9 inch x 5 inch loaf pan with non-stick spray.

2. Saute onions, garlic, and carrots in oil until soft. Remove from heat and allow to cool slightly before transferring to a separate bowl.

3. Combine the sautéed ingredients with the turkey, parsley, bread crumbs, eggs, salt and pepper and mix well.

4. Pack meat into prepared loaf pan, coat top with ketchup, and bake until cooked through to an internal temperature of 165° F.

Per Serving

Calories	220	Cholesterol	120	mg
Fat	10 g	Sodium	340	mg
Saturated Fat	2.5 g	Carbohydrates	10	mg
Trans Fat	0 g	Dietary Fiber	1	mg
Sugar	0 g	Protein	25	g

Recipe reprinted with permission from *Lunch Lessons* by Ann Cooper and Lisa M. Holmes (Harper Collins, 2006).

Staff Development

Inadequate staff training is a primary reason for the failure of some healthful dining programs. To keep momentum high, both kitchen and service staff must buy into the program's philosophy wholeheartedly.

Training for the back-of-the-house staff should include:

- Basic nutrition information explaining any changes. When staff members understand why changes are being made, they are better able to execute them.

- Portion control and ingredient-measuring techniques for standardized recipes.

- Across-the-board reductions in salt, fat and sugar in cooking.

- Switching to reduced-sodium sauces and heart-healthy oils.

- Proper cooking techniques and the need for conscientious application every time a dish is prepared.

- Translating customers' special requests into specific menu items (such as broiling fish instead of sautéing, frying or cooking a la minute).

- Importance of careful ingredient and technique control, especially while preparing foods for patrons with food allergies, intolerances or on special diets.

Training for the front-of-the-house staff should emphasize basic nutrition information as well as information about cooking techniques and ingredients. With this background, wait staff can respond to guests' individual needs and communicate special requests to the kitchen staff. There should be a designated individual who can answer questions on nutrient values and ingredients.

Some diners have allergies, intolerances or medical conditions that can be triggered by food choices. The patron who asks if there is cream in the soup or if a menu item has nuts requires a correct response. Sometimes, busy servers do not bother to check, especially if the food item is new to the menu. An incorrect response can lead to a medical emergency.

An effective training program should teach servers their many responsibilities, including how to sell menu items.

- Start by hiring job applicants who have the potential to be effective servers and sales people. Look for candidates who are friendly, personable, good at listening and persuasive. You should be able to ascertain many of these qualities during a job interview.

- As part of training, ensure that servers know about each menu item, including ingredients and preparation method. Provide opportunities for new staff members to taste each menu item. Employees who are informed about menu items will be able to give more knowledgeable answers to customer questions and thus boost sales.

- Consider having new employees learn the ropes by shadowing or trailing experienced servers. Start the shadowing experience on the right foot by selecting your best employees to serve as trainers. Compensate and recognize trainers with higher wages or some other incentive, such as gift certificates.

- Before new servers hit the floor, have them do a test run by serving experienced staffers or managers. Provide feedback on their performance, including their selling skills.

- Remember that training is a continuous process. Use pre-shift meetings to remind employees about selling techniques, to notify them about menu items you particularly want to sell and to provide food tastings.

Having a registered dietitian with culinary experience available to an operation provides credibility and reliability for any healthful dining initiative. A dietitian can be a source of accurate information for staff, management and marketing and also can help to generate local support by encouraging his/her clients and colleagues to enjoy healthy meals at your restaurant. Registered dietitians can also work with chefs to develop more healthful menu items and provide nutrient calculations for the menu and additional information as required by law. They can review recipes, cooking techniques and procedures and create lists of foods suitable for guests seeking vegetarian or gluten-free options, who must avoid common allergies or who have other health concerns.

Making a Nutrition Claim

Any restaurant (defined by the government as a place that serves food ready for consumption, including typical sit-down and carryout venues, as well as institutional foodservice, delicatessens and catering operations) that uses nutrient content claims or health claims on its menu must comply with Nutrition Labeling and Education Act (NLEA) regulations. [3] These regulations also apply to menus that use symbols – such as a heart, an apple or a checkmark – to signify healthful items.

Many of the nutrient and health claims used in food labeling (see Chapter 2) also apply to menus. A **nutrient claim** makes a statement about a specific nutrient or food component of a menu item or meal. It typically includes words such as "reduced," "free" or "low." Claims such as "low in fat," "sugar-free" or "cholesterol-free" are common on menus. For example, when an airline provides a special "low-sodium," "reduced-sodium," or "low-fat," meal, it is making a nutrient content claim. Not only must the meal meet the definition(s) for the claim(s), the airline must provide information on the nutrients that underlie the claim(s) – "low-fat," for example, means the meal contains only 10 grams of fat. This information must be provided by "reasonable means" such as a card identifying the meal as a special request or in a binder available from the flight attendants.

A **health claim** links the food or meal with health status or disease prevention and usually mentions a specific disease. Health claims are relatively uncommon on printed menus, but there are government-mandated rules for terminology. For example, a dish that is low in fat, saturated fat and cholesterol might carry a claim about how diets low in saturated fat and cholesterol may reduce the risk of heart disease. Health claims may appear on the menu in simple terms, such as "heart healthy."

The government strictly regulates health claims and has approved only those for which there is sufficient scientific support. These claims are also used on food labels (see Chapter 2). Some customers may be familiar with them. Foodservice operators are not permitted to make up their own health claims or alter the approved healthy claim statements in any way. For example, an operator cannot claim that a pomegranate blueberry smoothie is high in antioxidants and thus may help prevent cancer. There is no approved health claim for that relationship even if it is believed to be true.

When a nutrient or health claim is used, regulations require there be a reasonable basis for believing the food is qualified to make the claim. Although regulations allow foodservice operators some flexibility in establishing that reasonable basis, they must be prepared to show, on demand, that the menu claims are consistent with the definitions established under the NLEA. Foodservice operators may determine nutrient levels using computer databases, nutrient analyses, cookbooks or some other reasonable source that can provide assurance that the food or meal meets claim requirements.

The Food and Drug Administration (FDA) does not subject restaurant foods to chemical analysis to determine whether nutrient levels are properly declared. Rather, FDA will assess whether the restaurant's basis for a claim or other nutrition information is or is not reasonable. For example, if a restaurant claims a meal is "low-fat," FDA may look at the recipe, nutrient calculations and any other information used by the restaurant in determining whether the meal meets the definition of "low-fat" – that is, containing no more than 3 grams of fat per 100 grams of food.

The FDA offers operators a number of ways to present nutrient data information to patrons. Information is required only for nutrients for which a claim is made. For example, if the menu makes a claim about the

Claim It. Prove It.

If a menu uses any of the following words or symbols representing these words, documentation is required.

- Free
- Low
- Reduced
- Light/Lite
- Provides/Contains/ Good source of
- High/Excellent source of/ Rich in
- Lean/Extra-lean
- Fresh
- Natural
- Healthy

cholesterol content of an item, the operator must provide information on the amount of cholesterol but does not have to provide information about the item's calorie, fat or vitamin content. Of course, it would be helpful to guests if all nutrition information is available.

The nutrient information does not have to be in a special format, such as the Nutrition Facts label found on food products; it simply must be available – for example, in a brochure, on a poster or in a notebook. A statement from a server, such as "a low-fat meal contains less than 10 grams of fat," is the equivalent of full nutrition labeling. As a backup, a restaurant should also have nutrition information in writing to ensure that whatever servers communicate is accurate. It makes sense that restaurants know what they are serving from a nutrition perspective, even if they are not required to share this information with customers or guests or choose not to do so.

Where Does 'Fresh' Fit?

Although the word "fresh" is not a nutrient claim, federal regulations include a definition of what constitutes a "fresh" food item. Many foodservice establishments use the term fresh without knowing its legal definition – a food that is raw, has never been frozen or heated, contains no preservatives other than approved waxes or coatings, and may be washed with mild acid to clean. (Irradiation at low levels is allowed.) The term "fresh" also can be used to describe a product such as fresh milk or freshly baked bread.

FDA's regulation specifies that "fresh frozen" or "frozen fresh" means the food has been quickly frozen while still fresh (i.e., recently harvested when frozen). Appropriate blanching before freezing is permitted.

A Generational Study: The Evolution of Eating from The NPD Group shares that Millennials and Gen Z are embracing more fresh food choices than Baby Boomers, who focused on convenience foods. [4] Foodservice operators see "fresh" as a way to differentiate themselves from the competition.

Calculating Nutrient Data

Providing nutrient data for recipes is a common practice today as restaurants, cookbook authors, culinary demonstrators and food media respond to consumer demand for information on the healthfulness of food. On the surface, gathering these data may seem like a simple process. For example, a recipe for fruit salad containing a specified amount of select fruits per portion involves calculating the nutrient contribution of the edible portion of each fruit, totaling the nutrient values and dividing by the number of servings. This nutrient calculation is fairly straightforward. Few are so easy. Accurate nutrient calculations require more than simply inputting numbers from a database based on an ingredient list. Recipe calculation also calls for understanding how ingredients will react and the nutritional implications of various cooking techniques.

Even though nutrient calculations involve specific measurements and deliver precise-looking data, the numbers are approximate at best. Many factors – including seasonal variations, soil conditions, animal diet, storage conditions, cooking methods and variety of product used – affect the nutrient content of ingredients and the final product. Many restaurants hire registered dietitians with culinary nutrition expertise and experience to calculate nutrient data accurately.

Sometimes, to meet a nutritional goal, the amount of fat, salt or sugar used in a recipe must be adjusted or a pan size must be changed to yield more cuts and thus smaller portions. Sometimes a cooking method must be revised. With any change, a recipe must be retested and recalculated.

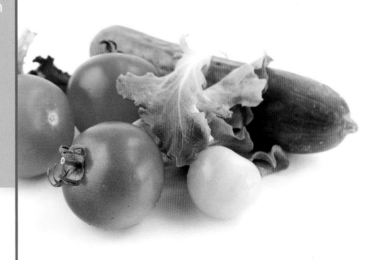

Analysis versus Calculation

True or chemical **nutrient analysis** refers to an assay of select nutrients done by laboratory analysis using incinerated ash or chemical extraction to determine the actual content of various components. Newer techniques are used for the extraction of bioactive chemicals. Each analytical laboratory has specific procedures for sample management and collection as well as procedures for quality assurance and control. The procedures usually include collecting samples from different batches and obtaining values of the blended samples.

Chemical nutrient analysis is typically used when precise data are essential; when the analysis will be entered into databases to be widely used; when nutrition claims will be made; when there are gaps in nutrient data; or when it is impossible to obtain data by calculation. While the advantage of this method is accuracy, the disadvantages are expense, collecting the appropriate number and type of samples, and the time needed to perform laboratory analyses. Although a nutrient analysis will report exactly what is in the sample(s) provided, because of seasonal variations and variations in cooking techniques from sample to sample, even with excellent quality control, the resulting data are still, at best, estimates, although they are far more accurate than calculated values.

Most foodservice operators will use computerized databases for estimating the nutrient content of foods. This procedure is commonly called **nutrient calculation**. Some practitioners refer to the process as nutritional analysis by calculation or nutrient analysis by database. Many nutrient databases are available. Nutrient calculation software offers the advantages of ease, speed and reduced cost, but is less accurate than true nutrient analysis. Certain additional skills, including culinary expertise, are necessary to ensure optimal results. Operators should keep files of all nutrient calculations - the source of the data, the person calculating, and the date of the calculation. When recipes are modified they need to be recalculated.

Only a few studies have compared the calculated and analytic nutrient values for foods. Differences between calculated and actual analytic results may reflect the effects of different types of cooking equipment, surface area of food contact exposure, length and temperature of cooking, and the volume of the product.

Standardization

The first step in calculating nutrient data is standardizing the recipe. It is important to be specific both with ingredients and amounts. For example, the ingredient "chicken" should specify with or without skin and bones, white or dark meat, and cooking method. If a recipe calls for 1 cup of fresh spinach, the calculator must know or decide if it is raw whole-leaf spinach with or without stems, baby spinach or mature leaves. When using a database and determining which item to select that most closely resembles a certain ingredient, calculators must look for key terms in the definition of the item. They also may weigh the ingredient and compare it to the weight or volume of a similar ingredient in the database. Experienced nutrient calculators maintain files detailing the weights of many foods in various forms so that they know, for example, how many grams of a vegetable in various cuts equal a cup or other measure of volume. A very common error is to confuse weights and measures. One cup of a food by measure can weigh as little as 2 ounces or as much as 10 ounces by weight. Recipes often include weights and measures of different ingredients - 1 teaspoon salt, 2 pounds chopped onions among other listed ingredients..

Seasonings, especially high-sodium ingredients such as salt, should be listed by amount, not "to taste" or "as needed." Saying "salt to taste" gives the calculator no information to determine sodium content. (Omission of seasoning in a calculation creates a false impression and is wrong; however, it is acceptable to note that salt may be omitted to reduce the sodium content of the recipe.)

Since the goal is a truly accurate report of nutrient content, the calculator may want to prepare the recipe or observe its being prepared to clarify exact ingredients and amounts. Chefs may add oil and seasonings to food (and to flat grills) during cooking and then make final flavoring and seasoning adjustments. As a result, they often have no idea how much oil or salt they actually use. In this case, it may be necessary to put generous premeasured weighed amounts of oil and salt on the mis-en-place tray, watch the chef prepare the food, and then measure the amount of oil and salt left after the dish is prepared. For calculation purposes, the difference between "before" and "after" is the amount actually used in the recipe. In addition to the amount of salt used, it is also important to clarify the type of salt. Kosher salt may have less sodium per teaspoon than regular table salt.

Cooking Method

It is important to remember that items in an ingredient list may not be the same in the finished product, and it is the finished product that must be calculated. A thorough understanding of food preparation and cooking methods is often necessary, especially when not all ingredients in a recipe will be consumed. For example, when a chicken breast is marinated prior to grilling and the unabsorbed marinade is discarded, only the absorbed marinade is calculated. A larger surface area will absorb more marinade (chicken tenders versus chicken breast), as will a product that is more porous (mushrooms versus red peppers). If the food is cooked on a grill, some marinade will burn off. In addition, sodium in the marinade will extract liquid from the product being marinated.

A nutrient calculation for stock made with beef bones and mirepoix (a combination of carrots, celery and onion) that is later discarded must account for nutrients that have been infused into the stock (with less sodium). In this situation, the calculation can substitute a laboratory-analyzed value of the most similar product, perhaps a canned stock. Special consideration is also needed in calculating the nutrients in pureed and strained fruits and vegetables. For example, strained sauces must be adjusted for fiber and other nutrient losses. A registered dietitian with culinary expertise might estimate a percentage of loss or estimate remaining fiber based on values of other strained sauces. Examples such as these illustrate that a high level of culinary expertise is necessary to make adjustments for food preparation and cooking methods when calculating the nutrient content of a recipe.

Sub-Recipes

Determining the per portion nutrient contribution of sub-recipes is usually a more complex task than calculating the value of one recipe with several components that are plated and served together as one dish. This step in the nutrient calculation process can also require culinary expertise beyond what packaged software offers.

Some recipes have several sub-recipes. For example, many fine restaurants serve a main item on a bed of something, surrounded by a small amount of one or more sauces and topped with an edible garnish. The dish as served may use varying amounts of each sub-recipe. Consequently, a sauce sub-recipe may make 16 servings of 1 tablespoon each, while the bed of vegetables or salad sub-recipe makes enough for 8 servings. In this case, it is necessary to determine the single-serving portions of each sub-recipe and then total the values for 1 serving of the main dish fully plated. A photo of the plated food can be used to confirm the amount of sauce served per portion and is always provided with the standardized recipe.

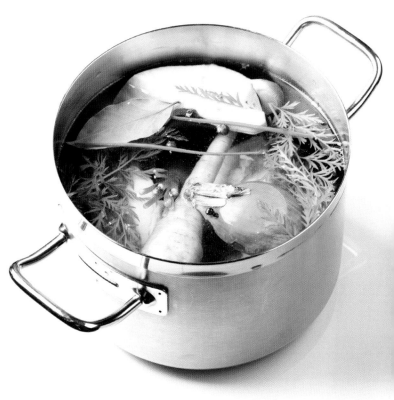

Yield

Yield is used to calculate per portion nutrient content. A very large volume of ingredients that yields only 4 or 6 servings or a low volume of ingredients that is meant to serve many will raise a red flag to an experienced calculator. This situation often requires that the full recipe be prepared, the yield weighed and measured, and the number of portions reevaluated. Yields may be determined by:

- Preparing the recipe, then measuring volume and determining the number of servings
- Using the yield given by the standardized recipe
- Adding the volumes of the served ingredients in prepared form (if there are multiple ingredient components)
- Measuring container size (e.g., 1 gallon) that holds finished product

Yield is best determined by an actual weight or measure of the finished product. Results can be inaccurate when weights and/or volumes of raw ingredients are used to determine yield. Combinations of ingredients and cooking methods significantly alter yield volume. For example, when reducing a sauce or baking a cake, moisture is lost, thus reducing final yield weight and increasing nutrients per portion.

If the recipe calls for a specific weight of raw meat to be added and cooked, and data exist for the nutrient content of cooked meat, one must apply a yield factor to the amount of raw meat needed in order to determine the amount of cooked meat that will result, and then calculate the nutrient content of that amount. Understanding cooking method is also necessary for determining nutrient values. For example, a sautéed entrée is usually served in a sauce made from the drippings remaining in the pan. Sometimes rendered fat will be poured off before the pan is deglazed, and a sauce will be prepared by reducing added liquid (stock, wine or juice) and seasonings. The amount of fat removed must be subtracted from the calculation. The reduced liquid will lower volume but not calories. Some of the calories from alcohol, however, such as a wine or brandy used to deglaze a pan, may burn off during cooking, depending on cooking time and total volume of liquid. These losses must be estimated and subtracted.

Basic Rules for the Yield Factor Method

- Use the form and portion of the food as served.
- Select raw if not heated or cooked.
- Select cooked if cooked before serving, using the database food code for the cooked ingredient.
- Convert or adjust the amount of the raw ingredient in the recipe by using a yield factor.

Where to Get Help

Foodservice operators, especially those who are required to provide calorie and nutrient information for the first time, may need assistance to generate accurate, defensible data. Many operators will want to work with a registered dietitian nutritionist (RDN) with culinary expertise. Your local or state dietetic association, the Food & Culinary Professionals Dietetic Practice Group (**www.foodculinaryprofs.org**) or The Academy of Nutrition and Dietetics (**www.eatright.org**) can help find someone to assist you in determining the nutritional composition of existing menu offerings and perhaps modifying offerings to enhance the healthfulness of the total menu. Onsite help, perhaps with observation to clarify techniques and standardize recipes, may be warranted.

There are also services that employ individuals experienced in calculating nutrient values. This approach works only if recipes are tested and standardized and requires substantial communication to clarify techniques, volumes and yield for proper calculation. For difficult-to-calculate items or when accuracy is essential, the best option is nutritional analysis not calculated values.

The only book on the subject is *Recipe Nutrient Analysis: best practices for calculated or chemical analysis* by Catharine Powers and Cheryl Dolven. This resource will provide guidance on the basics of recipe nutrient calculation and answer questions like: how much marinade is absorbed before cooking? How much fat is absorbed in deep frying? How do you calculate salt absorption in pasta cooking? This book provides the latest research needed to answer these and other essential questions and share the best practices from leaders in the foodservice nutrition industry. *(Disclosure: Powers is also an author of this book.)*

Recipe Nutrient Analysis

Presenting Nutrient Data

Given the ease and power of computerized nutrient calculation, resulting data are often carried out to several decimal points. The specificity of these numbers creates a false sense of accuracy and confidence in the numbers. All nutrient calculations are estimates; numbers calculated for recipes should be rounded according to the Food and Drug Administration's (FDA) rounding rules for product labels. In addition, nutrient calculation information should always include a statement that the values are an estimate based on calculations from whatever databases were used along with the professional judgment of the person who performed the calculation.

The following table summarizes FDA's rounding rules.

Guidance for Industry: Food Labeling

Nutrient	Increment Rounding	Insignificant Amount
Calories **Calories from fat** **Calories from saturated fat**	< 5 calories - list as 0 ≤ 50 calories - round to nearest 5-calorie increment > 50 calories - round to nearest 10-calorie increment	< 5 calories
Total fat **Saturated fat** **Trans fat** **Polyunsaturated fat** **Monounsaturated fat**	< .5 grams - list as 0 < 5 grams - round to nearest .5-gram increment ≥ 5 grams - round to nearest 1-gram increment	< .5 gram
Cholesterol	< 2 milligrams - list as 0 2-5 milligrams - report as "less than 5 milligrams" > 5 milligrams - round to nearest 5-milligram increment	< 2 milligrams
Sodium **Potassium**	< 5 milligrams - list as 0 5-140 milligrams - round to nearest 5-milligram increment > 140 milligrams - round to nearest 10-milligram increment	< 5 milligrams
Total carbohydrate **Dietary fiber**	< .5 grams - list as 0 0 < 1 gram - report as "contains less than 1 gram" or "less than 1 gram" ≥ 1gram - round to nearest 1-gram increment	< 1 gram
Soluble and insoluble fiber sugars **Sugar alcohol** **Other carbohydrate**	< .5 gram - list as 0 < 1gram - report as "contains less than 1 gram" or "less than 1 gram" ≥ 1gram - round to nearest 1-gram increment	< .5 gram

Guidance for Industry: Food Labeling *continued*

Nutrient	Increment Rounding	Insignificant Amount
Protein	< .5 gram - list as 0 < 1 gram - report as "contains less than 1 gram" or "less than 1 gram" or report as 1gram if .5 gram to < 1 gram ≥ 1 gram - round to nearest 1-gram increment	< 1 gram
Nutrients other than vitamins and minerals that have RDIs as a % DV	Round to nearest 1% DV increment	< 1% DV

Vitamins and minerals (% DV)	< 2% of RDI may be listed as:
	  a) 0
	  b) 2% DV if actual amount is 1% or more
	  c) an asterisk that refers to statement "Contains less than 2% of the Daily Value of this (these) nutrient(s)"
	  d) for Vit A, C, calcium, iron: statement "Not a significant source of _____ (listing the vitamins and minerals omitted)"
	≤ 10% of RDI - round to nearest 2% DV increment
	> 10% - 50% of RDI - round to nearest 5% DV increment
	> 50% of RDI - round to nearest 10% DV increment
		< 2% RDI

Beta-Carotene (% DV)	≤ 10% of RDI for vitamin A - round to nearest 2% DV increment > 10%-50% of RDI for vitamin A - round to nearest 5% DV increment > 50% of RDI for vitamin A - round to nearest 10% DV increment	

Note: To list nutrient values to the nearest 1-gram increment, for amounts falling exactly halfway between two whole numbers or higher (e.g., 2.5 grams to 2.99 grams), round up (e.g., 3 grams). For amounts less than halfway between two whole numbers (e.g, 2.01 grams to 2.49 grams), round down (e.g., 2 grams).

When rounding % DV for nutrients other than vitamins and minerals, when the % DV values fall exactly halfway between two whole numbers or higher (e.g., 2.5 to 2.99), the values round up (e.g., 3 %). For values less than halfway between two whole numbers (e.g., 2.01 to 2.49), the values round down (e.g., 2%).

Adapted from A Food Labeling Guide: Guidance for Industry; US Department of Health and Human Services, Food and Drug Administration-Center for Food Safety and Applied Nutrition. January 2013. **https://www.fda.gov/downloads/Food/GuidanceRegulation/GuidanceDocumentsRegulatoryInformation/UCM265446.pdf**

Round and Round and Round

The nutrient calculation report indicates that a recipe contains 277.62 calories, 464.49 milligrams of sodium, 39.221 grams of protein and 5.811 grams of fat per serving. The specificity of these numbers suggests a high degree of accuracy. To avoid the impression of unwarranted accuracy and to make nutrition labeling easier for customers to read and understand, foodservice operators should follow FDA's rounding rules. The above values should be listed as 280 calories, 460 milligrams of sodium, 39 grams of protein and 6 grams of fat.

Opportunities for Chefs

Nutrition is big business. Providing healthful choices to your guests can increase your bottom line and guest loyalty. How you communicate your nutrition message to guests can influence how healthful items are purchased, promoted and positioned. Additionally, federal regulations and laws mandate that the foodservice industry provide nutrition information. Calculating nutrient data is a challenging task for foodservice operators. Consulting a registered dietitian nutritionist with culinary expertise can help ensure accuracy of nutrient data.

Learning Activities

1. Using a nutrient calculation program, calculate the nutrient content of three recipes.

2. Identify a health-related cause and develop an action plan for supporting it and getting visibility for your establishment's participation.

3. Investigate the nutrient content of three chain restaurant concepts. (This information is commonly available on the company website.) What percentage of items have more than 500 calories per portion? Which items would you identify as healthful?

For More Information

- Powers C, Hess MA, Kimbrough M. *How accurate are your nutrient calculations? Why culinary expertise makes a difference.* J Am Diet Assoc. 2008;108(9):1418-22.

- USDA Food Composition Databases (USDA National Nutrient Database for Standard Reference and USDA Branded Food Products Database). Available at **https://ndb.nal.usda.gov/ndb/. Accessed April 11, 2018.**

- U. S. Food and Drug Administration. *Guidance for Industry: A Labeling Guide for Restaurants and Retail Establishments Selling Away-From-Home Foods - Part I.* Currently under revision. Available at **https://www.fda.gov/Food/GuidanceRegulation/GuidanceDocumentsRegulatoryInformation/ucm053455.htm.** Accessed April 11, 2018.

- U. S. Food and Drug Administration. *Guidance for Industry: A Labeling Guide for Restaurants and Retail Establishments Selling Away-From-Home Foods - Part II* (Menu Labeling Requirements in Accordance with 21 CFR 101.11). April 2016. **https://www.fda.gov/Food/GuidanceRegulation/GuidanceDocumentsRegulatoryInformation/ucm461934.htm.** Accessed April 11, 2018.

- U. S. Food and Drug Administration. *Claims That Can Be Made for Conventional Foods and Dietary Supplements.* Updated January 2018. **https://www.fda.gov/food/labelingnutrition/ucm111447.htm.** Accessed April 11, 2018.

- U.S. Food and Drug Administration and U.S. Department of Health and Human Services. *Food Labeling Guide.* Available at **https://www.fda.gov/downloads/Food/GuidanceRegulation/GuidanceDocumentsRegulatoryInformation/UCM265446.pdf.** Accessed April 11, 2018.

Selected Free Nutrient Calculation Software

- USDA Food Composition Databases, **https://ndb.nal.usda.gov/ndb/**

- **MyFoodRecord.com**

- **CalorieKing.com**

- CondéNet, **www.nutritiondata. com**

- **Fitday.com**

Chapter Twelve

Food for Healthy Living

Learning Objectives | *After completing this chapter, you should be able to:*

- Plan menus that are appropriate and nutrient rich for children and adolescents

- Identify issues specific to menu planning for aging adults

- Explain meal planning for athletes

- Discuss nutritional menu planning for weight management

- Plan healthful menus for vegetarians and vegans

- Describe dietary practices, restrictions and rationale for eating behaviors of people of the world's major religions

- Describe basic requirements for kosher meal preparation

- List foods permitted and foods to be avoided for halal meals

Everybody eats – but not everybody has the same needs and expectations when it comes to the foods they choose. Age, lifestyle, weight concerns and religion/culture affect how people incorporate food into their daily lives. In this chapter, experts from around the country – our Essentials Experts – have contributed their knowledge and practical advice about serving children, aging adults, athletes, vegetarians, dieters and patrons with strong religious and cultural food traditions. A boost in flavor here and a portion adjustment there may be all it takes to appeal to some guests. Others, however, have more complicated requirements and strict rules dictating what they can and cannot eat. Knowing the special needs of patrons is step one. Meeting those needs is what sets the successful chef apart from others.

Meeting the Needs of Children

Essentials Expert

Catharine Powers, MS, RDN, LD, co-author of this book, has worked with school nutrition programs around the country and is chair of the Culinary Institute of America's Healthy Kids Collaborative. She was project manager for the Institute of Child Nutrition's award-winning *Cooks for Kids* video program and *Culinary Techniques for Healthy School Meals* training program.

Whether served at home, in a restaurant or at school, children's food should be healthful and their meals well balanced. Too many children don't get enough of the nutritious foods that growing minds and bodies need. Some eat only a few foods over and over again. Others eat too many highly processed, high-fat and/or high-sugar foods. While it is primarily the responsibility of parents and caregivers to provide a healthful diet to children, schools also have a role as most children have one, and sometimes two, meals a day at school. Chefs can play an important role by providing food options that are interesting, nourishing and expand children's food experiences.

Nearly one in three American children is overweight or obese and thus at risk for a lifetime of obesity and serious diseases associated with obesity. And even overfed children can be undernourished. Most American children do not regularly eat enough foods that promote optimal health and growth. Per capita consumption of vegetables and fruits has declined 7% over the past 5 years. [1] Only 15% of teens in grades 9 through 12 consume at least 3 servings of vegetables per day. [2] Overall, almost all children consume too much sodium, and four out of five children consume saturated fat in excess. [3]

The *Dietary Guidelines for Americans 2015-2020* identified shortfall nutrients for children as vitamins A, C, D, E, and calcium, folate, magnesium, potassium and fiber [4]. Increasing intakes of vegetables (particularly dark-green and orange vegetables), legumes, fruits (particularly whole fruits), whole grains, fluid milk and milk products, meat and beans will help address these shortfall nutrients. Researchers have found that the majority of children, especially dark-skinned children, do not get enough vitamin D to build healthy bones. Dark-skinned children are vulnerable because the melanin that makes skin dark blocks ultraviolet rays that the body uses to make vitamin D. Consequently, additional sources of vitamin D, particularly fortified milk, are important for these children and their families as well. [5]

Key Nutrition Points

- Children need to eat every 4 to 6 hours. Make sure both snacks and meals are nutrient-rich.

- At least half of the grain products children eat should be whole grains. Serve whole-grain cereals and breads often and encourage use of whole grains whenever possible. Limit refined grains such as white breads and white rice.

- Children ages 2 to 8 years should drink 2 cups/day of fat-free or low-fat milk or equivalent milk products such as cheese or yogurt. Children age 9 and older should drink 3 cups/day of fat-free or low-fat milk or equivalent dairy products. Use cheese and yogurt in cooking, mixed dishes and salads, and smoothies.

- Total fat intake should be between 30% and 35% of calories for children ages 2 to 3 and between 25% and 35% of calories for children and adolescents ages 4 to 18. Most fats should come from polyunsaturated and monounsaturated fatty acids found in fish, nuts and vegetable oils. Just as for adults, food for children should limit saturated fat and eliminate trans fats.

- Many children don't consume enough dietary fiber. Adding whole fruits, dried fruits, vegetables, legumes, nuts and whole-grain products to the diet increases fiber intake.

- Avoid excessive calories from added sugars. While an occasional soft drink is okay, these beverages are not healthful and may train the brain to seek more sweets. Sweetened foods that provide few nutrients reduce diet quality and contribute to weight gain.

- Lack of iron can affect behavior, mood and attention span. Serve iron-rich foods such as lean meat, enriched cereals and legumes. Ground meats (in meat sauces, chili, meat balls and burgers) are easier for young children to chew. A source of vitamin C, such as red or green peppers or citrus fruit, increases the amount of iron absorbed from enriched grains, eggs and vegetables.

Best Choices

- Use primarily whole foods such as fruits, vegetables, legumes, lean meats, poultry and fish, whole grains, and low-fat milk and dairy products.

- Serve roasted, grilled or poached foods such as baked apples, grilled shrimp and scallops, and roasted potato strips.

- Serve fruits whole or cut to provide more nutrients and fiber. Place apple and orange wedges, a small bunch of grapes, a few cherries, or berries on plates to add color, texture and boost fruit intake.

- When serving juices, choose 100% juice rather than sweetened fruit drinks. Add 2 ounces of juice to 6 ounces water or sparkling water for a refreshing, healthful and lower calorie option.

- Serve vegetables – carrot or jicama sticks, zucchini or summer squash coins, blanched green beans or sugar snap peas, bell peppers or edamame – as healthful crunchy meal enhancers.

- Provide dips and sauces that are appealing to kids. Allow them to select from several sauces with their meal to encourage eating more fruits and vegetables. Include complementary sauces with menu items.
  - **Savory**: mild salsa, sweet and sour, barbecue, cheese, hummus, Asian dipping sauces, chutney, fruited vinaigrette, tzatziki (Greek cucumber sauce), ranch dip and peanut butter
  - **Sweet**: small amounts of caramel, chocolate, fruit purees, chutney

- Include nutrient-dense beverages with each meal, such as low-fat milk or 100% fruit juice. If sweetened beverages are served, make them lightly sweetened.

- Provide healthful side dishes as an option. Include seasonal fruits, vegetables, whole grains and legumes to add variety, color and new taste experiences to meals. Be specific in menu descriptions.

- Serve whole-grain breads, buns, crackers, tortillas, wraps and pitas when possible.

- Make low-fat milk or equivalent dairy products available at meals and with snacks. If white milk or plain yogurt is not popular, try flavored milk or fruited yogurt.

- Use brown rice and other whole grains. Use whole-wheat breadcrumbs for breaded items.

- Serve graham crackers and oatmeal raisin or other cookies with some healthful ingredients.

- Many children enjoy California rolls, Thai spicy rolls and other "wrapped" vegetables.

- Serve legumes in entrées, side dishes and soups.

- Include dried fruits and nuts in cooking or as snacks.

Foods to Limit

Generally, the foods to limit for children are the same as for adults making healthful choices. Limit portion size by serving kid-sized portions in a small cup, bowl or container. Try to limit:

- Fried foods
- Foods containing trans or saturated fats
- Refined grains, white rice
- Breads, cereals, crackers, pasta and pretzels made from refined flour
- Soft drinks, slushies and other highly sweetened beverages (liquid candy)
- Foods with added sugar
- Foods high in sodium
- Processed foods containing artificial colors, flavors and additives

casebycase | Farm-to-School Flourishes in Georgia

Donna Martin, RD, is school nutrition director for the Burke County school system in Waynesboro, Georgia. She oversees a staff of 60 employees who serve meals to more than 4,000 students in five schools, including pre-kindergarten.

Burke County, the second largest county in the state, is rural, impoverished and for all practical purposes, a food desert. Donna, a past president of the Academy of Nutrition and Dietetics and the first school nutrition director to hold that office, explains that she was attracted to school food service because of its health promotion opportunities.

In 2010, Congress authorized the funding of $5 million annually for farm-to-school competitive grants designed to improve student access to local foods and support experiential food education. Donna jumped at this opportunity. As a result, Burke County won a grant and launched its own farm-to-school program. "I worked with the county's extension office to get a list of farmers, large and small," Donna explains. "We invited them for lunch to see what we do."

The program sources fresh fruits and vegetables from 17 local farms. Beef for spaghetti sauce comes from nearby Washington, Georgia, and eggs from Statesboro. School menus list the source of foods. "We take the students and staff to visit farms so they can see how farming works," Donna says. "They appreciate food more when they see how hard farmers work to grow and harvest it. In our schools, farmers are rock stars!"

Fruit and vegetable consumption has doubled since the farm-to-school program launched. When schools introduce a new vegetable, local grocery stores are forewarned so they can stock up on it and meet demand as parents learn from their children.

"When the resources became available, I wasn't sure the farm-to-school program would work for us," Donna says, "but we were willing to try. I just knew we had to do something to help these kids."

Each year, USDA awards competitive farm-to-school grants to be used for training, supporting operations, planning, purchasing equipment, developing school gardens, developing partnerships, and implementing farm-to-school programs. In fiscal years 2019 and 2020, USDA will release approximately $7.5 million to help reach more communities seeking to incorporate local products into school meal programs, integrate agricultural education into the classroom, and cultivate and expand school gardens. For more information, visit USDA Grants and Loans That Support Farm-to-School Activities at **https://fns-prod. azureedge.net/sites/default/files/ f2s/GandLfact-sheet.pdf**.

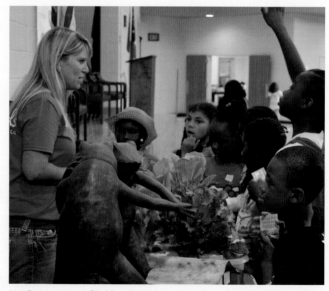

Lisa Dojan, owner of Fishheads, explains to students how she grows aquaponic lettuce for the farm-to-school program. Her farm is called Fisheads because she grows heads of lettuce in water containing fish whose "poop" provides fertilizer.

Tips for Chefs

Children have more taste buds than adults. As a result, they often dislike very strong-flavored and highly salted foods. This increased sensitivity to flavor along with a biological preference for sweet foods is part of the reason children often have strong food likes and dislikes, repeatedly requesting favorite foods and rejecting others. Children often enjoy brightly colored, mild-flavored foods such as corn. Crisp and chewy foods develop a child's chewing skills.

While parents play the primary role in providing healthful foods for their children, chefs can help by making the foods children should have more available and accessible. Eating away from home also provides opportunities for children to try foods not usually served at home. All segments of the food-service industry need to move beyond the narrowly focused traditional children's menu of breaded, fried chicken tenders, macaroni and cheese, burgers and pizzas. Children need a greater variety of food than what is provided at popular foodservice outlets.

- Offer a variety of food that appeals to different age groups and preferences.
- Serve small bites and hand-held food items.
- Use child-sized utensils and unbreakable plates.
- Minimize choking hazards for young children by avoiding foods that are round and about the size of a nickel such as grapes and cherry tomatoes. Remove pits from fruits and be sure fish is boneless.
- Be aware of common allergens. Peanut butter is popular, but peanuts are a common allergen. (See information on allergens in Chapter 13.)
- Serve foods and use flavors children know. Sweet flavors are most appealing to children. Some children also enjoy salsas and dips with a little heat and spiciness.
- Serve appropriate portions. Make half-size muffins, pancakes, meatballs, etc.
- Use healthful cooking techniques like grilling, baking and steaming, while minimizing fried items. For example, serve grilled chicken or chicken skewers rather than fried chicken fingers.

- Introduce new options in familiar ways – jicama or sugar snap peas with a dip, grilled cheese on whole-wheat bread, mashed butternut squash or an interesting-shaped pasta tossed with roasted vegetables.
- Serve colorful, nutrient-rich foods that add eye appeal – for example, broccoli, red peppers, edamame and cantaloupe.
- Put produce on every plate, making fruits and vegetables the side dish of choice.
- Add variety to children's menus by offering half portions of foods from the regular menu.
- For sandwiches, offer low-fat deli meat and sliced lean turkey, chicken or pork or reduced-fat cold cuts. Add extra vegetables, such as tomatoes, roasted red peppers or sliced cucumbers.
- Put healthful appetizers from the regular menu on the children's menu to provide interesting options beyond traditional kid-friendly offerings. Many children enjoy a shrimp cocktail or small crab cake as a healthful entrée.

For More Information

- Action for Healthy Kids, **www.actionforhealthykids.org**
- American Culinary Federation, Chef and the Child Foundation, **www.acfchefs.org**
- Culinary Institute of America, Healthy Kids Collaborative, **www.ciahealthykids.com**
- Fuel Up to Play 60, **www.fueluptoplay60.com**
- Institute of Child Nutrition, **www.theICN.org**
- School Nutrition Association, **www.schoolnutrition.org**
- U.S. Department of Agriculture, Food and Nutrition Services, Child Nutrition Programs, School Meals, **www.fns.usda.gov/cnd**
- U.S. Department of Agriculture, Food and Nutrition Services, Team Nutrition, **www.teamnutrition.usda.gov/Default.htm**

From the Kitchen
Rebecca J. Polson, CC, SNS
Culinary Supervisor, **Minneapolis Public Schools**

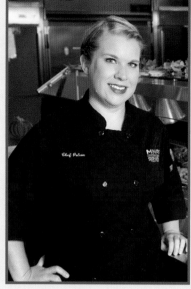

I started my cooking career later in life, and so was able to get past all the classical techniques and learn to just cook from the heart, serving food that makes people happy. Now I bring that love to thousands of schoolchildren every day. With kids, it's important to keep food approachable. Having lived overseas and traveled the world, I like to bring different flavors to familiar dishes. People are always more willing to try them this way.

When it comes to nutrition, especially in-school nutrition, I find myself assuming not just the role of chef, but also role model (in what I eat) and educator (in what they eat). By using high quality ingredients such as our farm-to-school produce and introducing students to flavors from around the world, we are changing palates, while educating students on the benefits of a well-balanced diet. By creating these healthy habits now, they'll continue to grow and live out a long and prosperous life.

Rebecca J. Polson, CC, SNS is the culinary supervisor for Minneapolis Public Schools in Minnesota. She began her career in the foodservice industry in 2011 after graduating from Johnson & Wales University-Charlotte Campus with a culinary arts degree. She also holds a bachelor's degree in merchandising and business from Florida State University. She has worked as line cook at James Beard award-winning Bern's Steakhouse, and run a test kitchen as research and development chef for restaurant chain Beef 'O' Brady's, as well as bar chain The Brass Tap. She now brings her culinary skills and passion for great food to Minneapolis Public Schools serving over 35,000 meals each day.

Curried Sweet Potato Salad
Servings: 20

Rebecca J. Polson, CC, SNS,
Culinary Supervisor, Minneapolis Public Schools

Sweet potatoes, peeled, ½ inch dice	4	pounds
Mayonnaise	1	cup
Curry powder	1	tablespoon
Lime juice	1	tablespoon
Lime zest	from 1	lime
Brown sugar, light	2	tablespoons
Kosher salt	½	teaspoon
Black pepper	½	teaspoon
Red onion, ⅛ inch dice	½	large
Cilantro, fresh, chopped	¼	cup
Cashews	½	cup
Dried cranberries	½	cup

1. Place sweet potatoes in a large pot and cover with salted, cold water. Cover, bring to a boil, reduce to a simmer and cook until tender, about 10-12 minutes. Do not overcook.
2. Drain sweet potatoes and place in the refrigerator until cool.
3. While potatoes are cooling, combine mayonnaise, curry powder, lime juice, lime zest, brown sugar, salt and pepper.
4. Fold sweet potatoes, dressing, onions, cilantro, cashews, and cranberries together. Refrigerate for 30 minutes. Allow flavor to meld.
5. Garnish with additional cilantro, if desired.

Per Serving

Calories	200	Cholesterol	5 mg
Fat	10 g	Sodium	125 mg
Saturated Fat	1.5 g	Carbohydrates	26 mg
Trans Fat	0 g	Dietary Fiber	2 mg
Sugar	5 g	Protein	2 g

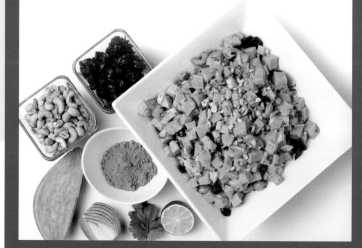

Meeting the Needs of Aging Adults

Essentials Expert

Becky Dorner, RDN, LD, FAND is one of the nation's leading experts on nutrition and aging and long-term health care. She has more than 30 years' experience as a speaker, consultant and author. Becky Dorner & Associates, Inc., publishes and presents continuing education programs and information on healthy aging and nutrition care for older adults. Her other company, Nutrition Consulting Services, Inc., which employs registered dietitian nutritionists and nutrition and dietetic technicians, registered, has provided services to healthcare facilities in Ohio since 1983.

Chefs feed aging adults everywhere, not only in restaurants and in healthcare communities such as skilled nursing facilities, assisted living facilities, and retirement and senior communities, but also on cruise ships and in resorts and other food outlets. Chefs also play a critical role in providing the 250 million meals served yearly at senior centers and to Meals on Wheels recipients in their homes. As the population ages, these opportunities will increase. Approximately 10,000 Americans turn 65 each day [6], and the percentage of the US population is projected to increase from 13% in 2010 to more than 20% in 2030 [7]. Life expectancies continue to increase especially at the older ages. Demand for long-term services and supports such as home and community-based care and services, assisted living and nursing facilities will increase as approximately 70% of older adults (65+) will need these services at some point during their lifetime [8].

Key Nutrition Points

- The nutrition concerns of aging adults are often driven by the onset of chronic diseases and the inability to participate in the normal activities of daily living.

- More than 80% of people age 65 or older have one or more chronic conditions that are affected by nutrition and/or food choices. As they age, Americans are likely to be concerned about sodium, cholesterol, fiber, trans fats and concentrated sweets.

- Aging adults are looking for healthy alternatives as research indicates that better nutrition, physical and mental activity can prevent or delay many chronic diseases.

- According to a 2014 report from the CDC, approximately 25% of people over 65 years of age are diagnosed with diabetes [9] and require some dietary modifications.

- Older adults need more nutrient-dense foods to meet nutritional requirements in fewer calories. In each decade after reaching adulthood, the body requires fewer calories to maintain a healthy weight. Some people with chronic diseases and conditions, however, may require additional calories, protein or other nutrients. For example, those who have pressure ulcers (commonly known as bed sores) may need up to 50% more calories and protein than those who do not.

- Many older adults are on therapeutic diets, but individualized and often liberalized diets are recommended for those who live in healthcare facilities. Promoting enjoyment of food and enhancing quality of life are important goals. Overly restrictive diets may reduce food intake and cause unintended weight loss, which can have devastating health effects [10, 11, 12].

- Malnutrition is a major concern that increases risk of mortality, hospitalization and length of stay, probability of readmission to the hospital and cost of care, while decreasing quality of life [13].

- Chewing and swallowing problems may require altering the consistency of a food and/or liquid to make it safer and easier to swallow.

- Since appetite may be small, pay attention to nutrient density. Smoothies, puddings and healthful muffins pack several nutrient-dense ingredients into a single serving.

Chefs are needed in settings that serve older adults, such as continuing care retirement communities, nursing facilities, assisted living facilities and independent living facilities. Many of these healthcare communities are moving toward "person-centered dining," which focuses on the desires of the individual by providing more choices in meal times, tablemates, food and dining styles. These facilities emphasize individual choice and offer alternative dining styles such as buffets, family-style dining and restaurant-style dining.

Improving food quality and service in healthcare communities is an area where chefs can really shine. Sanitation and food safety are also major issues due to the many regulatory guidelines that must be met in order to prevent foodborne illness in this potentially susceptible population. Chefs and dietitians make a great team in these settings and can work together for the benefit of all the older adults they serve.

Becky Dorner, RDN, LD, FAND
Becky Dorner & Associates, Inc.

Best Choices

The best choices for the older person's menu are what he or she can and will eat. Ask older people what their favorite foods are and their answers may surprise you! Don't assume aging people prefer bland food. With age, taste buds become less sensitive and it takes more spices and seasoning to perceive flavor. More flavorful foods can increase enjoyment and appetite.

- A well-rounded diet that generally meets *Dietary Guidelines* and *MyPlate* recommendations is best for older adults (plenty of vegetables, fruits, whole grains, lean meats and low-fat dairy, with moderation in sodium, fat and sugars). Healthy older adults can follow the same guidelines as other adults.

- Foods high in fiber and fluid are needed to aid elimination. Anyone increasing fiber in his/her diet should also drink plenty of fluids.

- Provide a vitamin C source daily and a vitamin A source three to four times per week. Foods such as red bell pepper, cantaloupe, spinach and butternut squash provide good sources of vitamins A and C and also help boost immunity.

- A typical meal pattern is three meals a day with between-meal and bedtime snacks. However, some older adults prefer small, frequent meals.

- What an older person will eat depends on activity level, ethnic and regional preferences, life history, and the presence or absence of health issues. Each person is unique and foods should be individualized based on preferences and needs. Seasonings, textures and portion sizes may need to be adjusted based on preference.

- A daily multivitamin or multivitamin with minerals may be recommended based on individual needs and the amounts and types of foods usually eaten. Supplementation with calcium and vitamin D may be recommended, especially when someone does not drink milk regularly or gets little exposure to sunshine. Vitamin B_{12} is another nutrient that may need to be supplemented in older adults.

- Many adults, regardless of age, may enjoy a glass of wine or beer at the start of a meal to help reduce stress, increase appetite and meal enjoyment. This is only allowed if approved by the individual's physician as alcohol can cause negative interactions with some medications and may be contraindicated with certain diseases and conditions.

- Because dental problems are common among older people, easy-to-eat foods that are relatively soft, moist or bite-sized are frequently preferred. Corn cut off the cob, meat loaf and other thinly sliced tender meats, soups and stews, soft vegetables, sauces and gravies, custards and puddings, and cut fruit make eating easier and may enable aging guests to eat without assistance.

Other Considerations

- Health issues of individuals may create the need to limit foods high in salt, fat, cholesterol or sugar. Use aromatics and seasonings without excessive sodium to intensify flavors. Work closely with a registered dietitian nutritionist to ensure personal needs are met.

- The immune system can be compromised with age, so it is important to follow best practices in food sanitation and safety. Cook food thoroughly and refrigerate it properly. Avoid serving risky foods such as raw oysters or uncooked eggs.

- Individuals with chewing and swallowing difficulties should avoid bite-size portions that can lodge in the throat and cause choking.

Tips for Chefs

- Older guests are quite likely to have questions about food intolerances, dietary restrictions, food preparation techniques and ingredients. Servers should be trained to communicate specific needs to the kitchen staff.

- Eating "early" and low-budget dining are common requests among older adult diners. Small portions, economical offerings and early dining options can add a new group of regular patrons, and they will have finished eating by the prime dining time.

- Older customers have smaller appetites. Be prepared for them to ask for smaller portions or to take leftover food home to use as another meal.

- Dental problems can make chewing difficult, and some older adults have swallowing problems, but healthful foods should not be limited unless the individual really cannot eat them.

For More Information

- Academy of Nutrition and Dietetics for research and information on nutrition and aging/older adults, **www.eatright.org** and **www.eatrightpro.org**

  - Position of the Academy of Nutrition and Dietetics: Food and Nutrition for Older Adults: Promoting Health and Wellness. **http://www.eatrightpro.org/resource/ practice/position-and-practice-papers/ position-papers/food-and-nutrition-for- older-adults-promoting-health-and-wellness.**

  - Position of the Academy of Nutrition and Dietetics: Food and Nutrition Programs for Community-Residing Older Adults. **http:// www.eatrightpro.org/resource/practice/ position-and-practice-papers/position- papers/food-and-nutrition-programs-for- community-residing-older-adults.**

  - Position of the Academy of Nutrition and Dietetics: Individualized Nutrition Approaches for Older Adults in Health Care Communities. **http://www.eatrightpro.org/resource/ practice/position-and-practice-papers/ position-papers/individualized-nutrition- approaches-for-older-adults**

- Becky Dorner & Associates, Inc. free information and resources on healthy aging and nutrition care for older adults, including publications, menus and recipes, and continuing education programs, **www.beckydorner.com**

  - Dorner, B. *Diet Manual: A Comprehensive Nutrition Care Guide*. Naples, FL: Becky Dorner & Associates, Inc; 2016. Dorner B. Policy & Procedure Manual: Food and Nutrition Guidelines for Health Care. Naples, FL: Becky Dorner & Associates, Inc; 2016.

  - *Making Mealtime Magic with Person Centered Dining*. Naples, FL: Becky Dorner & Associates, Inc; 2013.

  - Enhancing Nutritional Value with Fortified Foods: A Resource for Professionals. Available to members (membership is free): **http:// www.beckydorner.com/membersonly**

- Centers for Medicare & Medicaid Services (CMS), **www.cms.gov**

- State health departments for regulations on nursing homes and assisted living facilities (including food safety, sanitation and nutrition)

Meeting the Needs of Athletes

Essentials Experts

Jacqueline R. Berning, PhD, RD, CSSD, is associate professor and chair of the Biology Department at the University of Colorado at Colorado Springs. Jacqueline is board certified as a specialist in sports dietetics. She is sports dietitian for the Cleveland Indians and Colorado Rockies.

Nancy Clark, MS, RD, CSSD, counsels both competitive athletes and casual exercisers. Her successful private practice is located in Newton, Massachusetts. She focuses on nutrition for exercise, wellness and the management of eating disorders. Her clients run the gamut from Olympians to high school/college athletes, to "ordinary mortals," fitness exercisers and weekend warriors. She is Team Nutritionist for the Boston Red Sox and the author of *Nancy Clark's Sports Nutrition Guidebook*.

Whether feeding the casual exerciser or the professional athlete, there are some important points to keep in mind. Depending on the intensity and frequency as well as the type of activity, an athlete may require 3,000 to 6,000 calories per day. The optimal number of calories depends on age, body composition and environmental conditions. Healthful high-calorie foods are best for football and ice hockey players, as well as growing student athletes who want to maintain or increase their weight and muscle mass. In contrast, gymnasts, figure skaters, lightweight rowers and dancers must remain slim, so they seek healthful, low-calorie but high-satiety foods.

For people who exercise intensely for 90 minutes or more per day, refueling during exercise can be beneficial. Marathon runners, elite athletes and recreational sports participants who practice and train on a regular basis should pay extra attention to replenishing fluid and nutrient losses to maintain optimal blood sugar levels and maximize performance.

Key Nutrition Points

- All types of athletes should start every day with breakfast.
- Athletes need to eat evenly sized meals across the day for sustained energy.
- Serve a lean protein source at each meal combined with a source of carbohydrate (grain, fruit, starchy vegetables, such as potatoes).
- Carbohydrates from food (used to maintain blood sugar or stored as glycogen in the muscles) and fat are the primary fuel sources for exercise. For most athletes, 55% to 65% of calories should come from carbohydrates. Thirty percent or less of calories should come from fat. Protein needs are 1.2 to 1.7 grams of protein per kilogram of body weight, depending on the type of athletic activity, with the higher amount needs for weight-conscious athletes who are restricting calories.

- Hydration is critical. Athletes must drink plenty of beverages daily. It is recommended that athletes drink .6 ounces of fluid per pound of body weight per day. For example, a 150-pound person should drink 90 ounces of fluids (.6 x 150) daily. While weight-conscious athletes will want calorie-free beverages, athletes trying to maintain or gain weight will want juice, flavored milk, smoothies and shakes.

- Pre-game (pre-competition) meals should consist of foods that offer easily digested carbohydrates and lean proteins, such as pasta with tomato sauce and grilled chicken. Athletes wanting a hearty meal should eat it about 3 or 4 hours before competition, to allow time for food to clear the stomach before the event. During the hour before the event, some athletes might want another light meal, for example yogurt with fruit; oatmeal or granola with low-fat milk; a banana and peanut butter; or a smoothie made with low-fat yogurt, fruit and wheat germ. Avoid high-fat protein foods such as cheeseburgers or fried chicken. Offer plenty of beverages.

- The goal of a post-competition or post-workout meal is to replenish nutrients lost during exercise. Replacing lost fluid is an essential part of recovering. Good choices include water, juices, chocolate milk, fruit smoothies, and high-water-content fruit such as watermelon, grapes and oranges.

- Replacing the sodium, potassium and electrolytes lost through sweating is easy enough to do with food. Supplements are generally not recommended. Recovery foods high in essential electrolytes include potatoes, yogurt, orange juice, bananas and soup.

- The goal of recovery nutrition is to convert the body from a **catabolic state** (breakdown of muscle cells) to an **anabolic state** (building up of muscle cells). Immediately after exercise, the window is open for rapid nutrient delivery to muscle cells. Recovery is a three-step process:

  1. a meal or snack immediately after training,

  2. a meal approximately 1 hour later, and then

  3. frequent snacking on wholesome foods.

  Recovery meals and snacks should contain carbohydrates (45 to 75 grams) and lean protein (15 to 25 grams). Ideas for a snack immediately after exercise include chocolate milk, fruit smoothie made with a Greek yogurt base, trail mix or sandwiches. The recovery process is not complete until the athlete eats a meal within 30 minutes after training.

Best Choices

Most athletes need a carbohydrate-based diet focused on whole grains, fruits and vegetables. The need for protein may be high as well, so a consistent intake of protein and carbohydrates throughout the day is desirable along with a small amount of healthful fat. Female athletes often need more iron-rich foods, and vegetarian athletes need foods to compensate for any dietary shortfalls. Excellent choices include:

- Whole-grain pasta, bread and cereals
- Oatmeal
- Hearty stews
- Fruit smoothies
- Wild rice or brown rice
- All types of fruits
- Lean protein sources
- Cottage cheese
- Salads with lower-calorie dressings
- Fluids for hydration – plain and flavored low-fat milk and mineral waters, fruit juice and fruit spritzers

- Yogurt and frozen yogurt
- Iron-fortified breakfast cereals
- Chili with beans
- Baked lasagna
- Cornbread
- Bread or rice pudding

Foods to Limit

- Limit fried foods and high-fat foods that fill the stomach but leave the muscles unfueled.
- Limit foods with minimal nutritional value.

Tips for Chefs

Generally, athletes are not picky eaters; they are usually starving after exercise. New research on recovery nutrition shows, however, that eating a good carbohydrate source and a bit of protein can help an athlete recover faster if the foods are consumed shortly after exercise. Portable snacks that do not need refrigeration help in the recovery process. [14, 15]

For More Information

- Clark N. Nancy Clark's *Sports Nutrition Guidebook*. 5th ed. Champaign, IL: Human Kinetics; 2014.

- Karpinski, C, ed. Rosenbloom, CA, asst. ed. Sports Nutrition: A Practice Manual for Professionals. 6th ed. Chicago: The Academy of Nutrition and Dietetics; 2012.

- Dunford M, Doyle A. *Nutrition for Sport and Exercise*. 4th ed.Florence, KY: Wadsworth Publishing; 2018.

- Fink HH. Mikesky, AE, Burgoon, LA. *Practical Applications in Sports Nutrition*. 5th ed. Sudbury, MA: Jones and Bartlett; 2017.

- Thomas DT, Erdman KA, Burke LM. *Position of the Academy of Nutrition and Dietetics, Dietitians of Canada, and the American College of Sports Medicine: Nutrition and Athletic Performance*. JAND. 2016; 116(3): 501-528.

Banana Bread
Yield: 12 slices

Nancy Clark, sports nutritionist, Chestnut Hill, Massachusetts, says that this is her all-time favorite banana bread recipe. Banana bread is popular for carbohydrate loading and for snacking during long-distance bike rides and hikes. Add some peanut butter and you have a delicious, energizing sandwich.

Bananas, large, well-ripened	3	
Egg or	1	
Egg whites	2	
Canola oil	2	tablespoons
Milk, low-fat	⅓	cup
Sugar	⅓	cup
Salt	1	teaspoon
Whole-wheat flour	¾	cup
All-purpose flour	¾	cup
Baking soda	1	teaspoon
Baking powder	½	teaspoon

1. Preheat the oven to 350° F
2. Mash bananas with a fork.
3. Add egg, oil, milk, sugar, salt. Beat well.
4. Gently blend the flours, baking soda and baking powder, then add to the banana mixture and stir until moistened.
5. Pour into a 4" x 8" loaf pan that has been lightly oiled or sprayed with vegetable oil or lined with wax paper.
6. Bake for 45 minutes or until toothpick inserted near the center comes out clean.
7. Let cool for 5 minutes before removing from the pan.

Per Serving

Calories	150		Cholesterol	35	mg
Fat	3.5	g	Sodium	330	mg
Saturated Fat	0.5	g	Carbohydrates	28	mg
Trans Fat	0	g	Dietary Fiber	2	mg
Sugar	12	g	Protein	4	g

Source: Reprinted with permission from *Nancy Clark's Sports Nutrition Guidebook* 5th ed. (Human Kinetics Publisher, 2014)

Peanutty Energy Bars
Yield: 16 bars

Also from Nancy Clark: A delicious alternative to commercial products, this energy bar is perfect for traveling, hiking or biking. Variations include using cashews and cashew butter and/or a variety of dried fruits such as cranberries, cherries, blueberries or mangos.

Salted, dry-roasted peanuts	½	cup
Roasted sunflower seed kernels	½	cup
Raisins or other dried fruits	½	cup
Uncooked oatmeal	2	cups
Toasted rice cereal	2	cups
Peanut butter, crunchy or creamy	½	cup
Brown sugar, packed	½	cup
Light corn syrup	½	cup
Vanilla	1	teaspoon
Toasted wheat germ (optional)	¼	cup

1. Mix together peanuts, sunflower seeds, raisins, oatmeal, toasted rice cereal and wheat germ. Set aside.
2. Combine peanut butter, brown sugar and corn syrup. Microwave on high for 2 minutes. Add vanilla and stir until blended.
3. Pour the peanut butter mixture over the dry ingredients and stir until coated.
4. Press into a pan coated with vegetable spray (either a 8" x 8" or a 13" x 9" pan). Let stand for about an hour and then cut into 16 squares or bars.

Per Serving

Calories	230		Cholesterol	0	mg
Fat	9	g	Sodium	110	mg
Saturated Fat	1.5	g	Carbohydrates	33	mg
Trans Fat	0	g	Dietary Fiber	3	mg
Sugar	15	g	Protein	6	g

Source: Reprinted with permission from *Nancy Clark's Sports Nutrition Guidebook* 5th ed. (Human Kinetics Publisher, 2014)

Weight Management

Essentials Experts

Cheryl Forberg, RD, is a James Beard award-winning chef, a New York Times bestselling author and the former nutritionist for NBC's "The Biggest Loser," where her role is to help overweight contestants transform their bodies, health and ultimately, their lives. As a culinary expert and registered dietitian, she has shared cooking and nutrition tips with the contestants for eight seasons.

Marilyn Majchrzak, MS, RD, is the recently retired corporate menu development manager at Canyon Ranch in Tucson, Arizona. She was at Canyon Ranch for many years and was responsible for coordinating menu development with the chefs for all Canyon Ranch properties and projects.

Over the last 20 years, the problems of overweight and obesity in the United States have grown to epidemic proportions. Two-thirds of Americans are overweight or obese. The latest data from the National Center for Health Statistics show that 35% of U.S. adults age 20 and older – more than 60 million people – are obese. [16] Most Americans are either trying to lose weight (55%) or maintain their weight (22%) while 3% are trying to gain weight. [17] James O. Hill, MD, PhD, director of the Center for Human Nutrition at the University of Colorado Health Sciences Center and founder of the National Weight Control Registry, has found that the average American adult gains weight gradually – 1 to 2 pounds each year. This gain reflects eating about 100 calories more each day than needed to maintain weight. That means that all most adults need to do to prevent gaining weight is eat 100 fewer calories each day or exercise enough to burn 100 calories. [18] The solution might be as simple as lightening up a favorite coffee drink with nonfat milk, reducing the fat used in sauce preparation, trimming fat from meat, baking crispy foods instead of frying, or skipping soft drinks and switching to sparkling or plain water or low-fat milk. Other useful strategies are to simply reduce portion sizes or skip desserts or snacks if they are regularly eaten.

The World Health Organization considers obesity to be one of the top 10 causes of preventable death worldwide. [19] Overweight or obese individuals are at a higher risk for coronary heart disease, stroke, type 2 diabetes, certain types of cancers, hypertension (high blood pressure), sleep apnea and respiratory problems, osteoarthritis and other health problems.

When it comes to weight loss, there's no lack of diets promising fast results. But fad diets, which often eliminate foods or food groups that provide essential nutrients, can be unhealthy and tend to fail in the long run. Weight loss programs that promote fasting and special cookies or soups may result in quick weight loss, but they cannot be sustained. The key to achieving and maintaining a healthy weight isn't about short-term dietary changes. It's about a lifestyle that includes healthy eating and regular physical activity to achieve and maintain a healthy weight. Ensuring that the number of calories consumed is about equal to the number of calories the body uses for maintenance and activity will maintain that healthy weight.

Because genetics, amount of muscle mass, age and other factors influence a person's metabolic rate, different people need different levels of calories to lose, gain or maintain weight. Many Americans are fairly sedentary and do not exercise regularly, so their calorie needs are quite low. If they are not mindful of what they eat, they will gain weight. If they continue their same eating and exercise patterns as their metabolic rate decreases, they will gain weight.

Healthy weight management is about small steps that add up. Little changes in eating and activity level have a more positive impact on health than drastic changes, if for no other reason than it is easier to stick with smaller changes over time. Extreme diets, diets requiring purchasing "special" foods or products, and fast and intensive exercise regimens may work well at first, but lost weight rarely lasts.

The American public has long been obsessed with weight-loss programs and diet books. Plans come and go, but the truth is that any program that results in fewer calories consumed than needed to maintain weight will result in weight loss. Lack of exercise in conjunction with a low-calorie diet will cause the loss of both fat and muscle. People claim success on diets high in carbs, low in carbs, high in fat, low in fat, liquid diets, raw diets, home-delivered foods, frozen entrées and on and on. Most diets ultimately fail, however, because the dieter returns to his or her former eating habits and the lost weight returns, often plus more. The only weight-loss diets that seem to work in the long run are those that focus on portion size, include all food groups, reduce empty-calorie foods, increase nutrient-rich foods and incorporate healthy eating habits that can be sustained. WeightWatchers® is an example of such a program. It includes lifestyle changes that increase its success for long-term weight control.

Increasing physical activity and addressing behavioral and psychological issues that lead to emotional overeating are also important to long-term weight loss and maintaining desirable weight. People who lose weight and keep if off successfully usually exercise daily and are physically active.

Body Mass Index

Body mass index (BMI) can be a useful measure of overweight and obesity and is calculated from height and weight. It is an estimate of body fat and a good gauge of risk for diseases that can occur with more body fat. The higher your BMI, the higher the risk for certain diseases such as heart disease, high blood pressure, type 2 diabetes, breathing problems, and certain cancers. (See Appendix E for a BMI table.)

BMI Categories	BMI
Underweight	Below 18.5
Normal	18.5–24.9
Overweight	25.0–29.9
Obesity	30.0 and Above

Because athletes and people with lots of muscle mass, and relatively little body fat, can have a high BMI, this measure is not appropriate for them. Other techniques, such as bioelectrical impedance and certain body measurements, including waist circumference, are more useful in determining disease risk for them.

Do the Math

Managing a healthy weight can be a challenge, and the causes of obesity are complex, but the body's energy balance is straightforward. Maintaining weight is a matter of balancing calories consumed (from food and beverages) with calories expended (through exercise and maintaining body functions). Consuming more calories than the body needs results in weight gain in the form of stored energy or body fat. Consuming fewer calories than the body needs results in weight loss because the body will take energy from stored fat.

A pound of body fat is about 3,500 calories of stored energy. In other words, eating 3,500 more calories than the body needs results in the body's storing a pound of fat. Losing a pound of body fat entails eating 3,500 calories less than the body needs. Most successful weight loss is achieved at a rate of 1 to 2 pounds per week. Losing 1 pound of fat per week means eating 500 calories less than the body needs each day (3,500 calories divided by 7 days = 500 calories per day). An adult who needs 2,500 calories per day to maintain his or her weight would eat 2,000 calories per day (2,500 calories - 500 calories =2,000 calories) and lose about a pound a week or one could reduce intake by 100 calories per day and lose about one pound per month.

It is generally recommended that daily calorie intake not dip below 1,500 to 1,800 calories. When people consume too few calories, it is a challenge to get the vitamins, minerals, fiber and protein the body needs each day. And it is difficult to sustain a low-calorie diet when hunger sets in because of severe dietary restriction. The body will adapt to fewer calories and try to maintain itself to protect from starvation. The result can be that even fewer calories are needed to maintain weight.

As people age, particularly after age 50, metabolic rate slows and fewer calories are needed each following decade. The need for fewer calories makes maintaining or losing weight more challenging.

casebycase | Canyon Ranch Nutrition Basics

For the past 30 years, nutrition has been an exciting and integral part of the food and culinary program at the legendary Canyon Ranch. "We don't believe in dieting or in 'watching what we eat,'" explains Marilyn Majchrzak, MS, RD, recently retired corporate menu development manager at Canyon Ranch in Tucson, Arizona. "It's all about adopting a healthy weight philosophy – a lifelong strategy that involves understanding your own personal needs for food and being physically active enough so that weight management becomes achievable, sustainable and permanent," she says. "We believe in balance, moderation and savoring all the pleasures of eating well. We believe in food that nourishes the body and soul."

Canyon Ranch's corporate chef Scott Uehlein, who trained at the Culinary Institute of America, concurs. "Healthful cooking is real world cooking," he says. "Extreme diets are unsustainable – for chefs and customers. We stick to our basic philosophy: balance."

Canyon Ranch chefs work with a staff of nutritionists to ensure that every meal that comes out of the kitchen meets an exacting set of nutritional standards. "We start with fresh, clean and wholesome foods," says Marilyn. "At Canyon Ranch, fresh means foods that are local and regional, seasonal, and from sustainable sources. We define "clean foods" as free from pesticides and herbicide residues, hormones and antibiotics, unnecessary additives and preservatives, contaminants, and food-borne pathogens. Wholesomeness," she continues, "captures that old-fashioned sense of goodness. All really fresh food that's been cleanly grown and handled is wholesome. Eating it is an excellent way to support your health, manage your weight and live healthier longer."

"Guests at our resorts can 'self-monitor' their food intake," Scott explains. "At all our destination resorts, we have a comprehensive list of all the ingredients in everything we serve. People with special dietary needs can see exactly what they are eating."

Key Nutrition Points

Here are some key nutrition points from Canyon Ranch.

- Optimize protein portions to address individual needs and upsize nutrient-dense carbohydrates like vegetables, fruits and whole grains.

- Use a wide variety of plant ingredients. Vegetables, fruits, whole grains, beans, nuts and seeds, and herbs and spices are not only delicious and satisfying but also have the most power to prevent disease.

- Emphasize fiber from a wide variety of plant foods. The good news about fiber's health benefits appears to be never-ending.

- Use minimal added sugar and no artificial sweeteners. Canyon Ranch recipes call for a variety of natural sweeteners in minimal quantities, including cane sugar, honey and molasses.

- Provide meals and snacks that include protein, carbohydrate and small amounts of healthy fat. This combination satisfies both nutritional needs and appetite. Canyon Ranch chefs strive to balance each meal, including vegetarian options, with some protein-rich food. Protein offerings include beans plus soy foods, fish, eggs, low-fat dairy products, and the leanest cuts of poultry and red meat.

- Use healthy fats in moderation. Canyon Ranch chefs use special care in selecting fats and oils that are beneficial to health. Preferred choices are extra virgin olive oil and expeller-pressed canola oil, both rich in flavor and antioxidants. Also emphasize omega-3 fatty acids (found mainly in fish and flax seeds) and fats from other plant sources, including avocado and nuts. Minimize saturated fats and never use trans fats. Use cooking techniques such as braising, sautéing, grilling, broiling, baking and stir-frying.

- Season foods with an array of herbs and spices. Keep a careful eye on sodium, however, because most Americans regularly consume more salt than recommended. The goal is to allow the natural flavors of the food to shine. Canyon Ranch chefs prefer sea salt, which is a little lower in sodium and higher in other minerals than table salt.

Best Choices

- Serve plenty of real food that is fresh – lots of fresh fruits and vegetables, whole grains, lean proteins such as pork loin, chicken and turkey, occasional lean red meat, fish, lean dairy products, vegetable proteins such as beans and legumes, and good fats – avocado, flax, nuts, seeds and olive oil.

- If fresh produce is not available or affordable, frozen fruits and vegetables are good substitutes. Nearly any fruit and vegetable is better than no fruit and vegetable.

- Serve all food in moderate and appropriate portions.

- Prepare food with minimal fat and limit added sugar and salt.

- Foods that are cooked with healthful cooking techniques

Foods to Limit

- Refined grains like white rice, all-purpose flour and pasta
- Foods or ingredients high in sugar including granulated sugar, soft drinks, etc.
- High-fat cheeses, dairy products and sauces
- Foods with trans and/or saturated fats
- Fried foods unless used sparingly as a garnish
- Sugar and highly sweetened foods and sauces
- Salt and high-sodium sauces, prepared foods and condiments
- Cream-based soups, sauces and desserts and high-fat salad dressings
- Highly processed foods
- High-fat meats and processed meats
- Processed fat-free products
- Large portions
- Beverages containing alcohol (beyond one per day)

The quality of calories is just as important, if not more so, than the quantity.

Cheryl Forberg, RD
Nutrition advisor to television's "The Biggest Loser"

Help or Harm? Low-Calorie Sweeteners and Beverages

Diet beverages are widely available, and the general assumption has been that they are better than high sugar beverages for people who want to lose weight. While drinking a reasonable amount of diet soda, such as a can or two a day, isn't likely to cause harm, diet beverages are not a health drink. A few studies have suggested that low-calorie sweeteners may cause cravings for more sugar and/or lead to weight gain, but these studies have not changed the overall scientific consensus that low-calorie sweeteners can aid in weight management if the diet beverage replaces a sugared beverage that would ordinarily be consumed. While diet beverages do not have calories, they also do not have vitamins, minerals and phytochemicals that are in other beverage options.

A review of studies conducted over the past two decades has shown that low-calorie sweeteners can help with weight loss and/or maintenance if they are part of a healthy diet and exercise regimen. Certainly diet beverages and other sugar-free products that use low-calorie sweeteners are useful for people who have diabetes or other medical reasons to reduce sugar intake.

A study published in *Stroke*, a journal produced by the American Heart Association, drew on the health data of 82,000 women enrolled in a long-term study of women's health. Women who drank two or more artificially sweetened drinks had a 23% higher risk of strokes in general, and a 31% higher risk of strokes involving clotting in smaller blood vessels in the brain. They were also 29% more likely to suffer from heart disease and 16% more likely to die from any cause than other women in the study. [20]

Concerns about the potentially negative effect of carbonated beverages on bone health and concerns about artificial colors and flavors persist. Numerous other beverages choices are healthier, provide necessary liquids along with nutrients and are better for your guests, especially for children.

Tips for Chefs

- Many guests will have personal beliefs about dieting and what they want to fit into their diet regimen. Offer a variety of healthful choices that are low to moderate in calories.

- Offer skim milk, low-fat or fat-free salad dressing, sugar substitutes, diet soft drinks, unsweetened teas and other foods as options that dieters may expect – and delight them with plenty of other healthful options.

- If guests are on fad diets, low-carb, raw or other regimens for weight control, offerings should include some options suitable for them.

- Offer heart vegetables soups and salads that contain legumes and lean meats with light dressings.

- Look critically at the menu: Are there broth-based and vegetable soups without cream? Are there interesting salads that do not contain bacon, cheese, croutons or other high-fat ingredients? Are portions appropriate and not excessive? Are there a few desserts that are moderate in sugar and fat? Are half or smaller portions available? Are there whole-grain breads, rolls or crackers? Are there healthful olive oil dips or vegetable-based spreads for breads? Are raw, steamed, grilled or roasted vegetables available and abundant? Are there interesting options that feature legumes, seafood, poultry and lean meats? Do vegetarians have a reasonable selection? Is fresh fruit available as an appetizer, salad or dessert option? Are healthful cooking techniques used throughout the menu?

For More Information

- *Chemical Cuisine*, a guide to food additives when packaged foods are a more convenient choice, **www.cspinet.org**

- *Eat Wild*, guide to grass-fed and organic meat, poultry and dairy products including a list of suppliers of pasture-raised products, **www.eatwild.com**

- *Eating Well* magazine provides reliable current information on food and nutrition for home cooks and culinary professionals.

- Forberg C. *Flavor First: Cut Calories and Boost Flavor with 75 Delicious, All-Natural Recipes*. Flavor First Publishing; 2016.

- Forberg C. *The Biggest Loser Simple Swaps: 100 Easy Changes to Start Living a Healthier Lifestyle*. New York: Rodale; 2009.

- Institute for Agriculture and Trade Policy, Guides to Healthy Choices, **www.iatp.org**

- Krieger E. *You Have It Made: Delicious, Healthy, Do-Ahead Meals*. New York: Houghton Mifflin Harcourt. 2016.

- Local Harvest, sourcing local foods and community supported agriculture, **www.localharvest.org**

- Mullen MC, Shield J. *Academy of Nutrition and Dietetics Pocket Guide to Pediatric Weight Management*. Chicago, IL: Academy of Nutrition and Dietetics; 2nd, ed. 2017.

- Rolls B, Hermann M. *The Ultimate Volumetrics Diet: Smart, Simple, Science-Based Strategies for Losing Weight and Keeping It Off*. New York: HarperCollins Publishers; 2012.

- Uehlein S. *Canyon Ranch: Nourish Indulgently Healthy Cuisine*. New York: Viking Studio; 2009.

Cold Watermelon Ginger Soup with Mango

Serves: 10 servings, 3/4 cup each

Chef Scott Uehlein,
Formerly Corporate Executive Chef, Canyon Ranch, Tucson, Arizona

Watermelon, cubed 2 quarts	about 4	pounds
Ginger, minced, fresh	2	tablespoons
Green chili, chopped	¼	cup
Lime juice, fresh	¾	cup
Evaporated cane juice	⅓	tablespoons
Sea salt	½	teaspoon

Garnish

| Mango, diced, fresh | ¾ | cup |
| Cumin, whole seed | 1 | teaspoon |

1. Place all ingredients except for garnish in a blender container and puree until smooth. Strain through a sieve.

2. Place ¾ cup soup in a bowl and top with 1 tablespoon diced mango and a pinch of whole cumin seed.

Per Serving

Calories	60	Cholesterol	0	mg
Fat	0 g	Sodium	200	mg
Saturated Fat	0 g	Carbohydrates	16	mg
Trans Fat	0 g	Dietary Fiber	1	mg
Sugar	12 g	Protein	1	g

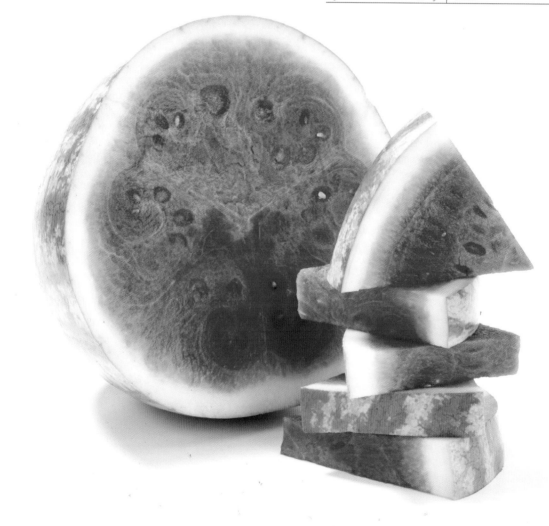

Seared Beef Tenderloin with Tomato Confit, Kale and Sage Polenta

Chef Scott Uehlein,
Formerly Corporate Executive Chef,
Canyon Ranch, Tucson, Arizona

Serves: 10, 1 filet with ¼ cup Tomato Confit,
⅓ cup Sautéed Kale and ⅓ cup Sage Polenta

Tomato Confit   Yield: 2 ½ cups

Roma tomato concasse	2 ½	cups
Olive oil, extra virgin	2	tablespoons
Sea salt	1	teaspoon
Black pepper, freshly ground	½	teaspoon
Garlic cloves	2	minced
Fresh thyme, chopped	2	tablespoons

Beef Tenderloin

Beef tenderloin filets	10 (2 ½ pounds)	4-ounce
Sea salt	½	teaspoon
Black pepper, freshly ground	½	teaspoon

Sautéed Kale   Yield: 3 ½ cups

Shallots, sliced	¼	cup
Kale, fresh, stems removed	2 (2 pounds)	bunches
Olive oil, extra virgin	1	tablespoon
Sea salt	1	teaspoon
Black pepper, freshly ground	½	teaspoon
Water	½	cup
Cider vinegar	⅓	cup

1. Preheat oven to 300° F.

2. Toss all ingredients for Tomato Confit together on a baking sheet. Roast for 20 to 30 minutes or until vegetables are cooked through and slightly caramelized.

3. Preheat grill or broiler.

4. Lightly season beef tenderloin filets with salt and pepper. Grill tenderloin filets for 3 to 5 minutes on each side or to desired doneness.

5. In a large sauté pan over medium heat, sauté shallots in olive oil. Add kale leaves, salt and pepper. Add water to steam and soften vegetables. Finish with vinegar.

6. Serve each beef tenderloin topped with ¼ cup Tomato Confit. Serve with ⅓ cup Sautéed Kale and ⅓ cup Sage Polenta.

Sage Polenta   Yield: 3 ¾ cups
Serves: 10- ⅓ cup each

Onion, finely minced	½	cup
Unsalted butter	2	tablespoons
Soft corn, cut from the cob	½	cup
2% milk	3 ¾	cups
Polenta	¾	cup
Sea salt	½	teaspoon
Black pepper, freshly ground	Pinch	
Evaporated cane juice	1	tablespoon
Parmesan cheese, grated	⅓	cup
Sage, fresh, chopped	1	tablespoon
Chives, fresh, chopped	2	tablespoons

1. In a large saucepan, sauté onion in butter over medium heat until translucent. Add corn and sauté briefly, about 30 seconds.

2. Add milk and bring to a boil. Using a wire whip, lightly whisk in polenta, salt, pepper and evaporated cane juice. Cook until thickened, about 3 minutes.

3. Add cheese, sage and chives and stir until cheese is melted.

Per Serving

Calories	320	Cholesterol	90	mg
Fat	14	g	Sodium	460	mg
Saturated Fat	4	g	Carbohydrates	13	mg
Trans Fat	0	g	Dietary Fiber	3	mg
Sugar	2	g	Protein	36	g

Meeting the Needs of Vegetarians

Essentials Expert

Jill Nussinow, MS, RD, aka The Veggie Queen™, is an expert in vegetarian, vegan and pressure cooking. In the past 25 years, she has taught thousands of people about the joys and delights of eating fresh, in-season plant foods. She is a speaker, writer and consultant on plant-food related topics.

According to The Academy of Nutrition and Dietetics and most health authorities, well-planned vegetarian diets are healthful and nutritionally adequate. People choose to become vegetarians for many reasons – including health, environmental, animal welfare, religion and ethics. Family or friends influence some people to become vegetarians.

Vegetarians are becoming more and more common as restaurant guests, in schools and on college campuses. In a Vegetarian Resource Group 2016 national poll conducted by Harris Poll, 3% of the U.S. population was identified as vegetarian and about half of those as vegan. [21] In that poll, thirty seven percent of the population always or sometimes eat vegetarian meals when eating out. About five percent always eat vegetarian or vegan meals when eating out. [22] All foodservice operators need to be creative in meeting these guests' preferences.

Generally, there are six different types of vegetarians:

- *Strict vegetarian* or *vegan*: Excludes all animal products including meat, poultry, fish, eggs, milk, cheese and other dairy products as well as ingredients from animal sources such as gelatin.
- *Lacto-vegetarian*: Excludes meat, poultry, fish and eggs but includes dairy products.
- *Lacto-ovo vegetarian*: Excludes meat, poultry and fish but includes eggs and dairy products. Most vegetarians in the United States fall into this category.
- *Raw vegan*: Includes raw vegetables and fruits, nuts and nut pastes, grain and legume sprouts, seeds, plant oils, sea vegetables, herbs and fresh juices. Excludes all food of animal origin, and all food cooked above 118° F.

- *Flexitarian*: A mostly vegetarian diet with an occasional meat consumption – "semi" or sometimes vegetarian.
- *Pescetarian*: A mostly vegetarian diet that includes fish and shellfish but excludes mammals and birds.

Eating more raw foods is certainly healthful and an easy way to incorporate more whole foods. Eating raw often takes as much work if not more, as eating cooked food, especially if you are relying on sprouting, dehydrating and fermenting, all of which take advance planning. Consequently, few people have the patience or desire to do it regularly. For example, you cannot decide to serve house-made sprouts on the spur of the moment; it takes several days to grow them.

Chefs often rely on vendors to supply prepared ingredients, but they are typically more expensive. Preparing sprouts or fermented foods is relatively inexpensive and can add a certain modern panache to a restaurant dish, hence the interest in "microgreens," which are truly sprouts (grown in soil). Dehydrated foods are great for when there is abundance. In my opinion, there's nothing quite like eating kale chips as a special treat. But again, advance planning is needed.

Jill Nussinow, MS, RD
The Veggie Queen™

Note: If purchasing sprouts, smell them to be sure they have a clean, fresh odor. Refrigerate them for use within two days. Some foodservice operations have "cutting gardens" that supply fresh snipped herbs and sprouts.

Key Nutrition Points

It is important for all vegetarians to choose a variety of foods, including plenty of whole grains, fruits, vegetables, legumes, nuts and seeds. In other parts of the world where meat is not available or is too expensive, people have learned to rely on plant-based sources of protein. Italian, Chinese, Spanish, Mexican, Thai, Indian and Japanese cuisines have many popular foods that are already vegetarian or easily adapted.

Vegetarianism is not simply a matter of cutting out meat and animal products; it is choosing a healthful diet without meat or animal products. Nutrients that should be of concern for vegetarians include:

Protein

Protein is found in most plant foods as well as animal foods. The body will make its own complete protein if a variety of foods and enough calories are eaten during the day. See Chapter 5 for a complete discussion of protein. Vegetarians need good non-meat sources of protein. These include:

- Beans and other legumes
- Soy products
- Whole grains
- Nuts and nut butters
- Dairy products (except for vegans)
- Eggs (except for vegans and lacto-vegetarians)

Vitamin B$_{12}$

Vitamin B$_{12}$ is found in all foods of animal origin, including eggs and dairy products. An adequate intake of vitamin B$_{12}$ is generally not a concern for vegetarians who eat some dairy products or eggs. Strict vegetarians or vegans, however, may need to supplement their diet by choosing a fortified breakfast cereal or by taking a vitamin B$_{12}$ (cobalamin) supplement of no more than 100% of the Daily Value. Good sources of B$_{12}$ include:

- Vitamin B$_{12}$-fortified foods – nutritional yeast, soymilk, meat analogs or ready-to-eat cereals (be sure to check the label)
- Dairy products
- Eggs

Calcium

Dairy products are the best sources of calcium. If dairy products are not included in the diet, adequate amounts of calcium can be obtained from plant foods. Lacto-vegetarians can get plenty of calcium from cow or goat milk, yogurt and cheeses. Pescetarians can get calcium from canned salmon and sardines or other seafood with soft edible bones or shells. Some other vegetarian-friendly sources of calcium are:

- Fortified soymilk, rice milk or almond milk
- Fortified breakfast cereals
- Soy products (tofu processed with calcium, soy nuts)
- Dark leafy green vegetables (spinach, kale, collard greens, turnip greens, bok choy, mustard greens)
- Calcium-fortified juices
- Sesame seeds and sesame butter (tahini)
- Almonds and almond butter
- Molasses

Iron

Vegetarians should eat a variety of foods with iron to meet the daily requirements for this important mineral. Good vegetarian-friendly food sources of iron include:

- Iron-fortified breakfast cereals
- Soy products (tofu, soybeans, tempeh, soy beverages)
- Dried and canned beans, lentils and other legumes
- Dark green leafy vegetables (spinach, beet greens, turnip greens)
- Some dried fruits (dried apricots, prunes, raisins)
- Molasses

Iron content listed in food composition tables can be misleading because relatively small amounts of iron from vegetable (non-heme) sources is absorbed by the body while iron from red meat sources (heme) is very well absorbed and utilized. Consuming a good source of vitamin C (citrus fruits, orange juice, peppers, tomatoes, etc.) at each meal increases iron absorption from non-meat foods. (More information on iron and its utilization is in Chapter 7.)

Best Choices

- Legumes, lentils, beans, peas, etc. (good sources of protein, fiber, iron, calcium, zinc and B vitamins)
- Soy products including tofu, tempeh, soymilk, etc.
- Vegetables
- Dried fruits (check labels; the drying process influences iron content)
- Grains of all types, particularly whole grains with bran and germ to provide protein, B vitamins, zinc and complex carbohydrates including fiber
- Dairy products and eggs (for vegetarians who will eat these foods)

Foods to Eliminate

- Meat and meat by-products
- Poultry
- Fish and seafood
- Milk, cheese and dairy products (for some vegetarians)
- Eggs (for some vegetarians)
- Honey (for vegans)
- Gelatin that is animal-derived (agar and carrageenan are vegetable-based sources)
- All ingredients and food processing chemicals derived from animal sources

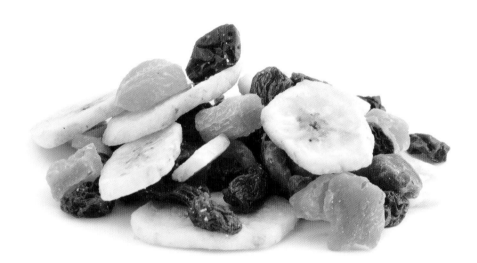

Tips for Chefs

- Chefs can show off their creativity with vegetarian and vegan appetizers, salads, soups, entrées and desserts. Generally, there should be a vegetarian option in each menu category plus at least one vegan entrée.

- Feature combination dishes that provide a variety of plant proteins to boost overall availability of protein – such as sandwiches on whole-grain bread and pita with hummus or portobello mushrooms and red peppers; red or brown rice with black beans; eggplant and sundried tomatoes on whole-grain pizza crust; bean and cheese burritos on whole-wheat tortillas; burgers made from beans or mushrooms; and beans in vegetable soups and in salads.

- Because meats, poultry, fish, etc. are not options for them, many vegetarians frequently serve pasta dishes at home. Chefs, however, should provide a variety of creative vegetarian options in addition to traditional pasta entrées.

- Canned beans typically have a lot of salt added to preserve texture. If liquid from the can is used, reduce the amount of salt in the recipe. If beans are drained, rinse them to reduce sodium.

- Roasted and grilled seasonal vegetables and fruit dishes, interesting salads, legumes and legume-vegetable combinations, hearty vegetable soups, ethnic foods without meat or dairy products, grain-vegetable combinations, flat breads or pizzas with vegetable toppings, and risottos and other grain-based dishes offer vegetarians options that may be popular with other guests as well.

- A combination of side dishes and garnishes from other menu items can make an interesting daily vegetarian offering.

For More Information

- American Test Kitchen editors. *The Complete Vegetarian Cookbook: A Fresh Guide to Eating Well With 700 Foolproof Recipes*. Vermont: American Test Kitchen. 2015.

- Berkoff N. *Vegan in Volume: Vegan Quantity Recipes for Every Occasion*. Baltimore, MD: Vegetarian Resource Group; 2000.

- Bittman M. *How to Cook Everything Vegetarian, 10th ed.* Boston: Houghton Mifflin, 2017.

- Davis B, Melina V. *Becoming Vegan: The Complete Guide to Adopting a Healthy Plant-Based Diet*. Summertown, TN: Book Publishing Company; 2014.

- Dragonwagon, C, *Bean By Bean: A Cookbook: More than 175 Recipes for Fresh Beans, Dried Beans, Cool Beans, Hot Beans, Savory Beans, Even Sweet Beans!*, 2012, Workman Publishing Company, New York.

- Madison D. *The New Vegetarian Cooking for Everyone*. Berkley, CA: Ten Speed Press; 2014

- Melina V, Davis B, Berry R. *Becoming Raw: The Essential Guide to Raw Vegan Diets*. Summertown, TN: Book Publishing Company; 2010.

- Natkin, M, *Herivoracious: A Flavor Revolution with 150 Vibrant and Original Vegetarian Recipes*. Boston, MA: The Harvard Common Press; 2012.

- Nussinow, J. *Vegan Under Pressure*. Boston, MA: Houghton Mifflin Harcourt; 2016.

- Nussinow J. *Nutrition Champs: The Veggie Queen's Guide to Eating and Cooking for Optimum Health, Happiness, Energy & Vitality*. Santa Rosa, CA: The Veggie Queen. 2014.

- Pant P. *The Indian Vegetarian Cookbook*. New York: Phaidon, 2018.

- Polenz K. *Vegetarian Cooking at Home with The Culinary Institute of America*. New York: John Wiley & Sons, Inc.; 2012.

- Stauch C. *Vegetarian Viet Nam*. New York: WW Norton Co, 2018.

- Vegetarian Resource Group, **www.vrg.org**

Black Bean Quinoa Burger

Serves: 10

Jill Nussinow, MS, RD
The Veggie Queen™, Santa Rosa, California

This recipe will likely work with any cooked grain or bean with slight adjustments in amounts. It is good served with a fruit or vegetable salsa. Use canned, drained and rinsed black beans. If prepared in advance, finish in a sauté pan or on a griddle.

Quinoa, cooked	¾	cup
Black beans, cooked	1	cup
Onion, chopped	¾	cup
Garlic cloves	3	
Fresh herbs such as parsley, basil or cilantro	¼	cup
Nutritional yeast	2	tablespoons
Salt, only if using fresh cooked, not canned, beans	½	teaspoon
Hemp seeds (optional)	2	tablespoons

1. Preheat the oven to 350° F

2. Put the quinoa, beans and onion in the food processor. Pulse a few times until slightly mixed. Add the garlic, herbs, yeast and salt, if using. Pulse again, adding 1-2 tablespoons bean liquid if it needs it. Stir in hemp seeds. Form into patties.

3. Bake on oiled baking sheet for 10 minutes. Turn over and bake another 10 minutes.

Per Serving

Calories	80	Cholesterol	0	mg
Fat	1	g	Sodium	280	mg
Saturated Fat	0	g	Carbohydrates	14	mg
Trans Fat	0	g	Dietary Fiber	3	mg
Sugar	1	g	Protein	5	g

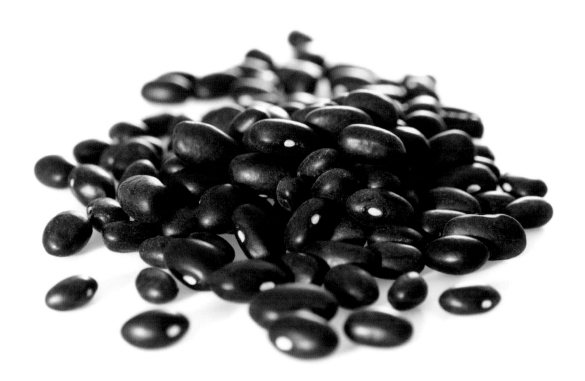

Religious Considerations

Chefs should understand the religious dietary practices of the communities they serve. For example, menus might be modified for Lent and other fast days when some guests will observe dietary restrictions. Many religions advocate vegetarianism; guests from these faith traditions can select from among vegetarian choices on a regular menu. Accommodating the dietary restrictions of observant Jews and Muslims requires substantial knowledge. Here our experts on kosher (Jewish) food and halal (Muslim) food practices share information for chefs to use to better understand the needs of these guests.

World Religions, Food Practices and Restrictions, and Rationales for Behavior

Religion	Practice or Restriction	Rationale
Protestants	Few food restrictions or fasting observations Moderation in eating and drinking, and exercise is promoted	God made all animal and natural products for humans' enjoyment. Gluttony and drunkenness are sins to be controlled.
Roman Catholicism	Meat restricted on certain days Fasting practiced	Restrictions are consistent on specified days of the church year.
Seventh-day Adventist	Pork prohibited and meat and fish avoided Vegetarian diet encouraged Alcohol, coffee and tea prohibited	Diet satisfies the practice to "honor and glorify God."
Mormonism	Alcohol and beverages containing caffeine prohibited Moderation in all foods Fasting practiced	Caffeine is addictive and leads to poor physical and emotional health. Fasting is the discipline of self-control and honoring God.
Eastern Orthodox Christianity	Restrictions on meat and fish Fasting selectively	Observance of holy days includes fasting and restrictions to increase spiritual progress.
Judaism (Orthodox; conservative, reconstructionist and reform Jews may or may not follow these dietary practices.)	Pork and shellfish prohibited Meat and dairy at same meal prohibited Meat only from hindquarter of animals; only kosher meat permitted Leavened food restricted during Passover Fasting on Yom Kippur	Land animals that do not have cloven hooves and that do not chew their cud are forbidden as unclean (e.g., hare, pig, camel). Kosher practice is based on the Torah.
Buddhism	Meat discouraged in favor of vegetarian diet Moderation in all foods Fasting required of monks	Natural foods of the earth are considered most pure. Monks of some sects avoid all solid food after noon.
Hinduism	Beef prohibited Other meat and fish restricted Alcohol avoided Numerous fasting days	Cow is sacred and can't be eaten, but products of the "sacred" cow are pure and desirable. Fasting promotes spiritual growth.

Religion	Practice or Restriction	Rationale
Islam	Pork and certain birds prohibited Alcohol prohibited Coffee/tea/stimulants avoided Fasting from all food and drink during specific periods	Eating is for good health. Failure to eat correctly minimizes spiritual awareness. Fasting has a cleansing effect on evil elements.
Rastafarianism	Meat and fish restricted Vegetarian diets only, with salts, preservatives and condiments prohibited Herbal drinks permitted Alcohol, coffee and soft drinks prohibited Marijuana used extensively for religious and medicinal purposes	Pigs and shellfish are scavengers and are unclean. Foods grown with chemicals are unnatural and prohibited. Biblical texts support use of marijuana and other herbs.
Baha'i	All foods allowed No alcohol in any form	Living simply and abstaining from alcohol and mind-altering drugs benefits spiritual development, reduces illness and has a good effect on character and conduct.
Jainism	Ascetic practices Vegans Avoid onions and garlic Avoid honey, eggs, figs Avoid root vegetables Generally, no eating after dark	Do no harm to any creature or to the environment. Onions and garlic increase sexual desire. Root vegetables are forbidden because insects are killed in their harvest. Eating after sundown might kill minute organisms that emerge after dark.
Sikhism	Halal and kosher meat forbidden Alcohol forbidden Simple, natural food preferred	Sikhs do not believe in ritual killing; thus, no halal or kosher meat is allowed. Consuming no alcohol or drugs promotes mental and physical fitness. Whether a Sikh eats meat or is vegetarian depends on personal interpretation of the writings of Guru Granath Sahib Ji. All food served in gurdwara (Sikh place of worship) is vegetarian.

Adapted from: Waibel RA. Religion and dietary practices. *Nutrition and Well-Being A to Z*, **www.encyclopedia.com/doc/1G2-3436200236.html**

Kosher

Essentials Expert

Tina Wasserman is the author of *Entrée to Judaism, A Culinary Exploration of the Jewish Diaspora* and the food authority for the URJ Reform Jewish movement for a decade. She is a highly respected food educator, lecturer and Jewish culinary historian. For more than 40 years, her hands-on approach to all facets of food has had broad appeal to students throughout the United States and Europe.

"The word 'kashrut,'" Tina Wasserman explains, "refers to the body of Jewish law dealing with what foods we can and cannot eat and how those foods must be prepared and eaten. Kashrut comes from the Hebrew root kaf-shin-reish, meaning fit, proper or correct. The more commonly known word **kosher**, also comes from this root and describes food that meets these standards."

According to the 2013 Pew Research Center Survey, *A Portrait of Jewish Americans*, 22% of American Jews report that they keep kosher in the home. [23] This number includes the vast majority of the Orthodox community as well as many Conservative, Reform and Reconstructionist Jews. Some keep kosher at home but will eat "kosher style" while dining out. This means that they will eat foods that are allowed by law but are not certified kosher (chicken or hamburger, for example), and they won't eat dairy products and meat products together on the same plate. Others will avoid breaking the laws of kashrut when dining out by eating a vegetarian dish or fish (not seafood that is unkosher) and dairy products. People who are strictly kosher will not eat in any facility that isn't supervised by a rabbi. They will not eat or drink from plates that have been used for non-kosher foods.

Many vegetarians (not vegans) pick kosher foods because a **pareve** label means no meat or dairy products are included as ingredients. Rules for the humane treatment of animals make kosher and halal attractive to individuals concerned about animal welfare. Kosher meat and other kosher foods must be inspected and certified by authorized rabbis who follow strict rules for sanitation.

Keep in mind, however, that a kosher label does not mean a food is a healthful choice. For example, the washing and salting of kosher poultry reduces the possibility of salmonella but increases sodium content. Many highly processed packaged cookies and snacks carry a kosher insignia. Deep fried foods may have all kosher ingredients

Key Nutrition Points

- Shellfish, fish without scales, and pork are not allowed.
- Kosher cuts of meat come only from the front of the animal above the sciatic nerve. Sirloin, tenderloin, rump roast, etc. are non-kosher cuts.
- If certified-kosher meat or poultry is used, always reduce the amount of salt in the recipe. The raw meat has been salted and rinsed to conform to Jewish dietary laws, and some salt remains.
- Do not include milk-based foods in recipes or meals containing meat. Dairy foods and meat foods may not be served at the same meal. For example, fried chicken is acceptable and so is macaroni and cheese, but serving them together at the same meal is not appropriate; chicken cannot be soaked in buttermilk before breading.
- Do not include chicken or beef base in a sauce that will contain butter or milk products.
- Different plates and eating and cooking utensils must be used for meat and dairy foods
- Dairy products, fish products and egg products may be served together according to most kosher authorities. Fish, eggs, fruits, vegetables and grains are neutral and can be served with either dairy or meat meals.
- Just about any ethnic cuisine can conform to keeping kosher.

- Thousands of products bear symbols indicating they are certified kosher. Look for a U within an O to represent the Union of Orthodox Rabbis or a K in a triangle to represent the Conservative Jewish Movement's stamp of approval. Other symbols exist, but these two are the most prevalent. Some very observant Orthodox Jews require the seal of specific certifying groups in addition to the circle U or K designation.

- Foods that are kosher and marked pareve have no milk or meat ingredients and can be used with either meat or dairy/milk meals. Mayonnaise (certified kosher) may be used for all food preparations if listed as pareve. Some non-dairy creamers contain thickeners made from gelatin (or animal products) and may be used only with meat meals if certified kosher. Cream or milk may be used only with milk/dairy meals.

- Adherence to Jewish dietary laws varies among people of the Jewish faith. Many do not adhere to any of the dietary laws and eat everything; some will not eat pork and/or shellfish; while others will eat only in kosher restaurants or homes and will eat only foods prepared and packaged in kosher kitchens. Kosher kitchens have strictly separated equipment, dishes and tools used to prepare dairy and meat products. Authorized rabbis must inspect these kitchens regularly.

Best Choices

- Fish and kosher chicken are the easiest to prepare given normal kitchen routine and recipes. Many favorites such as hamburgers (from kosher beef) are acceptable as well; however, cooking equipment must be used exclusively for kosher food.

- Vegetarian dishes using cheese (marked kosher) and tofu as the protein base do not have to be adjusted.

- Soy creamers and coconut milk are kosher substitutes for the cream in cream-style sauces.

- All oils are kosher.

- Vegetable oils may be used in all types of dishes.

- Serve plenty of fruits, vegetables and grains. All can be served with meat or dairy meals.

- Grilled, marinated meats (such as lamb chops or shish kabobs) and recipes that use small cubes of

meat are popular because many tender cuts of meat are not kosher. These cooking techniques tenderize tougher cuts.

- Sautéed, grilled, roasted or oven-fried chicken is popular as are fried cutlets (schnitzel).

- Prepare pizza with (kosher) meat but no cheese (or cheese pizza with no meat) or pasta with cheese but no meat. Either type of pizza may have vegetables. Kosher non-dairy, soy-based cheese substitutes are available.

- Use pareve margarine (no milk solids) and soy-based creamer instead of butter or cream in any meal containing meat and in making a béchamel or other sauces served with meat. Pareve non-dairy whipped topping, cream or coffee lightener may be used as well but note that non-dairy creamers are often sweetened and may need testing when used in place of cream in cooking.

Foods to Limit

Foods prohibited in the diets of those who keep kosher include all pork products, all shellfish and mollusks, fish without fins and scales (shark, sturgeon, catfish, octopus, squid, swordfish), cuts of meat from the hindquarters of animals (loin, sirloin, strip and porterhouse steaks, filet mignon, round, flank, etc.) and meat from animals that do not have cloven hooves and chew their cud (most game meats). Eating hare (rabbit), camel, birds of prey, reptiles, eel and insects is also forbidden. All meat that is non-kosher, that has not been slaughtered, salted, inspected and blessed by specially authorized rabbis, is not eaten. Most people who keep kosher eat foods that bear kosher symbols that ensure that food is appropriate. Some individuals who keep kosher will buy produce only from certain purveyors or restaurants (even kosher ones) because vegetables such as broccoli may have insects that would make these usually neutral foods unkosher.

In addition to selecting only kosher foods, the chef must be particularly careful to avoid serving any meat or meat-derived ingredient with a dairy meal or any dairy-based ingredient with a meat meal. Kitchen practices also require separate cooking equipment for meat and dairy food preparation and separate sinks for cleaning dishes and equipment.

Tips for Chefs

- A kosher kitchen has separate sets of utensils, dishes, etc. for meat/poultry and dairy/milk meals. Another set of dishes and utensils are used only for Passover. Kosher-certified cleaning products are required, but most detergents are certified. Disposables are often used to ensure that there has been no prior contact with either meat or milk meals.

- Unless a kitchen is strictly kosher and supervised by rabbis, chefs can serve only "kosher-style" food. In many situations, including catering, foodservice operators purchase prepared kosher foods in sealed containers to serve to kosher guests or customers.

- Read ingredient lists carefully. Look for kosher symbols on packaged foods. Remember that although there are kosher meats and kosher dairy products, they cannot be served together.

- Use vegetable broth when cooking foods for dairy meals.

- All foods in the same meal must be entirely meat or dairy. For example, if the entrée or salad contains meat, the dessert or salad dressing at that meal cannot contain any dairy products. Neutral foods can be served with either.

- For those who keep kosher, several hours must elapse between meat and milk meals; the time varies based on personal religious practices.

- Dried mushrooms or sun-dried tomatoes will add a salty or umami taste and may be used in place of small amounts of bacon or smoked meats in some recipes.

- Special dietary rules are observed on holidays – for example, fasting on Yom Kippur and eating only unleavened bread (matzos) during Passover.

For More Information

- Blau E, Deitsch T, Light C. *Spice and Spirit: The Complete Kosher Jewish Cookbook*. Brooklyn, NY: Lubavitch Women's Cookbook Publications; 1997.

- Marks, G. *Encyclopedia of Jewish Foods*. Hoboken, NJ: John Wiley & Sons; 2010.

- Nathan J. *Jewish Cooking in America*. New York: Alfred Knopf; 1994.

- Nathan J. *Joan Nathan's Jewish Holiday Cookbook*. New York: Schoken Books, Random House; 2004.

- Nathan J. *King Solomon's Table: A Culinary Exploration of Jewish Cooking from Around the World*. New York: Knopf; 2017.

- Orthodox Union, **http://oukosher.org/index.php/ common/article/ou_symbols**

- Rich TR. *Kashrut: Jewish Dietary Laws*, **www.jewfaq.org/kashrut.htm**

- Roden C. *The Book of Jewish Food: An Odyssey from Samarkand to New York City*. New York: Penguin Books; 1999.

- Saltsman A. *The Seasonal Jewish Kitchen: A Fresh Take on Tradition*. New York: Sterling Epicure; 2015.

- Star-K Kosher Certification, **www.star-k.org**

- Wasserman T. *Entrée to Judaism: A Culinary Exploration of the Jewish Diaspora*. New York: URJ Books and Music; 2010.

- Zeidler J. *The Gourmet Jewish Cook*. New York: William Morrow Cookbooks; 1999.

Chicken Fesenjan with Walnuts and Pomegranate Syrup

Serves: 10

Tina Wasserman, Author, *Entrée to Judaism:*
A Culinary Exploration of the Jewish Diaspora,
Dallas, Texas

This dish holds well and can be prepared in advance. The combination of nuts and pomegranate syrup is a traditional Middle Eastern flavor profile. This dish is excellent for guests who keep kosher. Serve it with Basmati rice or Israeli couscous. Most of the fat in this recipe comes from the walnuts, which are high in heart-healthy fats.

Walnuts, pieces	1 ⅓	cup
Onions, diced	2	medium
Olive oil	5	tablespoons, divided
Tomato paste	¼	cup
Pomegranate molasses or syrup	¼	cup
Honey	¼	cup
Lemon juice	2	tablespoons
Kosher salt	½	teaspoon
Black pepper	¼	teaspoon
Cinnamon	1	teaspoon
Water	½	cup
Chicken stock	1 ½	cup
Chicken, breast or thighs, skinless	10	each

1. Toast the walnut pieces in a 350° F oven until fragrant. Remove from oven and cool. Reserve ⅓ cup for garnish.

2. Sauté onion in 3 tablespoons olive oil. Chop onions and walnuts in a food processor to a coarse paste. Add the tomato paste, pomegranate molasses, honey, lemon juice, spices and water and process until mixed. Set aside.

3. Sauté chicken in remaining 2 tablespoons of oil. Brown chicken on both sides. Remove and hold.

4. Deglaze the pan with chicken stock. Add walnut-onion sauce mixture and stir. If necessary, adjust seasonings by adding more honey or lemon juice to the mixture to get a balanced sweet/sour taste. Return chicken to pan. Cover pan.

5. Put in 350° F oven for 35 minutes or until meat is tender. Baste chicken several times while cooking.

6. When serving, garnish with reserved toasted walnuts.

Per Serving

Calories	370		Cholesterol	85	mg
Fat	18	g	Sodium	180	mg
Saturated Fat	2.5	g	Carbohydrates	17	mg
Trans Fat	0	g	Dietary Fiber	2	mg
Sugar	13	g	Protein	35	g

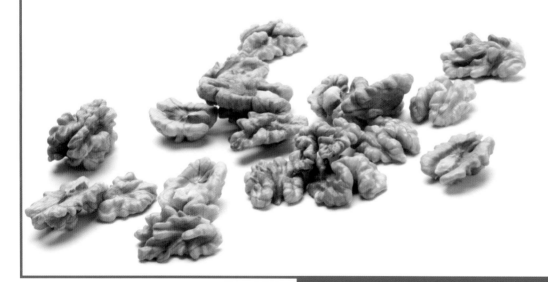

Halal

Because many chefs have limited knowledge of Islamic food practices and beliefs, our experts have explained them here in some detail.

Key Nutrition Points

Many Muslims are observant and adhere to the dietary restrictions that follow. Others of the Muslim faith, however, are far less stringent in adhering to dietary restrictions.

Requirements for Meat and Poultry

No pork is permitted in any form. Animals must be of an acceptable halal species, such as cattle and chicken. Animals and birds must be slaughtered by a Muslim of sound mind and blessed by pronouncing the name of Allah. A sharp knife must be used to severe the jugular vein, carotid arteries, trachea and esophagus, and blood must be drained out completely. The slaughtering must be done by hand with the complete removal of blood from the carcass.

Islam places great emphasis on humane treatment of all living things including animals. Meat that is not slaughtered in the Islamic manner is not suitable for Muslims. Because the rules for slaughter are similar, some Muslims eat kosher meat, although the rules of who does the slaughtering and the blessings differ. Any by-products of meat and poultry, such as beef fat or chicken broth, must come from an animal slaughtered in the Islamic way. Unlike those observing kosher rules, Muslims can eat meat and dairy together.

Vegetable soups that contain chicken or beef stock that are not halal are unsuitable for consumption by Muslims. Other ingredients that may be of animal origin include emulsifiers such as mono- and di-glycerides, which may be made from beef fat, lard or vegetable. If the source is not listed on the label as vegetable, the product is "mashbooh" (doubtful). Another ingredient of concern is glycerin or glycerol, which can be sourced from animals or plants; only the type from a vegetable source is permissible.

Those who observe the dietary tenets of Islam are usually aware which restaurants and grocery stores sell halal "zabihah meat." Some Muslims do not eat any meat or poultry when dining out, preferring instead to order vegetarian fare or seafood. Many halal meat products and other halal meat-based products are now available for foodservice and retail use. For information on how to obtain packaged halal-certified meat products, contact the Islamic Food and Nutrition Council of America at **www.ifanca.org**.

Requirements for Fish and Seafood

Due to the different schools of Islamic jurisprudence and certain cultural practices, some Muslims may not eat fish without scales such as catfish, while others will not eat mollusks and crustaceans, often referred to as "makrooh" (disliked). Various seafood flavors, such as shrimp flavors used in sauces, may be a concern.

Requirements for Eggs and Dairy Products

Milk and eggs from halal animals can be consumed without restrictions. The source of vitamins used in fortification can be questionable. Vitamin A sometimes includes gelatin as a carrier, which could be from pork or beef. If the source of the vitamin A is unknown, the vitamin is questionable, or mashbooh. Because gelatin is obtained after the animal is slaughtered, the animal must be Islamically slaughtered for that gelatin to be halal. Porcine gelatin can never be halal. Vitamin D is sometimes derived from lanolin; sheep's wool is an accepted source. Devout Muslims want to make sure that the source of vitamins, whether in milk or other products, is plant-based or synthetically produced. If synthetic, then the starting material should be non-animal.

Enzymes used during cheese making and whey products should be from microbial sources. Halal animal enzymes are rare; therefore, microbial enzymes used for cheese and whey are acceptable. Milk and egg products can become mashbooh if emulsifiers, mold inhibitors and other functional ingredients are from non-halal sources. For example, there may be vitamin A added to butter or gelatin in sour cream. Some cheeses and other dairy products are certified as halal and carry a crescent M logo on the packaging.

Plants and Vegetables

This category is inherently halal except for alcoholic drinks or other intoxicants. In addition, vegetables that are processed using equipment also used for meat can be cross-contaminated. Certain ingredients derived from animal sources, such as mono- and diglycerides or cysteine, make these vegetables unacceptable choices.

L-cysteine is an amino acid used in commercial bakery products. L-cysteine derived from human hair is not acceptable; however, some Islamic certifying groups consider duck feathers an acceptable source for this amino acid ingredient. Others allow only vegetarian sources of l-cysteine. For observant Muslims, monitoring processing and production methods is necessary to keep halal status intact.

Key Terms

Halal – permissible and lawful

Haram – prohibited

Mashbooh – doubtful

Makrooh – disliked or detested

Zabihah – meat slaughtered by a Muslim according to Islamic law

Islam is a religion that is a complete way of life. Islam is often connected with the people of Middle Eastern origin, but it is for all Muslims. Commandments on how to live life are found in the Quran (divine book from Allah) and the Sunnah of Prophet Muhammad.

Followers of Islam are advised to eat moderately; to eat only permissible and pure foods; to eat with three or five fingers; to wash your hands prior to eating; to invoke Allah's bounties prior to eating; to thank Him after eating; and to drink water while sitting down.

Food is central to our lives and society because it brings people together, creates harmony and creates a sense of belonging. For a Muslim, food brings all these good things along with nourishment. Food becomes an act of worship and a way to attain good deeds in Islam. The goal of life is to be obedient to Allah. The life of a Muslim revolves around what is permissible (halal) and what is prohibited (haram).

Miriam Majeed
Formerly with the Islamic Food and Nutrition Council of America

Sanitation and Cross Contamination

In food production, halal avoids cross-contamination of halal foods with non-halal or animal-based foods or ingredients. Certain equipment can be marked as "halal only." For non-meat products, equipment can be used for halal items after thorough washing. If meat items are being served in the same facility, it is best to use the same pans and equipment for halal and vegetarians, provided there is no alcohol or any other doubtful ingredients in the vegetarian dish.

Chemicals used for cleaning, including soaps and foams, should be checked to ensure they contain no animal products or alcohol. Check the Islamic Food and Nutrition Council of America, **www.ifanca.org**, for lists of food and cleaning products certified as halal.

Best Choices

- All fruits and vegetables
- Eggs
- Meat, poultry and dairy products, if certified as halal
- Vegetarian salads, soups and entrées
- Fish and seafood
- Grains
- Legumes
- Vegetable oils
- Sugar and sweeteners
- Herbs and spices

Foods to Limit

Foods that are "haram" (not permissible) include:

- Animals dead before slaughtering
- Blood or blood by-products
- Pork including all its by-products (for example, gelatin in any form)
- Animals not slaughtered according to halal rules
- Intoxicants of all types, including alcohol and drugs
- Carnivorous animals with fangs such as wolves, lions, dogs or tigers
- Birds with sharp claws (birds of prey) such as eagles, owls, falcons or vultures
- Certain land animals such as frogs or snakes

Alcohol is not permitted in any form, even if it may evaporate in cooking. Alcohol naturally present in fruits is acceptable in small amounts. Alcohol used for technical reasons, such as in vanilla or other flavor carriers, may be permitted. Certain halal-certifying organizations, such as the Islamic Food and Nutrition Council of America, maintain that a product should contain less than 0.1% grain alcohol. A Muslim cannot buy, sell, raise, transport, slaughter or derive benefit from swine or alcohol.

Once something is haram it cannot be halal no matter what science may show, no matter how clean that animal might become and no matter what justifications anyone might suggest. In addition, there is a gray area between halal and haram called "mashbooh," which can involve a simple ingredient such as whey in a chocolate candy bar. If the source of enzyme used during the whey production for that candy bar is unknown, the food is considered doubtful and should not be eaten.

Lentil Curry

Miriam Majeed, *Food Technologist, formerly with*
the Islamic Food and Nutrition Council of America, Park Ridge, Illinois

Yield: 7 cups
Serves: 10, ³/₄ **cup**

This recipe is suitable for halal, vegans, vegetarians and others. Serve over rice with pita or naan bread and a salad.

Red lentils	2	cups
Vegetable broth	6	cups
Oil, canola	¼	cup
Onions, diced	2	medium
Garlic cloves, diced or crushed	4	teaspoons
Ginger root, peeled and chopped	2	tablespoons
Curry powder	4	teaspoons
Red chili powder	½	teaspoon
Cumin, ground	2	teaspoons
Coriander, ground	2	teaspoons
Salt	1	teaspoon
Pepper	½	teaspoon
Tomatoes, chopped	1 can	(14 ½ ounces)

1. Heat vegetable broth in pot until boiling. Add lentils and boil for one minute. Reduce heat to a simmer and simmer lentils until they resemble a thick paste.

2. While lentils are simmering, heat oil in frying pan. Add onion, garlic and ginger. Sauté until soft. Add curry, chili, cumin, coriander, salt and pepper, sauté for 2-3 minutes. Add tomatoes and cook for another 3-5 minutes.

3. Add fried spice mixture into lentil paste, stir and cook an additional 15-20 minutes over very low heat.

Per Serving

Calories	220	Cholesterol	0	mg
Fat	7 g	Sodium	370	mg
Saturated Fat	0 g	Carbohydrates	29	mg
Trans Fat	0 g	Dietary Fiber	7	mg
Sugar	4 g	Protein	12	g

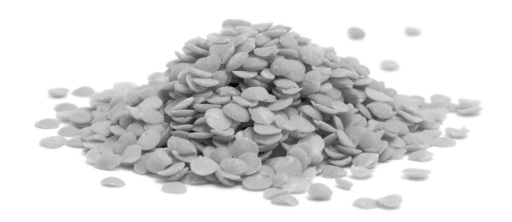

Tips for Chefs

- Sometimes customers will ask you to prepare foods in separate oil, change your gloves or use clean utensils to ensure that there has been no exposure to animal or non-halal products. Just do it.

- Muslims may request a scrambled egg if they are unable to determine the halal status of other foods on the menu.

- To provide adequate information to customers, chefs who serve Muslim patrons should keep product specification sheets.

- If you have questions about how to prepare halal, contact a halal-certifying agency that works with foodservice operators to help accommodate halal in the kitchen.

For More Information

- Helou A. *Feast: Food of the Islamic World*. New York: Ecco/Harper Collins, 2018.

- Hussaini MM. *Islamic Dietary Laws and Practices*. Bedford Park, IL: Islamic Food and Nutrition Council of America; 1983.

- Islamic Food and Nutrition Council of America, Halal Foodservice Kit, **http://www.ifanca.org/Assets/ PopularLinks/Halal%20Foodservice%20Kit.pdf**

- Maffei Y. *My Halal Kitchen: Global Recipes, Cooking Tips, and Lifestyle Inspiration*. Chicago, IL: Agate Surrey; 2016.

- Riaz MN, Chaudry MM. *Halal Food Production*. Boca Raton, FL: CRC Press; 2003.

- Regenstein JM, *The Cornell Kosher and Halal Food Initiative*, 2007 Impact Statement. Cornell University; 2007.

Opportunities for Chefs

Age, lifestyle and religious preference have a significant influence on the food people choose to eat. This chapter looked at the nutrition and basic menu planning requirements for children, aging adults, athletes, vegetarians, the weight-conscious, and people of the Jewish and Muslim faiths. Understanding the special needs of these groups gives you a head start in creating dishes and designing menus that appeal to the patrons you want to attract.

Learning Activities

1. Select a menu from a foodservice operation that you work in or visit frequently. Develop vegetarian options for each menu category.

2. You are catering a function for a religious group. Select a religion and plan the menu. Detail what type of function it is, how many people are attending and why you selected each menu item.

3. Develop five recipes for a spa. Include the following: breakfast item, appetizer, dessert, main course, salad and salad dressing.

Chapter Thirteen

Serving Guests with Special Health Needs

Learning Objectives | *After completing this chapter, you should be able to:*

- Explain nutritional meal planning for guests with special health needs
- Plan menus for guests with special health needs
- Apply the American Heart Association nutrition recommendations in planning and preparing menu for patrons with cardiovascular disease
- Explain the DASH diet for the control of hypertension
- Discuss the relationship between cancer and diet
- Identify best food choices and poorest food choices for those with diabetes mellitus and explain why
- Describe the digestive process and contrast three digestive diseases
- Differentiate food allergies, intolerances and aversions
- Identify the most common allergens and at least 10 foods that include each of them
- Explain what gluten intolerance is and the dietary restrictions required to control it

Glance across a crowded dining room, a bustling hospital or school cafeteria, or an elegant catered event. Any time, any place a group of people gather for a meal, you can be sure there are some diners trying to prevent or manage a chronic disease or trying to skirt a food allergy or intolerance. The one thing all these people have in common is the desire to have a satisfying, flavorful meal.

This chapter focuses on serving guests with some common special health needs. Nutrition experts from around the country – our Essentials Experts – have come together here not only to give you a better understanding of how food affects these conditions (for better or worse), but also to share practical menu planning, preparation and presentation techniques that will make your foodservice operation seamlessly inclusive to all people who want to enjoy a good meal, whatever their special health needs may be.

While the chef sets the tone, he or she is not the only person who creates a winning atmosphere. Servers play a key role, too, by demonstrating the operation's commitment to accommodating a patron's special health needs, being knowledgeable about ingredients and cooking techniques, and carefully communicating guests' special requests and concerns to the chef.

Our Diet and our Health – How Big Is The Problem?

There is no question that food affects one's health – both in the short term and over a lifetime. As the chart on page 313 shows, diet plays a part in most of the top seven leading causes of death – heart disease, cancers, strokes and diabetes. Additionally, obesity is associated with increased risk of heart disease, stroke, diabetes, some cancers, hypertension, osteoarthritis and gallbladder disease. Some of the primary dietary risk factors associated with these diseases include high saturated fat and trans fat intake, low whole-grain, fruit and vegetable intake, high sugar intake, high refined-grain intake and excessive sodium intake. The foodservice industry can play an important role in providing all guests healthful menu options. For those guests with specific dietary needs, this is often a valuable service.

More than one-third of adult Americans (92 million) suffer from some form of cardiovascular disease, and more than 830,000 adults die each year from heart attacks or strokes. [1] Coronary heart disease is the number one killer of both men and women.

Approximately 45 percent of adult Americans have high blood pressure or hypertension. [1] Because hypertension is without symptoms, many people are unaware they have it. If uncontrolled, hypertension can lead to coronary heart disease, heart failure, stroke, kidney failure and other health problems.

While cancer is the second leading cause of death in America, rates of new diagnoses and rates of death from all cancers combined have declined significantly during the last decade for both men and women in the United States. This downward trend is driven largely by declines in the rate of new cases and lower rates of death for the three most common cancers in men (lung, prostate and colorectal) and for two of the three leading cancers in women (breast and colorectal). New diagnoses for all types of cancer in the United States decreased, on average, almost 1% per year from 2007 to 2013. Cancer deaths decreased each year from 1993 to 2014. [2] These declines are surprising in light of the ongoing obesity epidemic and the relationship between weight and cancer.

According to the National Diabetes Information Clearinghouse, approximately 30 million people, or about 9.4 % of the population, have diabetes and another 84 million have pre-diabetes. Diabetes is the seventh leading cause of death in the United States, and complications from the disease can lead to other very serious health problems. Potential complications include heart disease and stroke, high blood pressure, blindness, kidney disease, nervous system disease, amputations, dental disease and complications of pregnancy. Diabetes is also a financial drain on the healthcare system with estimated direct and indirect costs of about $245 billion annually. [3]

Leading Causes of Death in the United States

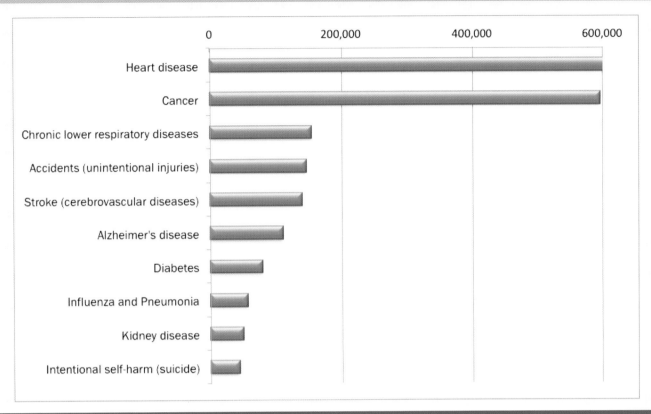

Source: National Vital Statistics Reports, **https://www.cdc.gov/nchs/data/nvsr/nvsr66/nvsr66_05.pdf**

Cardiovascular Disease

Essentials Expert

Penny M. Kris-Etherton, PhD, RD, FAHA, distinguished professor of nutrition at Pennsylvania State University, is a leading researcher on cardiovascular nutrition. Penny served on the Dietary Guidelines Advisory Committee and on the Institute of Medicine Committee of The National Academies of Science to establish macronutrient Dietary Reference Intakes. She is a recognized leader in the American Heart Association and the National Lipid Association.

Cardiovascular disease (CVD) is a group of diseases related to the heart and blood vessels. Many factors increase risk for cardiovascular disease, including heredity, cigarette smoking, physical inactivity, obesity, high blood pressure, and a diet high in saturated fat and trans fats and low in vegetables, fruits and whole grains. Guests, whether looking for foods that will help control cardiovascular diseases or wanting meals that will decrease risk of heart disease, appreciate foodservice operations that provide a wide range of flavorful, appealing foods that meet their unique dietary needs. Culinary professionals have a key role in developing foods that are lower in saturated fat and trans fats and providing flavorful vegetables, whole grains and fruits.

Arteries become blocked due to a buildup of plaque on their inner walls. This process, known as *atherosclerosis*, affects almost everyone to varying degrees. The major dietary causes of plaque formation are saturated fats and trans fats. Obesity, diabetes and hypertension (related to high salt intake) also greatly increase risk factors for cardiovascular disease. Foodservice menu items are often high in calories, salt, saturated fat, trans fat and cholesterol – the very nutritional factors that individuals with cardiovascular disease need to limit. In addition, many foodservice menus offer few sources of soluble fiber, which is an important addition to diets low in saturated fat and cholesterol. Soluble fiber binds some of the cholesterol from food and digestive secretions and increases elimination of cholesterol from the body.

Key Nutrition Points

Patrons with cardiovascular disease, as well as those trying to prevent it, rely on the chef to create healthful dishes. Key menu-planning points for this audience are the same as those for planning a well-balanced diet in general.

- Include plenty of low-calorie menu items and fewer high-calorie items. People with cardiovascular disease are often overweight or obese and need fewer calories.
- Offer smaller portions. Portioning is the simplest way to manage calories. Be mindful of high-fat sauces and dressings.
- Use healthful cooking techniques for most offerings. Limit fried foods and reduce portion sizes of all fried foods offered.
- Use fat moderately throughout the menu. Substitute other cooking methods for frying wherever possible. If frying is necessary for some foods, serve a small portion as an accompaniment or garnish with foods prepared more healthfully.
- Use less heart-unhealthy fats and oils (butter, cream, bacon fat, meat drippings, saturated margarines and shortenings).
- Use only heart-healthy oils such as olive, grapeseed or canola oils. Use specialty oils (liquid at room temperature) such as nut, herb or spice-flavored oils to incorporate healthy fats in the diet and add flavor while decreasing salt. Other oils recommended by the *Dietary Guidelines* include safflower oil, sunflower oil, corn oil, soybean oil, peanut oil, and cottonseed oil.
- Unrefined whole-grain foods contain fiber that can help lower blood cholesterol and create a feeling of fullness that helps manage weight.
- Serve more and a greater variety of fruits and vegetables and higher-fiber foods. Pay particular attention to seasoning them without a lot of fat or salt.

- Provide more options for patrons to lighten up calories and fat – for example, light mayonnaise, light dressings or less dressing on salads, vegetable-based pasta sauces, and smaller main course options and dessert portions.
- Serve a bread basket with a variety of whole grain breads, bread sticks and rolls, including some that have vegetables, nuts and/or seeds in or on them.
- Use plenty of fat-free, 1% fat and low-fat dairy products.
- Use fruits and vegetables to increase the volume of the portions served without significantly increasing the calories.
- Look for ways to increase food volume, such as incorporating air in recipes. Souffles, angel food cake, meringues and foams have volume without a lot of added calories.

Types of Cardiovascular Disease

Cardiovascular disease is an umbrella term for conditions that affect the heart (cardio) and the arteries (vascular).

- *Arteriosclerosis* is a chronic disease in which thickening, hardening and loss of elasticity of the arterial walls result in impaired blood circulation. It develops with age and with conditions such as hypertension, high blood cholesterol and diabetes.
- *Atherosclerosis* is a type of arteriosclerosis in which plaque causes the clogging or hardening of arteries or blood vessels. *Plaque* is an accumulation of substances including cholesterol, fibrous tissue and calcium.
- *Coronary heart disease*, the progressive reduction of blood supply to the heart muscle due to narrowing or blocking of a coronary artery, can lead to a heart attack.
- *Hypertension*, or high blood pressure, is the elevated force of blood pushing against the walls of arteries as it flows through them.
- *Ischemic stroke* is the sudden death of brain cells in a localized area due to inadequate blood flow caused by pieces of plaque creating a blockage in a blood vessel.

- Include heart-healthy meatless dishes such as appetizers, entrées and side dishes.
- Find ways to include more legumes in the menu.
- Focus on nutrient-rich foods like sweet potatoes instead of white potatoes, berries instead of apples, and spinach salad instead of iceberg lettuce salad.

The American Heart Association's Life's Simple 7 Steps

For ideal cardiovascular health:

1. Don't Smoke
2. Maintain a Healthy Weight
3. Engage in Regular Physical Activity
4. Eat a Healthy Diet
5. Manage Blood Pressure
6. Take Charge of Cholesterol
7. Keep Blood Sugar at Healthy Levels

The American Heart Association recommends eating a wide variety of nutritious foods daily. Even simple, small changes can make a big difference in living a better life. As part of a healthy diet, adults consuming 2,000 calories daily should aim for:

- **Fruits and vegetables:** At least 4 to 5 cups a day
- **Fish (preferably oily fish):** At least two 3.5-ounce servings a week
- **Fiber-rich whole grains:** At least three 1-ounce equivalent servings a day
- **Sodium:** Less than 1,500 milligrams a day (1 teaspoon salt contains 2,300 milligrams of sodium)
- **Sugar-sweetened beverages:** No more than 450 calories (36 ounces) a week

Other recommendations:

- **Nuts, legumes and seeds:** At least 4 servings a week
- **Processed meats:** No more than 2 servings a week
- **Saturated fat:** Less than 7% of total energy intake

Source: American Heart Association, **http://mylifecheck.heart.org/Multitab.aspx?NavID=3&CultureCode=en-US**

Best Choices

Moderation and variety are keys to planning, preparing and serving heart-healthy foods. Be creative when planning menu items for guests with cardiovascular disease. Remember that everyone benefits from heart healthy foods – not only those with heart disease. Prevention of heart disease should be a goal for everyone.

- Emphasize fruits and vegetables in menu planning. Make vegetables so scrumptious that patrons will order more. Add more grilled and roasted vegetables; they are delicious and colorful and open up a new world of options for patrons. Incorporate vegetables and fruits in appetizers, entrées, side dishes, breads and desserts. Experts at the 2010 Worlds of Healthy Flavors program at the Culinary Institute of America said that doubling produce usage should be a leading goal of the foodservice industry. [4]

- Serve a variety of whole grains that are naturally low in fat and high in fiber. Include whole-grain breads, rolls and crackers, brown rice, quinoa, barley and cereals. Use flaxseed, wheat germ and oatmeal as ingredients. Even a 50% or 75% whole grain is a better choice than a refined grain. Explore legume and nut flours for healthier crackers and flatbreads.

- While fish and poultry are good lean proteins, they are not the only answer to keeping fat and calories under control. Also offer lean lamb, bison, beef and pork. Offer fish dishes (not fried). Use omega-3-rich fish such as salmon, mackerel and herring. Walnuts and flax seeds also are sources of omega-3 fatty acids.

- Serve moderate portions: 4-ounce entrées of lean meat cuts; 5 to 6 ounces of poultry; 6 to 8 ounces of fish. Portions of heart-healthy foods can be larger than less healthful items.

- Serve legumes, peas, beans, lentils and soy products as protein sources. They are low in fat and contain no cholesterol. Feature plant proteins prepared using high-flavor techniques from various world cuisines. These foods add health benefits including fiber and reduce food costs.

- Serve low-fat and nonfat dairy products and use them liberally as ingredients.

- As noted, use plant oils that are healthy and un-saturated, such as those from canola, soy, peanuts, olives, fish, nuts, seeds, avocados and whole grains.

- Shift the balance in composite salads by replacing or using only small amounts of croutons, cheese, bacon and dressings. Avocado is high in heart-healthy fat, so it can be used moderately.

- Serve balsamic vinegar, olive oil, marinara sauce, pesto, hummus or bean dips for bread, rather than butter.

- If ground meat or sausage is used, choose lower-fat, lower-salt varieties and use small portions.

- Use plenty of egg whites and moderate amounts of whole eggs. (Egg yolks are rich in cholesterol.) Pair eggs with healthful ingredients such as whole grains, low-fat dairy products, vegetables, nuts, seeds, legumes and healthful fats.

- Offer at least one low-calorie or fat-free salad dressing and dress all salads lightly.

Foods to Limit

Calorie-dense foods should be served in small portions. Limit:

- All fried foods – chips, doughnuts, fried vegetables, fried chicken or fish, French fries, etc.

- Use small amounts of cheese, croutons or fried anything on salads.

- Soups, dips and sauces made with cream or sour cream or roux-based thickeners.

- Bacon, hot dogs and sausage. Substitute Canadian bacon, turkey sausage or lean pork to cut fat and sodium.

- Rich sauces and cream-based soups. Substitute broth-based, vegetable and soups with legumes.

- Limit alfredo and creamy sauces on pasta and substitute tomato or vegetable-based sauces.

- Prime grade or high-fat cuts of meat such as short ribs, brisket, spare ribs and rib-eye.

- Doughnuts, sweet rolls, croissants, biscuits and other high-fat breads.

- Refined grains and added sugars, including table sugar, sweetened beverages and syrups

- Butter, lard, high-fat dairy products, hydrogenated oils or shortenings, and coconut, palm, cotton-seed and palm kernel oils.

- Organ meats, such as liver and especially foie gras.

Sources of Soluble Fiber

- Apples, pears, bananas, berries, prunes
- Broccoli, carrots
- Legumes, soy products, peas, beans
- Oats, barley
- Potatoes, yams and root vegetables

Tips for Chefs

Chefs have an important opportunity to make a difference in the cardiovascular health of Americans. Here are a few tips:

- Reduce unhealthy fats and salt to the lowest level that yields excellent flavor and functionality. Use healthy fats prudently so as not to markedly increase calories.

- Use reduced-sodium sauces (soy sauce) and bases routinely.

- Pay attention to sodium, saturated fat, trans fat and total calories. Offer more plant-based entrées with fruits and vegetables, whole grains and legumes.

- Don't be afraid of seasonings when preparing lean or low-fat food items. Boost flavors with aromatic herbs or spices that do not add salt.

- Encourage shared desserts or offer mini-desserts. Include fruit as a dessert option.

- Use a range of cooking techniques for fruits such as poaching, grilling and roasting.

- Use smaller plates, bowls and glasses to serve food and beverages so moderate portions do not look skimpy.

For More Information

- American Heart Association, **www.americanheart.org**

- American Heart Association. The New American Heart Association Cookbook, 9th Edition. New York: Harmony Books/Crown Publishing Group; 2017.

Hypertension

Essentials Expert

Georgia Kostas, MPH, RD, LD, is a consulting nutritionist, speaker, author and president of Georgia Kostas & Associates, Inc. in Dallas, Texas. She is a cardiovascular and preventive medicine registered dietitian who focuses on weight management, wellness and health promotion through nutrition and fitness. In her 25 years as director of nutrition at the Cooper Clinic, she has counseled more than 25,000 people. Georgia is an innovator who believes the chef–dietitian team is key to demonstrating that healthy can be delicious.

Blood pressure is the force of blood pushing against the walls of arteries as it flows through them. When blood pressure is measured, two numbers are reported: systolic and diastolic pressures. **Systolic** is the pressure created when the heart beats while pumping blood. **Diastolic** is the pressure created when the heart is at rest between beats. Blood pressure numbers are written with the systolic number above or before the diastolic – for example, 120/80 mmHg. (The mmHg stands for "millimeters of mercury," the units used to measure blood pressure.) Healthy resting blood pressure is 120 over 80 or below.

Larger colorful veggie portions show people how a plate can be full and the meal filling and pleasing with the same favorite foods in adjusted portions. Patients tell me they tire of yellow squash and zucchini and want to see more veggie options on menus. I believe red and green foods should be on every plate! I tell my patients, "Red and green keep your arteries clean." I also suggest delectable sharp cheeses in small amounts. If you use cheese creatively for flavor, you can use less and have a powerful taste!

Georgia Kostas, MPH, RD, LD
Georgia Kostas & Associates

Blood Pressure Levels in Adults

Blood Pressure Category	Systolic mm Hg (upper number)		Diastolic mm Hg (lower number)
Normal	Less than 120	and	Less than 80
Elevated	120 – 129	and	Less than 80
High Blood Pressure Stage 1	130 – 139	or	80 – 89
High Blood Pressure Stage 2	140 or higher	or	90 or higher
Hypertensive Crisis (consult your doctor immediately)	Higher than 180	and/or	Higher than 120

Source: American Heart Association, https://www.heart.org/en/health-topics/high-blood-pressure/understanding-blood-pressure-readings#.VtRM-7JwrKUk

High blood pressure can be caused by many factors including genetics, smoking, stress, weight, diet and inactivity. The body's sodium level is a major factor regulating blood pressure. Sodium helps maintain fluid and electrolyte balance in the body and also helps regulate heartbeat. While some dietary sodium (about 200 milligrams per day) is essential for life and health, dietary excesses create problems.

Reducing sodium in the diet generally reduces blood pressure, but the American public really enjoys sodium-rich foods. Culinary professionals are challenged to prepare lower-sodium, flavorful foods that can help diners control their sodium intake. Chefs are the experts on developing flavor in foods while reducing dependency on salt and high-sodium ingredients. Because much of our sodium comes from processed foods, chefs have an advantage when using less-processed foods and ingredients.

Recent compelling research indicates that all American adults, with or without hypertension, can reduce their blood pressure by reducing sodium intake by 1000 mg a day. This is an excellent initial sodium reduction target. Our taste buds can adapt to a healthier sodium intake while cardiovascular events may be reduced. The American Heart Association maintains that sodium reduction is warranted due to cardiovascular benefits beyond hypertension. AHA warns that excessive sodium leads to blood thickening and blood vessel dysfunction, taxing arteries and the heart.

Key Nutrition Points

- The report of the 2015-2020 *Dietary Guidelines for Americans* advises Americans to try to consume no more than 2,300 milligrams of sodium per day. The American Heart Association recommends 1,500 milligrams daily to further reduce one's risk of cardiovascular events or strokes, for those over age 50 and/or those at higher risk. [1]

- The American Medical Association recommends a minimum 50% reduction in the amount of sodium in processed foods, fast food products and restaurant meals to be achieved over the next decade. [5]

- While some foods are naturally rich in sodium, most sodium in the typical diet comes from salt (sodium chloride) added during food processing or preparation. More than 75% of sodium in the American diet comes from processed food. [6]

- The DASH (Dietary Approaches to Stop Hypertension) eating plan is a heart healthy, nutrient-rich diet based on research supported by the National Heart, Lung and Blood Institute. Adherence to the DASH diet requires eating whole, fresh or frozen foods and only a few processed products, which provides a sodium intake of less than 2,300 milligrams/day. Research supporting the DASH diet shows that individuals can reduce blood pressure further if they limit sodium to 1,500 milligrams per day. Following the DASH diet for six weeks can lower systolic blood pressure 8 to 14 points (mm Hg) – as much as medications! [7]

- Some restaurant main courses contain more than 3,000 milligrams of sodium per serving, more than twice the recommended daily limit in one food item.

- Because high blood pressure increases the risk of chronic diseases that contribute to healthcare costs, reducing sodium has become a major public health issue. With research showing the benefits of reducing dietary sodium and with increased regulatory pressures, the foodservice industry needs to find ways to meet the challenge of reducing salt and other sodium sources in food. [4]

Daily Nutrient Goals Used in the DASH Studies
For a 2,100-Calorie Eating Plan

Total fat	27% of calories
Saturated fat	6% of calories
Protein	18% of calories
Carbohydrate	55% of calories
Cholesterol	150 milligrams
Sodium	2,300 milligrams
Potassium	4,700 milligrams
Calcium	1,250 milligrams
Magnesium	500 milligrams
Fiber	30 grams

Source: What Is the DASH Eating Plan? **http://www.nhlbi.nih.gov/health/resources/heart/hbp-dash-how-plan-html**

National Salt & Sugar Reduction Initiative

The National Salt and Sugar Reduction Initiative (NSSRI) is a partnership of over 100 local, state and national health organizations The New York City Health Department launched the initial phase of this effort, the National Salt Reduction Initiative (NSRI), in 2009 and set targets for reduced sodium levels in packaged and restaurant foods. Between 2009 and 2015, there was a 6.8 percent reduction in sodium levels in the food supply, demonstrating the feasibility of this model.

The NSSRI applauds the restaurants that have committed to reduce salt in their menu items to meet the NSSRI restaurant food targets and encourages all restaurants and foodservice companies to follow their example. The following companies have agreed to work toward restaurant food targets:

- Au Bon Pain
- Bertucci's Italian Restaurant
- Starbucks Coffee Company
- Subway®
- Uno Chicago Grill

The following are a few of the companies that have agreed to pursue one or more NSSRI targets for packaged food:

- Boar's Head Provisions Co.
- Butterball
- Campbell Soup Company
- Goya Foods
- Hain Celestial
- Heinz
- Kraft Foods
- McCain Foods
- Red Gold, Inc.
- Unilever

Targets for sodium levels in various food categories set for 2014. No menu item should be more than 1,200 milligrams sodium/serving.

Soup	280 mg sodium/100 grams
Hamburgers	330 mg sodium/100 grams
Sandwiches	370 mg sodium/100 grams
Cheese pizza	390 mg sodium/100 grams

Source: National Salt & Sugar Reduction Initiative. **https://www1.nyc.gov/site/doh/health/health-topics/national-salt-reduction-initiative.page**

The DASH Diet: Dietary Approaches to Stop Hypertension

Foods	Recommended Servings
Whole grains	6 - 8 per day (each is ½ cup or 1 slice bread)
Fruits and vegetables	8 - 10 per day (4 - 5 cups total)
Fat-free or low-fat dairy	2 - 3 per day (2 - 3 cups total)
Lean meat, poultry, fish	6 ounces or less per day
Nuts, seeds and beans	4 - 5 per week (½ cup beans or 1 ounce of nuts is 1 serving)
Fats and oils	2 - 3 small servings per day (2 - 3 teaspoons)
Sweets	5 or fewer per week
Sodium	1,500 or 2,400 milligrams per day (1,500 milligrams recommended for individuals with hypertension)

Source: DASH Eating Plan, www.nhlbi.nih.gov/health/public/heart/hbp/dash/new_dash.pdf

Best Choices

- Limit or substitute lower-sodium versions of America's "top ten" salty foods consumed: bread/rolls, pizza, cold cuts and cured meats (bacon, ham, sausage, etc), poultry (injected with salt water solution), soups, sandwiches, cheese, pasta dishes, meat dishes and snacks

- More unprocessed foods that are naturally low in sodium (fruits, vegetables, whole grains and dry beans)

- Fresh or frozen vegetables. Avoid canned vegetables with added salt.

- Desserts with fruits as the base. Fruits are naturally high in potassium and antioxidants, and low in saturated fat, trans fat, cholesterol and sodium. Use dried fruits, nuts and nut flour to add flavor and texture without a lot of added sugar.

- Plain rice or brown rice, noodles, and whole grains not seasoned with mixes that contain sodium but rather with sautéed mushrooms, onions, dried fruits, nuts and herbs

- Fresh and frozen fruits, including sorbets and fruit ices

- Most beverages, except tomato and other vegetable juices and sports drinks

- Low-fat or nonfat dairy products

- High-fat foods and ingredients in moderation. Switch the balance from a rich dessert with a fruit garnish to bite-sized desserts or a fruit dessert with a small cookie, meringue or brownie.

- Fresh foods and packaged foods that are unsalted, no salt added, sodium-free or low-sodium

- Healthful cooking techniques

- Foods low or moderate in calories to assist with weight control

- Herbs, spices, aromatics, and lemon juice and zest to season foods without salt

Potassium and High Blood Pressure

The *Dietary Guidelines* report that potassium intake is low enough to be a public health concern for both adults and children. The guidelines recommend choosing foods that provide more potassium, which is found in vegetables, fruits, whole grains, beans and peas, and milk and milk products.

Dietary potassium can lower blood pressure by blunting the adverse effects of sodium. Other possible benefits of eating a diet rich in potassium include a reduced risk of developing kidney stones and decreased bone loss. The recommended intake for potassium for adults is 4,700 milligrams per day. Available evidence suggests that African Americans and individuals with hypertension especially benefit from increasing their intake of potassium.

Foods to Limit

- Salt and seasoned salts
- High-sodium ingredients such as spice blends, soy sauce, MSG (monosodium glutamate), anchovies, olives and capers, pickles, steak sauce, barbeque sauce, Worcestershire sauce, most Asian sauces, and any ingredient that is pickled, brined, smoked or cured
- All processed foods (including processed cheese) that are high in sodium. Choose natural sharp cheeses that can be used in smaller amounts.
- Salted or cured foods, such as ham, bacon, hot dogs, olives, corned beef and smoked salmon
- Breaded fish, poultry and meats
- Prepared mixes for stuffing and breading
- Broths or bases containing salt or sodium in any form
- Most cheeses (check labels), canned soups, snack foods, chips, crackers, salted nuts and popcorn
- Dried soup mixes and bouillon cubes

Tips for Chefs

- Use plenty of fresh lemon juice (reduces bitterness), citrus, wine, vinegars, fruit such as grapes, vegetables such as garlic, mushrooms, onion and peppers.
- Omit or reduce salt used in food preparation. Pay particular attention to enhancing flavor without sodium-rich ingredients. Focus on flavors from spices, herbs and aromatics and on flavor-building techniques from world cuisines.
- Describe healthful foods in ways that stimulate the senses. Try the "stealth health" strategy – present healthful, full-flavored foods but don't label them as "healthy" on the menu. Have nutrition information available upon request.
- Use lots of fresh herbs, unsalted seasoning blends, spices and aromatic ingredients to boost flavor without salt, including Kitchen Bouquet® and Angostura Bitters®.
- Prepare food with olive oil or canola oil when possible. Corn, peanut and other oils are also unsalted.
- Have oil and vinegar, fruit juice, or fruit infusions available for making an unsalted salad dressing.
- Always read labels and check for listed sodium content.

For More Information

- How to Understand and Use the Nutrition Facts Label, **www.fda.gov/Food/LabelingNutrition/ ConsumerInformation/ucm078889.htm**
- National Heart Lung and Blood Institute, **www. nhlbi.nih.gov**
- Your Guide to Lowering Blood Pressure with DASH, **www.nhlbi.nih.gov/health/public/ heart/ hbp/dash/new_dash.pdf**
- Your Guide to Lowering Blood Pressure, **www.nhlbi.nih.gov/health/public/heart/hbp/ hbp_low/hbp_low.pdf**
- *American Heart Association Low-Salt Cookbook*, 3rd edition. New York: Clarkson-Potter Publisher; 2006.
- Kostas G. The Cooper Clinic Solution to the Diet Revolution: Step Up to the Plate! Dallas: Good Health Press; 2009. **www.georgiakostas.com**

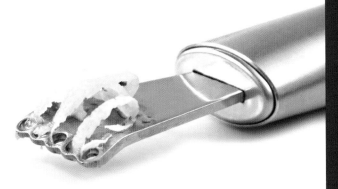

Cancer

Essentials Expert

Karen Collins, MS, RDN, CDN, FAND, is nutrition advisor to the American Institute for Cancer Research, located in Washington, DC. She specializes in nutrition's role in reducing cancer risk, supporting health of cancer survivors and promoting heart health. Karen encourages healthy eating as a nationally syndicated nutrition news columnist, speaker and consultant. She has authored and co-authored several book chapters and journal reviews for health professionals summarizing research on nutrition and cancer prevention and has been featured in more than 2000 media segments. Having conducted a long-time private practice in nutrition counseling, Karen emphasizes the importance of making healthful eating realistic and enjoyable. It always delights Karen when people say, "I love coming to your parties, because it's such fun to see how you make healthy eating so delicious and yet 'normal'!"

Cancer is actually many different diseases caused by many different types of abnormal cells. Thus, different kinds of treatments may be used. Because there are so many types of cancer, it is difficult to predict necessary dietary modifications. For those faced with cancer, the term "cancer survivor" is used from the time of diagnosis through the balance of life. However, nutrition issues can change during treatment or recovery, after recovery, or while living with advanced cancer. Maintaining good nutritional status is important in all phases of cancer, and chefs can help guests with cancer to enjoy their meals.

"From the moment of cancer diagnosis, people are often inundated with advice from family, friends and what they see in the media," says Karen Collins. Today's research shows that healthful diets can help cancer survivors fight cancer, continue in its treatment, and reduce the risk of recurrence and other long-term health risks. However, no single nutrient, food or diet can cure cancer. Furthermore, the principles of good nutrition for cancer survivors can be met in a variety of different ways, so there's no 'best' diet plan".

Eating patterns in which healthful plant foods take center stage are recommended to reduce cancer risk and are recommended for cancer survivors whenever possible. Some may choose to accomplish this through some form of vegetarian diet. Vegetarian diets include many healthful features and tend to be low in saturated fats and high in fiber, vitamins and phytochemicals (health-protective natural plant compounds). The American Cancer Society states, "No direct evidence has helped to determine whether consuming a vegetarian diet has any additional benefit for the prevention of cancer recurrence over an omnivorous diet high in vegetables, fruits, and whole grains, and low in red meats." [8]

For the cancer survivor, maintaining a healthy weight is extremely important. Being overweight or gaining excess weight during treatment increases the risk of recurrence or poor outcome, especially for those with prostate or post-menopausal breast cancer. Being underweight or experiencing unplanned weight loss is also a serious problem during cancer treatment. During treatment, the goal should be to maintain normal weight or perhaps gradually lose excess weight through a healthful lifestyle. Some people may need higher-calorie foods and small, frequent meals to meet their needs. When dining out, they may want to order small portions, share their food or take some food home for another meal. Others, however, may be focused on meeting nutrient needs without excessive calories to avoid unhealthy weight gain.

The many side effects of cancer treatment can cause a variety of problems. One issue is early satiety – getting full fast or being able to eat only a few bites at a time. Some cancer treatments cause nausea, dry mouth or sores in the mouth. Taste changes can be an issue as well. Food may taste like cardboard or metal due to medications that change the composition of saliva and alter the flavor of food. Radiation and other treatments can alter taste perception and the ability to swallow.

Key Nutrition Points

- Eating a diet rich in fruits and vegetables may reduce a person's risk for cancer because these foods are rich in antioxidants and a variety of natural plant compounds that protect cells from damage. Studies suggest that people who eat lots of vegetables and fruits have lower risk of developing some types of cancer.

- Studies show that antioxidants in pill form do not convey the same benefits as food sources of antioxidants.

- The health benefits of allium compounds found in garlic and onion family vegetables have been widely publicized. Garlic is linked with lower risk of colorectal cancer and is under study for potential to reduce risk of other cancers, but there is not enough evidence at this time to support a specific recommendation for its use.

American Institute for Cancer Research
Recommendations for Cancer Survivors

1. Be as lean as possible without becoming underweight.
2. Be physically active for at least 30 minutes every day. Limit sedentary habits.
3. Avoid sugary drinks, and limit consumption of energy-dense foods.
4. Eat more of a variety of vegetables, fruits, whole grains, and legumes such as beans.
5. Limit consumption of red meats (such as beef, pork, and lamb) and avoid processed meats.
6. If consumed at all, limit alcoholic drinks to two for men and one for women a day.
7. Limit consumption of salty foods and foods processed with salt (sodium).
8. Do not use supplements to protect against cancer.

And always remember, do not smoke or chew tobacco.

— *Reprinted with permission, American Institute for Cancer Research (*http://aicr.org*)*

- Studies have found a link between alcohol and increased risk of cancer of the mouth, throat, larynx, esophagus, liver, breast and colon. Generally, people living with cancer are advised to limit or avoid alcohol. Moderate consumption is 1 drink per day for women, and no more than 2 for men. Five ounces of wine, 12 ounces of beer, or one-and-a-half ounces of 80-proof liquor counts as one drink.

- There is little solid scientific evidence that total fat, type of fat, cholesterol, sugar, fluoride, organic foods, approved food additives or irradiated food has any specific effect on cancer incidence or recurrence. These substances may be positive or negative for other health reasons but are statistically unrelated to cancer risk.

- Maintaining a healthy weight plays a major role in reducing risk of cancer and can help improve outcome after cancer, including potential to reduce risk of recurrence. Being overweight or obese substantially raises the risk for endometrial (uterine), post-menopausal breast, ovarian, colorectal, esophageal, liver, pancreatic, gallbladder, kidney and advanced prostate cancers.

- Other ways to reduce cancer risk include avoiding all forms of tobacco and avoiding excessive exposure to ultraviolet rays from the sun and tanning beds.

- Physical activity is very important in preventing many cancers, decreasing risk of cancer recurrence and promoting better overall outcome after cancer.

- A healthful diet may help someone with cancer fight the disease and survive, but this is not the time to be overly restrictive. Serve whatever will please the guest and meet his/her unique needs.

Best Choices

Cancer survivors widely differ in calorie needs and appetite. Regardless, serve as many nutrient-rich foods as possible. Whole grains are more nutritious than refined grains and overall preferred, although cancer survivors who have digestive tract side effects from cancer or its treatment may need the lower-fiber refined grains. Fruits and vegetables are an excellent choice as part of every meal. They contain antioxidant and phytochemicals that may help prevent or slow down cancer by protecting cells from abnormal changes. A wide variety of fruits and vegetables is best in order to get the broadest possible array of protective nutrients and compounds. Some especially good choices include:

- **Fruits**: blueberries, blackberries, strawberries, raspberries, cranberries, grapes, cherries, apples, melon, oranges and pomegranates
- **Vegetables**: broccoli, cauliflower, cabbage, Brussels sprouts, kale (all cruciferous vegetables contain phytochemicals with cancer-fighting potential), onions, garlic, spinach, asparagus, peppers, peas, beets, squash, pumpkin, sweet potatoes and tomatoes

The person with cancer who is having difficulty maintaining weight needs nutrient-rich fluids with calories, such as fruit juice, smoothies, milkshakes or lattes made with whole milk. Nutrient-rich soup can also be an excellent way to provide fluids. Any liquid counts toward fluid intake. For example, tea (particularly green tea) and coffee are good fluids and also contain protective phytochemicals. Both caffeinated and decaffeinated teas and coffee are fine. Tea may protect against some cancers, though more research is needed. Old worries that coffee could promote pancreatic or other cancers have not been supported by new research. In fact, coffee is actually a plant and provides a rich source of phytochemicals and is linked to lower risk of some cancers.

Some people with cancer need very mild foods with very few spices because they have mouth sores. The acid in citrus and tomato sauces can cause pain for them. Icy foods may be soothing. In contrast, some who have damaged taste buds may enjoy extra

Nutrition-Related Challenges

During cancer treatment, and sometimes even after it is concluded, some cancer survivors face one or more problems that affect what they are able to eat and enjoy. Specific suggestions for dealing with each of these can be found in the resource listed below:

- Weight loss and loss of appetite
- Weight gain
- Diarrhea
- Constipation
- Nausea
- Vomiting
- Sore mouth, tongue and throat
- Dry mouth
- Difficulty swallowing
- Feeling full quickly
- Taste changes and food aversions
- Fluid retention
- Milk or lactose intolerance
- Fatigue

Adapted from: American Institute for Cancer Research, *Cancer*Resource™. Available in print or online at: **http://www.aicr.org/patients-survivors/cancerresource/cancerresource-intro.html. Accessed May 14, 2018.**

spice in their foods. Serve foods with a variety of spice-level options. Offer a balsamic vinegar reduction and a balsamic vinegar/sugar reduction to drizzle on vegetables and other dishes to add flavor and cut through the bad taste in the mouth caused by many cancer medications.

Some medications cause dry mouth, which makes it difficult to chew and swallow. Guests taking these medications need moist, semi-pureed or very soft foods with gravies or sauces. Soups, puddings, custards and flans, eggs, risotto, mashed potatoes and ice cream are easy to chew and swallow. Offer some high-calorie options for those who need to gain or maintain their weight.

Sugar Issues

A common concern during cancer treatment is whether "sugar feeds cancer." In fact, the constant supply of sugar in the blood stream is available to all cells, including cancer cells. Eating a chocolate chip cookie will not make cancer cells grow faster. When a person with cancer has little appetite, some sugar may help increase caloric intake.

For best nutrition, cancer survivors, like other people, are often advised to limit intake of foods high in added sugars. This includes honey, raw sugar and molasses as well as white sugar and high fructose corn syrup. However, it is not necessary to completely eliminate all sugars. Large portions of high sugar foods, especially eaten alone, can increase the body's production of insulin. High circulating insulin on a regular basis may promote cancer cell growth, at least among people who are overweight and sedentary or who have insulin resistance or diabetes in the family. Remember, a diet with lots of added sugar is not a healthful diet. High-sugar foods are usually low in important nutrients and full of empty calories, and often replace valuable health-promoting foods, so are not great choices for anyone.

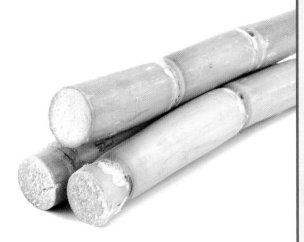

What About Soy in Plant-Based Meals?

With growing interest in plant-based eating for people with and without a history of cancer, questions about whether soy foods are safe for cancer survivors have been highly controversial, especially for those with estrogen-sensitive cancers. Like other legumes, soy foods contain nutrients and phytochemicals that promote good health and may help lower cancer risk, and many are good sources of dietary fiber. Soy foods also contain relatively unique phytochemicals called isoflavones. These compounds are classified as phytoestrogens ("plant estrogens") based on their chemical structure, and early laboratory studies raised concern that eating soy foods could be harmful for women at risk of or with a history of breast cancer. However, human research now provides clearer answers.

Human studies clearly and consistently show that eating up to three serving of soy foods a day does not pose risk, even for women with estrogen-sensitive breast cancer. Limited, but not conclusive, evidence suggests that soy foods might benefit breast cancer survivors. Individuals may have personally-specific discussions with their healthcare providers, which should be respected. Overall, however, cancer survivors who wish to include soy foods for protein and other nutrients as part of healthful, plant-focused eating can comfortably do so.

Moderate consumption of soy foods is considered one to two standard servings a day, and studies show safety of up to three servings a day. Examples of one standard serving include 1/3 cup tofu, 1/2 cup tempeh, 1/2 cup edamame or cooked soybeans, 1 cup soy milk or yogurt, and 1/4 cup soy nuts. (One serving averages about 7 grams of protein and 25 milligrams (mg) of isoflavones.)

Sources:
American Institute for Cancer Research, *Cancer*Resource™. Available in print or online at: **http://www.aicr.org/patients-survivors/cancerresource/cancerresource-intro.html**. Accessed May 14, 2018.

World Cancer Research Fund International. Continuous Update Project Report: Diet, Nutrition, Physical Activity, and Breast Cancer Survivors. 2014. Available at: **www.wcrf.org/sites/default/files/Breast-Cancer-Survivors-2014-Report.pdf**. Accessed May 14, 2018.

American Cancer Society -- Rock CL, Doyle C, Demark-Wahnefried W, Meyerhardt J, Courneya KS, et al. CA: A Cancer Journal for Clinicians. 2012; 62(4):243-74. Available at **http://onlinelibrary.wiley.com/doi/10.3322/caac.21142/epdf**. Accessed May 14, 2018.

Nechuta SJ, Caan BJ, Chen WY, et al. Soy food intake after diagnosis of breast cancer and survival: an in-depth analysis of combined evidence from cohort studies of US and Chinese women. *Am J Clin Nutr*. 2012;96(1):123-132.

Foods to Limit

- Eating more than 18 ounces a week of red meat increases colorectal cancer risk.

- Processed meats and lunchmeats are made with nitrates, smoke and/or salt. Processed meats, such as bacon and sausage, are even more strongly linked to colorectal cancer, and are recommended for use in only very limited amounts.

- Blackened char on meat or chicken contains compounds called heterocylic amines (HCAs), which can create cell damage that leads to cancer. Lowest levels of HCAs form in animal muscle protein when it is cooked slower, at lower temperatures and less well-done.

- Although sweets are not good sources of nutrients and may contribute to unwanted weight gain, it is not necessary for people with cancer to avoid all sugar.

- Eggs served to guests with cancer must be fully cooked. Do not serve foods with uncooked eggs (soft boiled, poached or in salad dressings or soft meringues) unless the eggs are pasteurized.

- Cancer survivors with weakened immune systems, especially likely during certain types of cancer treatment, need to be vigilant to avoid infection from foods that carry harmful bacteria. For these people, avoid sushi; any raw or undercooked meat, poultry, fish or shellfish; unpasteurized milk or juice; and raw honey. Food safety recommendations during these times call for avoiding salad bars and ensuring that fresh fruits and vegetables are carefully washed.

Addressing Taste Changes

People differ in which, if any, taste changes they experience during or after cancer treatment. Don't assume that everyone has these issues. However, since these changes can profoundly alter ability to enjoy food, if you inquire and find that a guest is experiencing one or more of these taste challenges, here are suggestions to add flavor and help your guests enjoy the meals you provide.

Lack of flavor:
Lemon; pickled vegetables; fruit marinades; cranberry; increased amounts of herbs and spices; hot sauce.

"Off" flavors:
Acidic ingredients and fruity or salty flavors may cut through unpleasant tastes: citrus or vinegar; fruit toppings; feta or Parmesan cheese; teriyaki-type sauces and other salty ingredients.

Metallic or bitter taste:
Onion, garlic, spices such as cumin; increased sweetness from some combination of sugar, honey, maple syrup; fruit sauce or salsa; sweet and sour type sauce; marinate meat and possibly poultry.

For people with a metallic taste, fish, poultry, eggs, cheese, beans and nuts are often better tolerated than red meat. Use fresh or frozen ingredients rather than canned and cook in glass or ceramic cookware. Bamboo skewers or chopsticks, or plastic eating utensils may be preferred.

Add sugar or other sweeteners or bold spices if someone experiences sour, bitter or salty tastes to make food more palatable.

Before turning to acid flavorings like citrus and vinegar, make sure that mouth or throat sores are not an issue.

Tips for Chefs

- Provide higher-calorie, nutrient-rich foods for cancer survivors who have trouble getting enough calories to maintain their weight. However, don't assume that all people in cancer treatment need high-calorie foods.

- For people who are having trouble consuming enough food to meet calorie needs, start by making the foods they can consume more concentrated in calories. Use calorie-dense ingredients like avocado, sweet potato, nuts and seeds, nut butters, tofu and other legumes, hummus and dried fruits. These can be pureed or ground to add to a wide variety of foods for thickening or other purposes, and in doing so provide valuable nutrients rather than calories alone.

- Offer smaller portions. It's not uncommon for people with cancer to experience early satiety – getting full quickly or being able to eat only a few bites at a time.

- Provide foods with a range of flavors. Cancer treatment may change taste perceptions and alter the flavor of food.

- Serve high-protein foods as a first course, when the guest's appetite is strongest.

- Those who fatigue through the day may have appetite that is strongest at breakfast, so offer a variety of foods rich in protein and other nutrients then.

- Odors are often bothersome to people with cancer. Try serving foods cold or at room temperature. Hot fragrant foods can sometimes aggravate nausea.

- Serve soft-textured foods for people with mouth, tongue and throat sores from cancer therapy.

- Adding sugar to some foods can help decrease salty, bitter or unpleasant tastes.

- Tart foods and beverages such as oranges and grapefruit, lemon sorbet, yogurt or lemonade may be appealing.

- Some people with cancer are on raw or juice diets. Although most scientific research does not support this practice, as with all guests, try to provide foods acceptable to their wishes.

- Be particularly careful to avoid serving people undergoing cancer treatment any food that carries increased risk of bacteria or other contaminants, since they may have compromised immunity. [See details about foods of concern noted above.]

For More Information

- American Institute for Cancer Research, http://aicr.org (and Healthy Recipes section at **http://www.aicr.org/healthyrecipes/**)

- Besser J, Grant B. *What to Eat During Cancer Treatment: More Than 130 Recipes to Help You Cope*. Atlanta, Georgia: American Cancer Society, 2018.

- Center for Disease Control, Division of Cancer Prevention and Control, **http://cdc.gov/cancer**

- Collins K. *Caring for Today's Cancer Survivor*. Today's Dietitian. 2014; 16(8):42. **http://www.todaysdietitian.com/newarchives/080114p42.shtml**

- Kushi LH, Doyle C, Mc-Cullough M, Rock CL, Demark-Wahnefried W, et al. *American Cancer Society Guidelines on Nutrition and Physical Activity for Cancer Prevention: reducing the risk of cancer with healthy food choices and physical activity*. CA: A Cancer Journal for Clinicians. **http://onlinelibrary.wiley.com/doi/10.3322/caac.20140/full** National Cancer Institute, National Institutes of Health, **http://cancer.gov**

- Oncology Nutrition Dietetic Practice Group of the Academy of Nutrition and Dietetics. *Eat Right to Fight Cancer (tips for dealing with side effects of various cancer treatments)*. **https://www.oncologynutrition.org/erfc/**

- Rock CL, Doyle C, Demark-Wahnefried W, Meyerhardt J, Courneya KS, et al. *Nutrition and Physical Activity Guidelines for Cancer Survivors*. CA: A Cancer Journal for Clinicians. 2012; 62(4):243-74. **http://onlinelibrary.wiley.com/doi/10.3322/caac.21142/full**

From the Kitchen
Melanie Bianca Stewart
General Manager at Gourmetfile, Personal Chef
Boca Raton, FL

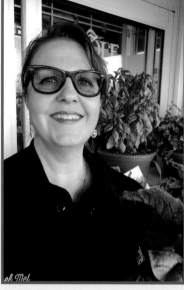

As a chef, I believe I have a responsibility to serve the very best dishes I can. A chef doesn't have much control over people's personal eating habits, but we can serve them healthy and balanced dishes, and inspire through creation and instruction. I always enjoy serving delicious, healthy plant-centric dishes to guests that may not be that familiar with plant-based cuisine and seeing their reactions.

At home and in the kitchen, I like to keep things simple. I try to always have some highly seasoned garlic olive oil on hand to season roasted vegetables, whole grain pasta and broccoli, or tuna filets. I make hummus and baba ghanoush every week for snacking, along with vegetables and pita or naan bread. I love Italian inspired dishes, and also Bragg Liquid Aminos for that perfect salty umami flavor–fresh, simple and deeply satisfying.

I always believe that we don't eat enough fruits and vegetables. In the store, for our wine dinners tastings I always incorporate fruits, vegetables and fresh herbs along with the rich foods we are famous for carrying. There needs to be balance in all things, and in all styles of eating.

Melanie Bianca Stewart is the General Manager of Gourmetphile, a rare wine and food shop in Boca Raton, Florida that carries hard to find wines, specialty cheeses, charcuterie, and unusual products from around the world. The shop offers weekly wine tastings with food pairings as well as private wine & beer dinners, which Stewart create menus for. Stewart is also a personal chef, and the variety of her clients' dietary needs has given her much insight and practice into preparing healthy, wholesome meals.

"Hint of Mint" Almond Pesto
Chef Melanie Stewart, *Gourmetphile*
Yield: about 2 cups

This pesto is very dense and rich. When using for spaghetti, be sure to reserve some of the pasta cooking water to thin out the pesto, which will create a smoother more luxurious sauce. This pesto can also be blended with mayonnaise or vegenaise to create a spread for sandwiches.

Sliced almonds, lightly toasted	1 ¼	cups
Garlic, peeled and chopped	1	clove
Flat leaf parsley	1	cup
Mint leaves	½	cup
Basil leaves	3	cups
Extra virgin olive oil	⅓	cup
Salt	½	teaspoon
Freshly ground black pepper	¼	teaspoon

1. Add the almonds to the bowl of a food processor. Pulse until the almonds resemble the texture of panko bread crumbs.

2. Add the garlic, salt and pepper. Pulse to break down the garlic. Add herbs and pulse until finely ground. With the machine running, slowly drizzle oil through the feed tube. Stop to scrape down the sides of the bowl and pulse again, to ensure all of the ingredients are blended.

3. Check for seasoning and adjust to your taste.

To store the pesto, place in a jar or container with a tight-fitting lid. Before sealing, add a thin layer of olive oil. This will protect the pesto and preserve its bright color. Store up to two weeks.

Per 2 Tablespoons

Calories	90	Cholesterol	0	mg
Fat	8 g	Sodium	75	mg
Saturated Fat	1.5 g	Carbohydrates	2	mg
Trans Fat	0 g	Dietary Fiber	1	mg
Sugar	0 g	Protein	2	g

Growing up with an Italian mom who made delicious food, Stewart was always drawn to the kitchen. From a young age, she loved to rummage in the fridge and cupboards and come up with her own creations. Swirling Hershey's syrup into Cool Whip was one of her favorite treats. Now she balances that sweet tooth by eating mostly vegetarian. Two of her favorite foods are avocado and kombucha.

Panna Cotta

Serves: 6, ½ cups

Donna Welhofen, MS, RD
retired, Senior Clinical Nutritionist,
University of Wisconsin Comprehensive Cancer Center, Madison, Wisconsin

Here is a base recipe for a dessert that can be adapted to varied nutritional needs. Changing ingredients will change the calorie, fat and sugar content according to the needs of your guests. Sugar, Splenda® or Splenda® Sugar Blend can be used for the sweetener. Dairy products range from fat-free half-and-half to heavy cream. The calories in the panna cotta can be as low as 80 or as high as 410 per serving.

Panna cotta is Italian for "cooked cream." It is very similar to the Scandinavian Swedish Cream. This smooth and creamy dessert can be served with nutrient-rich fruits such as blueberries, strawberries, cherries, peaches, plums or citrus fruit or with a simple fruit coulis.

Panna Cotta, base recipe

Unflavored gelatin	1	envelope
Water	2	tablespoons
Dairy	2	cups
Sugar	½	cup
Sour cream	1	cup
Vanilla extract	2	teaspoons

Reduced-calorie

Unflavored gelatin	1	envelope
Water	2	tablespoons
Whole milk	2	cups
Sugar or Splenda®	½	cup
Fat-free sour cream	1	cup
Vanilla extract	2	teaspoons

Reduced-calorie, fat-free

Unflavored gelatin	1	envelope
Water	2	tablespoons
Fat-free half & half	1	cup
Nonfat milk	1	cup
Sugar or Splenda®	½	cup
Fat-free sour cream	1	cup
Vanilla extract	2	teaspoons

Moderate calorie

Unflavored gelatin	1	envelope
Water	2	tablespoons
Half & half	2	cups
Sugar	½	cup
Sour cream	1	cup
Vanilla extract	2	teaspoons

High calorie

Unflavored gelatin	1	envelope
Water	2	tablespoons
Heavy cream	2	cups
Sugar	½	cup
Sour cream	1	cup
Vanilla extract	2	teaspoons

1. In a medium heavy saucepan, combine gelatin powder and water. Stir to soften gelatin. Add 2-3 tablespoons of dairy and stir to mix.

2. Add remaining dairy and sugar or Splenda.®

3. Cook over medium heat while stirring constantly until mixture comes to a boil. Remove from heat and cool until mixture comes to room temperature and just begins to set.

4. Add sour cream and vanilla. Stir to mix well.

5. Portion into individual ramekins or custard cups.

6. Cover and refrigerate until set and ready to serve.

Per Serving

	Calories	Fat (gm)	Sat fat (gm)	Trans fat (gm)	Cholesterol (mg)	Sodium (mg)	Carbohydrates (gm)	Dietary Fiber (gm)	Sugar (gm)	Protein (gm)
Base recipe	180	9	5	0	25	65	22	0	22	4
Reduced calorie with sugar	150	2.5	1.5	0	10.0	100	28	0	21	5
Reduced calorie with Splenda®	100	2.5	1.5	0	10	100	13	0	6	5
Reduced calorie, fat free with sugar	140	0.5	0	0	5	135	29	0	21	5
Reduced calories, fat free with Splenda®	80	0.5	0	0	5	135	14	0	6	5
Moderate calorie	240	16	9	0	45	60	21	0	18	4
High calorie	410	36	22	1	125	60	20	0	18	3

Diabetes

Essentials Expert

Maggie Powers, PhD, RD, CDE, is a research scientist at the International Diabetes Center at Park Nicollet, in Minneapolis. The author of *Handbook of Diabetes Medical Nutrition Therapy, Guide to Eating Right When You Have Diabetes, The American Diabetes Association's Forbidden Foods Cookbook*, and many other publications, Maggie is an internationally known diabetes educator. She is a leader in the American Diabetes Association, the American Association of Diabetes Educators and The Academy of Nutrition and Dietetics. Maggie has always been concerned about the "food" side of nutrition therapy. She says that "the best nutrition therapy recommendations don't mean a thing if someone cannot obtain healthy food and enjoy it. Nutrition therapy is based on one's ecology, the system they live in and all of its influences on behaviors. There is a science and art to providing nutrition therapy."

Diabetes mellitus is a chronic metabolic disease characterized by high blood glucose, also called blood sugar, and insufficient or ineffective insulin. By knowing what persons with diabetes want and need, foodservice professionals can help 26 million people enjoy better health. A primary goal of diabetes care is to help people with the disease attain and maintain a blood glucose level as close to normal as possible. Because carbohydrate is the food component that raises blood glucose levels, people with diabetes need to monitor the amount of carbohydrates they eat by balancing food intake with physical activity and insulin – either their own or injected insulin. Experts recommend distributing carbohydrates fairly evenly throughout the day – some at each meal and with snacks. People with diabetes should not skip breakfast and lunch and then eat a very large dinner. A quick, appetizing and easy-to-consume snack may be substituted for breakfast or lunch.

When foods, particularly carbohydrates, are eaten, they are digested and absorbed as glucose. Glucose is the energy source for all cells in the body. The body needs the hormone insulin to move glucose from the bloodstream into cells. Individuals with diabetes can increase or decrease blood sugar levels with more or less food and exercise. When blood sugar levels are too low, an individual with diabetes needs a quick source of sugar – often fruit juice. If blood sugar levels are too high, insulin may be injected to prevent medical emergencies.

The person with diabetes either makes too little insulin or is resistant to insulin produced. As a result, blood glucose levels get too high (**hyperglycemia**). This condition can be controlled with medications that boost insulin production, with injections of insulin or with medications that help control blood glucose levels. Early in the development of diabetes, some people can manage their blood glucose by food and exercise alone. Even when medications are added, food and exercise are still important parts of the diabetes management plan. Near-normal blood glucose levels help people feel better and may reduce or prevent the complications of diabetes.

Too much insulin, too little food or unplanned exercise can cause a low blood glucose level (**hypoglycemia**). When blood glucose is too low, a person may be hungry, irritable and feel very weak. This condition can be avoided by having a treatment plan that has been individualized for them so it fits into their food habits, meal times and exercise schedule.

Diabetes is a chronic disease that has several forms based on how much insulin is produced and the level of insulin resistance. Generally, **type 1 diabetes** occurs earlier in life and requires daily insulin injections or an insulin pump. **Type 2 diabetes** is much more common and, until recently, generally occurred later in life. It is reported that one in three children born today will develop type 2 diabetes. This type of diabetes may be controlled by diet, by diet and pills, or by diet and insulin injections. Being overweight and inactive increases the likelihood of developing type 2 diabetes. Early in the condition, small amounts of weight loss and improved food choices are sometimes enough to control blood glucose without medication.

Many people with diabetes use *Choose Your Foods: Food Lists for Weight Management* (2014) developed by the American Diabetes Association and The American Dietetic Association. (**See Appendix F: Food Lists.**) There are seven exchange lists, with foods grouped according to similar numbers of calories, carbohydrates, proteins and fats. The portion size of each food varies so that foods can be exchanged for each other in a predetermined meal plan. The exchange lists are very useful for chefs as a resource for nutrient content and information about food for guests with diabetes.

Another popular resource, *My Food Plan* (5th edition, 2014) developed by the International Diabetes Center, focuses primarily on carbohydrate counting, which some find easier to use than planning for all seven exchange groups. (**See Appendix G: Carb Counting**.) The list of carbohydrates includes single foods, mixed dishes, snacks and desserts. Portions (choices) are similar; each contains about 15 grams of carbohydrates. *My Food Plan* includes guidance for determining how many carbohydrate choices are best for each meal and snack. Food plans based on a vegetarian diet and several ethnic diets can be found on the International Diabetes Center website, https://idcpublishing.com/?c=home

Key Nutrition Points

- Many people with diabetes have 2 to 4 carbohydrate choices (servings) at each meal. One cup of berries (1 choice) and a sandwich made with 2 slices of bread (2 choices) equals 3 carbohydrate choices. A large bagel counts as 4 carbohydrate choices. Self-monitoring of blood glucose (or blood sugar) helps people with diabetes know if they are eating the right amount of carbohydrate.

- The overall emphasis is on healthful eating. Those with diabetes benefit from eating a variety of food with a basic healthful food plan emphasizing whole grains, fresh food and moderate serving sizes. Their diet should be low in saturated and trans fat since people with diabetes are at a higher risk for developing cardiovascular disease.

- People with diabetes need to manage their carbohydrate intake – how much they consume and when they consume it. Amount and types of food and eating at regular mealtimes are important.

- Healthy eating for people with diabetes is the same as healthful eating for all people and does not necessarily require special "diet" foods. Carbohydrate is the nutrient requiring particular attention. To assist those with diabetes, chefs should offer lower-carbohydrate alternatives, such as spaghetti squash (instead of pasta) with marinara or Bolognese sauce and sandwiches on bread rather than on oversized buns.

- Each person with diabetes should have a meal plan tailor-made to his/her individual needs, food preferences, medications and lifestyle – preferably planned with a registered dietitian, who may also be a certified diabetes educator. Some professionals recommend counting carbohydrates. Others use the exchange system with certain types and amounts of foods from various food groups at each meal and snack.

- In addition to controlling carbohydrates, people with diabetes should limit sweet, salty and high-fat food. People with diabetes are especially prone to cardiovascular disease and kidney disease.

- Generally, there is relatively little room for added sugar in a diet for a person with diabetes; sweetened food products should be limited because they take the place of more nutrient-rich carbohydrates.

- Sugar substitutes may be useful, especially in beverages. People with diabetes and those controlling their weight expect packets of sugar substitute to be available and appreciate desserts low in sugar. See Chapter 3 for information about sugar substitutes.

- Portions of food for those with diabetes should be quite modest. For those using food exchanges or carbohydrate counting, 1 serving is equal to 15 grams of carbohydrates, which is 1 ounce of bread, ½ English muffin, ½ tortilla, or ⅓ cup of rice or pasta. A modest 1 cup of plain pasta counts as 3 servings for someone with diabetes. The typical serving of meat should be a 3 to 4 ounce portion.

- People with diabetes can consume a delicious-looking dessert or have jelly on their toast and be well within their eating guidelines. Unfortunately, some people judge what someone with diabetes is eating based on outdated information.

- Some guests will decline a bread basket or ask for an open-faced sandwich to avoid consuming extra carbohydrates. Offering a salad with the dressing on the side or a steamed or grilled vegetable in place of potatoes is a thoughtful substitution. Including a broth-based soup on the menu gives the person with diabetes a food option when others are having a high-fat, high-carbohydrate appetizer.

Best Choices

There are very few differences between a diabetic diet and the healthy diet of someone without diabetes. Food for patrons with diabetes should be as enjoyable as food for any guest. Just be sure to have a variety of items on the menu that are low in calories, carbohydrates and fat so that guests with diabetes have a full range of choices. Generally, foods promoted in *MyPlate* are best choices for those with diabetes.

- Several food items or dishes that are low in carbohydrates should be available so guests with diabetes can manage their intake and still have choices within each menu category.

- The best food choices are those that don't have hidden fat or carbohydrate and thus allow the guest to make an informed choice. For example, many restaurants will make mashed potatoes with lots of added fat. A little extra fat is acceptable, but too often it can be quite high. It is helpful to offer simple foods – vegetables with no added fat (or less than 1 teaspoon per serving) and desserts with no added sugar such as fresh cut fruit. If the clientele includes many diners with diabetes, offering sugar-free gelatin with some berries would be a good menu addition.

- Foods prepared without added fat or with just enough fat to maintain a flavorful presentation are best. Because total calories are an important

issue for them, people with diabetes are encouraged to eat plenty of low-carbohydrate vegetables in salads, side dishes, entrées and soups. Fill the plate with low-carbohydrate vegetables such as green beans, broccoli or asparagus simply steamed, roasted or grilled.

- Because individuals with diabetes are frequently seeking a 3- to 4-ounce protein source, appetizers such as crab cakes or chicken skewers are good entrée choices.

Foods to Avoid

Virtually all foods can be worked into a diabetes food plan, even if in a small amount. There are some foods, however, that people with diabetes should avoid because they are easy to overeat and very high in carbohydrates. These foods include sugared beverages such as sodas, punches, ades, juices and sweet tea (containing regular sugar). People with diabetes are encouraged to avoid high-calorie foods and foods high in fat, especially saturated and trans fat.

People with diabetes who want to eat high-sugar foods such as regular jam, regular syrup or a dessert, can certainly do so and enjoy it, but they also must be aware of how much carbohydrate they are consuming and adjust for it in the same or other meals or snacks or alter their insulin dosage accordingly.

Tips for Chefs

- Be creative! Help your customers savor the taste of fresh food that blends textures and taste using lot of vegetables, legumes, fruit and whole grains. Offer "fillers" that don't add carbohydrates and fat.

- One of the most important steps you can take to help people with diabetes and anyone seeking healthful food is to reduce portion sizes. List the size or ounces of the piece of meat, chicken or fish so that guests know how much they are getting. Offer low-fat, low-calorie side dishes and salad dressings and sauces on the side so that guests can control the amount they use. Remember that people who have diabetes do not need special foods; however, they do need reasonable options from which to choose.

- Cook with as little fat and sugar as possible.

- Offer at least one green salad with interesting vegetables, fresh fruit, and herbs but without croutons, bacon and other high-fat ingredients. Have a low-fat dressing or oil and vinegar available. Dress salads lightly.

- Have fresh berries, sliced melon or other fresh, ripe, delicious fruits available as a dessert option. Fresh fruit is a good menu addition for those on almost any special diet, for those watching their weight and for kids.

- An appetizer of hummus with crudités – fairly low in carbohydrate and fat, crunchy and tasty – helps decrease hunger.

- Provide packets of a calorie-free sweetener so guests can sweeten beverages without adding sugar.

- If a hostess or server is told that a guest with diabetes must eat soon, react quickly. Bring a glass of fruit juice and ask what else to bring to avoid an emergency caused by low blood sugar.

For More Information

- American Diabetes Association, **www.diabetes.org**
- Mills, J. *1000 Diabetes Recipes*. Hoboken, NJ: John Wiley & Sons, Inc., 2011.
- National Center for Chronic Disease Prevention and Health Promotion, **www.cdc.gov/diabetes**
- National Institute of Diabetes and Digestive and Kidney Diseases, **www2.niddk.nih.gov**
- Powers M. *American Dietetic Association Guide to Eating Right When You Have Diabetes*. New York: John Wiley & Sons; 2003.
- Powers M, Hendley J. *Forbidden Foods Diabetes Cooking*. Alexandria, VA: American Diabetes Association; 2000.
- Warshaw H. *Diabetes Meal Planning Made Easy*, 5th ed. Alexandria, VA: American Diabetes Association; 2016.

Blueberry Cobbler

Yield: 12 servings

Carolyn Leontos, MS, RD, CDE

Professor Emeritus Retired,
University of Nevada Cooperative Extension, Las Vegas, Nevada

To accommodate individuals with diabetes who want fewer calories, bake with Splenda® or another non-nutritive sweetener that with-stands heat. Splenda® Sugar Blend adds some calories, but the sugar in the blend enhances the texture and color of the crust.

Blueberries, fresh or frozen	2	pounds
Flour, all-purpose	2	tablespoons
Splenda® or Splenda® Sugar Blend	³/₈	cup
or the equivalent amount of other non-nutritive sweetener	¾	cup
All purpose flour	1 ½	cups
Baking powder	1	tablespoon
Salt	¾	teaspoon
Splenda® or Splenda® Sugar Blend or the equivalent amount of other non-nutritive sweetener	3	tablespoons
1% milk	1 ¼	cups
Oil, vegetable	5	tablespoons

1. Preheat oven to 400° F.

2. Let blueberries thaw, if frozen. Mix 2 tablespoons flour and ¾ cup sweetener into the blueberries. Put blueberry mixture into individual ramekins sprayed with non-stick spray. Do not overfill, as mixture will bubble up in oven.

3. Mix 1 ½ cups flour, baking powder, salt and 3 tablespoons sweetener. Add milk and oil to flour mixture and mix just until dry ingredients are moistened. Mixture will be thin and lumpy. Spoon dough onto berry mixture. Bake 30-35 minutes until crust is golden brown.

Blueberry Cobbler made with Splenda®
Carb Choices: 1 ½
Diabetic Exchanges: ½ starch + 1 fruit + 1 fat

Blueberry Cobbler made with Splenda® Blend
Carb Choices: 2
Diabetic Exchanges: 1 starch + 1 fruit + 1 fat

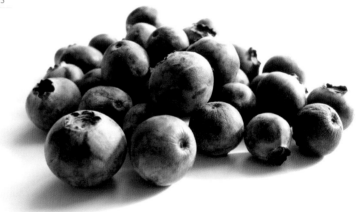

Per Serving

	Calories	Fat (gm)	Sat fat (gm)	Trans fat (gm)	Cholesterol (mg)	Sodium (mg)	Carbohydrates (gm)	Dietary Fiber (gm)	Sugar (gm)	Protein (gm)
with Splenda®	170	7	1	0	0	280	25	3	9	3
with Splenda® blend	190	7	1	0	0	280	30	3	14	3

Digestive Disorders

Essentials Expert

Leslie Bonci, MPH, RD, LDN, CSSD, is adjunct instructor in the school of dental medicine at the University of Pittsburgh and lectures extensively at universities and corporations. Leslie is a board-certified specialist in sports nutrition and she is the nutrition consultant for the Kansas City Chiefs , Carnegie Mellon University athletics and the Pittsburgh Ballet Theatre. She is the author of *Sport Nutrition for Coaches* and the American

Dietetic Association Guide to Better Digestion and co-author of *Run Your Butt Off, Walk Your Butt Off, the Active Calorie Diet and Bike Your Butt Off.* She is developing programs with chefs and master gardeners that focuses on helping kids and adults cultivate, investigate and appreciate a love for cooking and gardening with Camp Delicious and Root Camp.

Digestion is the process by which food and drink are reduced to smaller nutrient units that can be absorbed into the bloodstream and carried throughout the body to build and nourish cells and to provide energy. **Absorption** is the passage of these molecules through the walls of the digestive tract so the substances can enter the bloodstream and then enter cells. **Metabolism** is the chemical activity within cells that breaks down nutrients to provide energy, uses nutrients to build necessary compounds and tissues, and releases the end products.

Organs that make up the digestive tract are the mouth, esophagus, stomach, small intestine, large intestine (or colon), rectum and anus. Inside these hollow organs is a lining called the **mucosa**. In the mouth, stomach and small intestine, the mucosa contains tiny glands that produce digestive juices to help break down the food. The digestive tract also contains a layer of smooth muscle that helps break down food and move it along the tract. Two solid digestive organs, the liver and the pancreas, produce digestive juices that reach the intestine through small tubes called ducts. The gallbladder stores the liver's digestive juices until they are needed in the intestine. Parts of the nervous and circulatory systems also play major roles in the digestive system.

Digestive disorders include diseases such as diverticulitis, celiac disease, ulcers, gastric reflux (GERD), irritable bowel syndrome, hepatitis, ulcerative colitis, Crohn's disease, dyspepsia, functional heartburn and chronic constipation. Each affects different parts of the digestive system. In ulcerative colitis for example, the colon is inflamed but the small intestine works normally. Crohn's disease affects the small intestine, making it difficult to digest and absorb nutrients.

In all digestive disorders, alterations in taste, poor nutrient utilization, pain, decreased appetite and the inflammatory process can lead to weight loss and malnutrition. With recurrent diarrhea, the risk for anemia and vitamin deficiencies rises. Small, frequent meals of foods that can be tolerated minimize symptoms. Gastrointestinal problems tend to reduce the efficiency of nutrient absorption, so a nutrient-dense diet is advisable. Adequate liquids are necessary to prevent dehydration.

The Digestive Tract

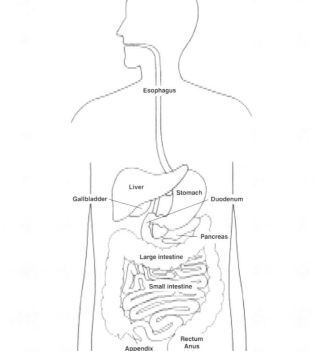

Source: National Institute of Diabetes and Digestive and Kidney Diseases, **http://digestive.niddk.nih.gov/ddiseases/ pubs/yrdd/index.htm**

Diverticulitis is an inflammation of small pouches in the lining of the large intestine. Fecal matter becomes trapped in these pouches if the diet does not have adequate fiber. Symptoms include abdominal cramping, painful spasms, distention, nausea and fever. The treatment is bowel rest with a temporary low-residue liquid diet followed by a low-fiber, low-residue diet. When symptoms disappear, high-fiber foods are introduced and lots of water is generally recommended.

Irritable Bowel Syndrome (IBS) is a common disorder causing abdominal pain, bloating and changes in bowel habits. Crohn's disease and ulcerative colitis are two types of IBS. In IBS, the colon is very sensitive and may contract causing pain and diarrhea, or it may fail to contract causing severe constipation and pain. Sometimes bacterial infections cause IBS.

Crohn's disease is an inflammation of the small intestine that makes digestion and the absorption of key nutrients difficult and painful. It causes bloating, diarrhea, abdominal pain and cramping and can lead to malnutrition, anemia and low levels of certain vitamins and folic acid. Although the disease is an immune reaction in the intestinal tract, avoiding certain foods that "trigger" the painful symptoms is important. With Crohn's disease, eating regular meals and additional snacks throughout the day ensures that an ample supply of key nutrients is getting into the digestive tract. Doctors usually recommend vitamin and mineral supplements to replenish losses. Once a person determines what foods cause symptoms to flare up, the troublesome foods can be avoided or prepared in a different manner.

People with *ulcerative colitis* (ulcerations in the colon/large intestine) should eat at regular times and eliminate alcohol, carbonated beverages, caffeine, dairy products and other foods that trigger reactions. Probiotics, such as yogurt, and adjusting levels of dietary fiber may be recommended, depending on symptoms.

Acid reflux, also called heartburn, or GERD (gastroesophogeal reflux disease), occurs when the sphincter between the esophagus and stomach relaxes and food comes back up after it has been

What are FODMAPs?

FODMAPs, an acronym that stands for Fermentable Oligosaccharides, Disaccharides, Monosaccharides and Polyols, are short chain carbohydrates and sugar alcohols that may be poorly absorbed by the body. These carbohydrates ferment in the large intestine during digestion, drawing in water and producing carbon dioxide, hydrogen and methane gas that cause the intestine to expand. This causes gastrointestinal symptoms such as bloating and pain that are common in gastrointestinal disorders.

FODMAPs are abundant in the diet and can be found in everyday foods such as: wheat, barley, rye, apples, pears, mango, onion, garlic, honey, kidney beans, cashew nuts, agave syrup, sugar free gum, mints and some medicines, to name a few. Up to 75% of those who suffer with irritable bowel syndrome will benefit from dietary restriction of FODMAPs.

There is emerging research that the FODMAP diet may be an effective therapy in the management of IBS symptoms. This does not present a cure, but a suggested dietary approach to improve symptoms and quality of life.

What is the low FODMAP diet?

The low FODMAP diet is a two to six-week elimination diet that involves removing high FODMAP foods from the diet to assess whether FODMAP rich foods are triggering GI symptoms. The low FODMAP diet is a learning diet with the goal of determining personal dietary triggers. After the low FODMAP elimination diet phase, a dietitian will guide on how to re-introduce FODMAPs, in a methodical manner, to assess tolerance to various FODMAP containing foods. Many people will find they can liberalize their FODMAP diet restrictions and only need to restrict some high FODMAP foods. The low FODMAP diet should be implemented with the help of a FODMAP knowledgeable dietitian to help a person navigate the many nuances of the diet and to develop a personalized, well-balanced eating plan.

mixed with stomach acids. Foods that tend to stimulate stomach acid production and increase heartburn include caffeinated and carbonated beverages, alcohol, spicy foods, black pepper, citrus fruits and juices, and tomato juice. All high-fat foods and chocolate tend to relax the sphincter, often causing heartburn. Eating small frequent meals and not eating close to bedtime can help reduce heartburn.

An *ulcer* is a sore, an open painful wound. ***Peptic ulcers*** occur in the stomach or upper part of the small intestine. For almost 100 years, it was believed that ulcers were caused by spicy foods, stress and alcohol. Now we know that peptic ulcers are caused by a particular bacterial infection (***Helicobacter pylori***), by certain medications or by smoking. Physicians Barry Marshall and Robin Warren received a Nobel Prize for this discovery in 1982. The formation of ulcers seems to require both H. pylori and over-secretion of stomach acids, which irritate the lining of the stomach. The treatment is typically antibiotics and antacids. Any food that specifically causes distress may be eliminated, but a bland diet is no longer the recommended treatment for peptic ulcers.

Key Nutrition Points

- Often foods that are too rich or very high in fat will cause digestive distress because there are not enough digestive enzymes or bile to break down the fat to molecules that can be absorbed.

- Very spicy foods can cause discomfort when they irritate the lining of the digestive tract.

- Too much acid, as in raw or lightly cooked tomatoes, can be a problem for some people. Using a tomato sauce instead of raw tomatoes may alleviate this problem.

- Individuals vary greatly in their ability to digest different types of food. This variability has to do with the amount of secretions (particularly digestive enzymes), the condition of the membranes within the digestive tract, and the presence of normal bacteria that help break down foods for absorption.

- When the amount of food eaten exceeds the digestive tract's ability to break it down efficiently, the result is gastrointestinal distress. Bloating, burping or belching, cramping and abdominal pain, gas and diarrhea are common symptoms of gastrointestinal distress.

- Getting enough fiber in the diet is important to promote regular elimination and also to help rid the body of excess cholesterol. If the body has difficulty breaking down food for any reason, gastrointestinal distress results and nutrients are poorly absorbed.

- Certain high-fiber foods, such as bran or flax seeds, may increase gas production and bloating. Gas-producing fiber is usually insoluble (mainly found in cereals or whole grains). Soluble fiber, mainly found in vegetables and fruits, is less likely to cause gastrointestinal distress. Certain foods, such as beans, cabbage, legumes (peas, peanuts and soybeans), and sometimes apples, melons, grapes and raisins may produce gas in the lower bowel. Bacteria in the colon ferment undigested particles of food, which causes flatulence (gas) and distress.

Best Choices

- Most Americans do not eat enough fiber. Adding high-fiber vegetables, fruits, grains, legumes, seeds and nuts to the menu is desirable – unless fibers cause distress.

- People with gastrointestinal diseases have especially sensitive digestive tracts. Small meals are usually best for them because large portions of food can trigger symptoms. Adequate protein intake is important; lean proteins are preferred.

- Live active cultures in buttermilk, yogurt and other foods promote gastrointestinal health and generally aid digestion. Use these foods as ingredients in cooking and when making smoothies, dips, sauces and salad dressings.

- Ginger is a gut-friendly spice and ginger tea is a soothing beverage that can alleviate nausea for many people with gastrointestinal problems. Freshly grated ginger and crystallized ginger add a lot of flavor and are versatile ingredients.

Foods to Avoid

- There is no scientifically proven diet for inflammatory bowel disease. Each person with IBS has his/her own trigger foods. The guest will know what foods he or she must avoid and should be able to order accordingly. Often-reported trigger foods include:

  - Alcohol-containing beverages
  - Butter, oil and other fats
  - Carbonated beverages
  - Coffee and tea
  - Chocolate
  - Cornhusks
  - Gas-producing foods
  - High-fiber foods such as raw fruits and vegetables and bran
  - Red meat and pork
  - Spicy foods
  - Nuts and seeds

- If a primary digestive disorder symptom is flatulence that causes pain, it helps to limit gas-causing foods. People with this problem generally know which foods to avoid – for example, cruciferous vegetables and legumes, specifically mature beans and peas.

- For some people, flaxseeds are an irritant. Other seeds and nuts can also irritate the villi in the lining of the intestines.

- Large volumes of food in the gastrointestinal tract can trigger symptoms such as bloating, abdominal discomfort and diarrhea.

Tips for Chefs

Guests with irritable bowel syndrome, Crohn's disease, celiac disease and other gastrointestinal disorders usually know which foods trigger symptoms and order foods accordingly. They may ask if foods have specific ingredients that they must avoid. Servers should be prepared to answer these questions.

For More Information

- Bonci L. *American Dietetic Association Guide to Better Digestion*. Chicago: The American Dietetic Association; 2003.

- International Foundation for Functional Gastrointestinal Disorders (IFFGD), **www.iffgd.org**

- *Mayo Clinic on Digestive Health*, 3rd ed. Rochester, MN: Mayo Clinic Trade Publishing; 2014.

- The National Institute of Diabetes and Digestive and Kidney Diseases, **www2.niddk.nih.gov**

- Raman M, Sirounis A, Shrubsole J. *The Complete IBS Health and Diet Guide.* Toronto, Canada: Robert Rose, 2011.

Wild Rice Salad

Yield: 8 cups

Provided by Leslie Bonci, MPH, RD, LDN, CSSD

Serves: 10 servings, ³/₄ cup each

Director of Sports Nutrition, University of Pittsburgh Medical Center
Recipe from Chefs Kevin Watson and Denise Pierchalski

This side dish or salad is colorful and has a variety of flavors and textures. The sweetness of the dried cherries balances nicely with the sourness of the salad dressing. The toasted pecans and sweet peppers add just the right crunch. This salad is perfect for most diets, including vegan, kosher and halal.

Vegetable broth	5	cups
Wild rice, rinsed	²/₃	cup
Short grain organic brown rice	1	cup
Pecans, toasted, chopped	½	cup
Dried cherries or sweetened cranberries	¾	cup
Scallions, light and dark green parts only, sliced thin	1	bunch
Red pepper, diced	1	each
Yellow pepper, diced	1	each
Zest of one orange	2	tablespoons

Dressing:

Dijon mustard	1	tablespoon
Shallot, minced	2	teaspoons
Garlic, minced	1	teaspoon
Brown sugar	1	tablespoon
Cider vinegar	¼	cup
Basil, fresh, chopped	2	teaspoons
Salt	½	teaspoon
Pepper	¼	teaspoon
Olive oil	¹/₃	cup

1. Bring 2 ½ cups of vegetable broth to a boil, add wild rice and simmer covered for about 40 minutes, stirring occasionally until rice starts to break open and becomes tender, add more liquid if needed. Remove rice to a sheet pan to cool.

2. Bring 2 ½ cups of vegetable broth to a boil, add brown rice and simmer about 30 minutes until liquid is absorbed, and remove rice to a sheet pan to cool.

3. In a large bowl combine pecans, cherries, scallions, peppers and orange zest. Add cooked wild and brown rice and mix well.

Dressing:

1. Combine Dijon mustard, shallot, garlic, brown sugar, vinegar, basil, salt and pepper in a bowl. Slowly whisk in olive oil. Pour dressing over salad and toss well.

2. Refrigerate salad until needed, serve at room temperature.

Per Serving

Calories	240	Cholesterol	0	mg
Fat	10 g	Sodium	170	mg
Saturated Fat	1.5 g	Carbohydrates	32	mg
Trans Fat	0 g	Dietary Fiber	3	mg
Sugar	8 g	Protein	4	g

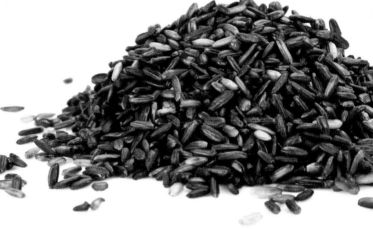

Food Allergies and Intolerances

Essentials Expert

Margaret Condrasky, EdD, RD, CCE, is associate professor of food science and human nutrition at Clemson University. She has written extensively and designed culinary nutrition seminars and refreshers, particularly for the American Culinary Federation. Marge works with industry chefs and product devel-opers. At the university she directs the CU CHEFS® (Clemson University's Cooking and Healthy Eating Food Specialists) instructional program and, in the academic arena, she focuses on the culinary scienc-es for undergraduates and graduate students.

Food allergies are relatively uncommon, affecting only about 6% of children and about 4% of adults. All told, only about 12 million Americans have food allergies, but the number is increasing. During the last decade, food allergies have become more common in children. Fortunately, most children outgrow them, especially allergies to milk, eggs and soy. Although only eight foods account for 90% of all food-related allergic reactions – milk, eggs, peanuts, tree nuts, fish, shellfish, wheat and soy – a growing allergen-consciousness is evidenced by the introduction of many new products created and labeled as allergen-free. [9]

A ***food allergy*** occurs when a food protein is at-tacked by the immune system. This attack triggers a sudden release of histamine, among other chemicals, and results in allergic reaction symptoms. These symptoms may be relatively mild (rashes, hives, itching, runny nose, watery eyes, headache, cramp-ing, swelling, etc.) or severe (trouble breathing, wheezing, loss of consciousness, etc.). A severe or life-threatening allergic reaction – when the airways swell closed and breathing is blocked – is called ***anaphylaxis*** or ***anaphylactic shock*** and can cause death if not treated immediately. Symptoms usually occur immediately but may appear up to two hours after ingesting an allergen.

If there is any indication that a guest is having an allergic reaction, call 911 immediately. Also check to see if the person is carrying the prescription drug epinephrine, typically as a pen-like device (EpiPen®). If so, administer the drug immediately. The device contains a spring-loaded needle that exits the tip of the pen. The medication should be injected into the person's outer thigh.

Because of the potential danger associated with an allergic reaction, people with food allergies must

Since chefs know so much about ingredients, they can equip themselves with awareness and techniques to help guests with food allergies enjoy wonderful meals. Individuals with food allergies or intolerances who would potentially enjoy dining away from home compose a virtually untapped market segment in the restaurant world. Chefs and foodservice estab-lishments can and should work to gain the trust and patronage of this group who will bring family and friends to places where they can dine safely.

Margaret Condrasky, EdD, RD, CCE
Clemson University

assess and evaluate their food choices carefully. They may ask a lot of questions about ingredients and cooking techniques. These are not idle queries. Servers should convey all of these concerns to the chef, and both serving staff and chefs should be prepared to answer all questions completely.

Even tiny traces of an allergen can trigger reactions in susceptible individuals. The only way to assure diners that a dish is safe to eat is to know what is in it. Often, a potential allergen is not obvious or not recognizable in foods. Sometimes allergens are in food processing ingredients, such as stabilizers or thickeners.

Cross contamination is one of the leading causes of food allergy reactions in restaurants. Clean utensils and work surfaces thoroughly before using them to prepare food for an allergic guest. Be especially careful of cutting boards, slicers and other kitchen equipment that may have been used before for an allergen-containing food. Traces of egg, flour or nuts may adhere to rubber gloves, parchment paper or a spatula. Garnishes or salad bowls with traces of crushed nuts, pasta water that was used to boil cheese-filled pasta, tongs used to turn fish then used to turn beef – all of these can lead to severe reactions in allergic guests who have carefully ordered foods they assume to be safe. Consider having a separate "allergy-free" station with dedicated equipment, a dedicated pot of boiling water to be used for gluten-free cooking, and cutting boards, mixers, etc., that are used only for allergy-free orders. Evaluate your menu and train servers to know which menu items are free of major allergens.

As part of an allergy response plan, maintain a notebook or file with ingredient lists of all menu items, including ingredients in outsourced foods. Make a list of menu items suitable for guests with specific allergens or intolerances. Include text on your menu that encourages guests to notify the serving staff about food allergies. During hours of operation, a restaurant should have at least one person on duty, ideally the manager, who can handle questions and special requests from guests with food allergies. Because so many ingredients may contain allergens, guests may request to read the list for themselves, rather than having a staff member interpret ingredients for them. This involvement places some of the responsibility for ascertaining the safety of foods on the customer.

Every food service operation should have a list of food offerings that are suitable for guests with common food allergies or intolerances. A dietitian, knowledgeable chef or manager should carefully evaluate each recipe and all ingredients (including prepared ingredients and condiments) and create a listing of offerings suitable for those on gluten-free, lactose-free, nut-free, soy-free, vegan and other common dietary restrictions. Servers may have general knowledge but need a resource to properly answer questions from diners. Servers should not be expected to know the very specific composition of recipe ingredients that may be harmful to some patrons. For example, some prepared salad dressings may contain peanut oil that can cause a severe allergic reaction in a person with a peanut allergy; many ingredients contain small amounts of gluten that can trigger reactions in very sensitive individuals.

Food Intolerance and Aversion

A food intolerance and food aversion are not the same. A *food intolerance* is characterized by unpleasant symptoms, such as stomach cramps or diarrhea that occur after consuming certain foods. People with a food intolerance can eat minimal amounts of the food in question without experiencing major symptoms. The amount of food tolerated varies greatly from person to person.

A *food aversion* is neither an allergy nor intolerance. It is an intense dislike that may cause a biological response (usually nausea). Aversions usually have psychological and/or physiological causes or effects. Many aversions are based on what foods are acceptable within one's culture. Sometimes aversions occur because a food made that person ill at an earlier time.

If an individual has a true food allergy or multiple allergies and tells staff, the chef or manager can respond that the kitchen is not able to serve that person safely. While awkward, it protects both the foodservice and the guest. Often, especially with children with severe allergies, a parent will bring prepackaged safe foods, while others choose from the regular menu.

Key Nutrition Points

- For the person with a food allergy, complete avoidance of the allergenic ingredient is critical.

- Reading labels, particularly ingredient lists, is essential.

- Encourage diners with special needs to call ahead to make sure you can accommodate them and encourage them to pre-order so the chef can check ingredients and use appropriate equipment for food preparation.

- Avoid cross contamination. Use clean equipment and clean spoons and measures for adding ingredients. For example, is the wok you are using to stir-fry vegetables the same wok just used for a stir-fry containing shrimp?

- Be sure the chef understands that foods for guests with allergies must be prepared using only the ingredients in the recipe directions. Creative adjustments such as adding a bit of flour to thicken or butter to enrich can cause a dangerous reaction in an allergic guest.

Milk Allergy

A ***milk allergy*** is an immune system response to the protein in milk. People with a milk allergy are likely to be allergic to goat, sheep and cows' milk and products made from them. Soymilk, rice milk and nut (almond) milk are useful alternatives if no other allergies are present. Each of these "milks" has a different nutrient profile and cooking and flavor characteristics.

Milk allergy is different from the more common lactose intolerance. People with ***lactose intolerance*** lack the enzyme lactase, which is required to digest lactose, a sugar in milk. They experience gas, bloating and abdominal pain. Many lactose-intolerant people drink dairy products with added lactase or take lactase tablets before they drink milk or eat foods containing milk or milk products. Individuals who do not drink milk early in life can stop making lactase and may become lactose intolerant later.

Many lactose-intolerant people can handle some but not much lactose without ill effects. They can enjoy cultured milk products like yogurt or kefir; hard aged cheeses like Cheddar, Colby, Swiss or Parmesan; and milk products found in very small quantities in food additives or preservatives.

Allergens Listed on the Food Label

The Food Allergen Labeling and Consumer Protection Act (FALCPA), which took effect January 1, 2006, mandates that the labels of foods containing major food allergens (milk, eggs, fish, crustacean shellfish, peanuts, tree nuts, wheat and soy) declare the allergen in plain language, either in the ingredient list or by one of these two statements:

- The word "Contains" followed by the name of the major food allergen – for example, "Contains milk, wheat"
- A parenthetical statement in the list of ingredients – for example, "albumin (egg)"

Allergenic ingredients must be listed if they are present in any amount, even in colors, flavors or spice blends. Additionally, manufacturers must list the specific nut (for example, almond, walnut, cashew, etc.) or seafood (for example, tuna, salmon, shrimp, lobster, etc.) used. Unfortunately, gluten is not included in FALCPA.

Source: U. S. Food and Drug Administration, **http://www.fda.gov/food/ingredientspackaginglabeling/foodallergens/ucm079311.htm**

Dairy Products to Avoid

All milk products must be excluded from the diet when there is a milk allergy.

Acidophilis milk

Butter

Buttermilk

Cheese

Cheese food

Coffee creamer

Condensed milk

Creamed soups

Custards

Evaporated milk

Ice cream

Margarine containing milk solids

Milk chocolate

Puddings

Sour cream

Whipped cream

Whole, skim and low-fat milk

Yogurt

Ingredients to Avoid

Ammonium caseinate

Binding agents

Butter flavorings

Calcium caseinate

Caramel or caramel flavorings

Carob

Casein

Casein hydrolysate

Ghee

Lactalbumin

Lactate

Lactic acid

Lactoferrin

Lactoglobulin

Lactulose

Malted milk

Milk protein

Non-dairy creamer (may contain casein)

Nougat

Protein hydrolysate

Rennet casein

Simplesse™

Skim milk solids

Sodium caseinate

Whey

Whey protein hydrolysate

Foods Commonly Containing Milk or Milk Products

- Baked goods, cakes and cookies
- Biscuits
- Bread
- Breakfast cereals
- Butter, alone, in or on foods
- Candy, fudge, milk chocolate and caramels
- Canned tuna (some brands contain casein)
- Cheese
- Cocoa mixes
- Crackers and cereals
- Cream sauces
- Custard
- Deli meats and cold cuts with casein as binder
- Egg substitutes
- Foods fried in batter
- Gravies
- Ice cream, gelato and sherbet
- Instant drink mixes
- Instant potatoes
- Hot dogs (unless kosher)
- Margarine
- Mayonnaise
- Pancakes and waffles
- Salad dressings
- Sausages
- Soups
- Sour cream
- Soy/vegetarian cheese
- Specialty coffees, latte, cappuccino
- Tofu
- Vegetables in cream or cheese sauces
- Whipped toppings
- Yogurt

Tips for Chefs

- Have soymilk, rice milk or almond milk in the kitchen to substitute for cow's milk.
- Use vegetable oil instead of butter when possible.
- Offer a tapenade or hummus as a spread for bread instead of butter.
- Kosher foods marked pareve contain no milk or dairy products; therefore they are acceptable for those with milk allergy or lactose intolerance.

Egg Allergy

Egg allergy, especially an allergy to egg whites, is more common in children than in adults and is likely to be outgrown over time. Strictly avoiding eggs and food containing eggs and egg products is the only way to prevent a reaction. It is not always easy to avoid these foods because many unexpected products contain eggs. For example, egg yolks are sometimes used to glaze baked items like pretzels or bagels. Eggs also may be used as a foaming agent in beer, lattes or cappucinos.

Always check the label for ingredients before you use a product. In addition, check the label each time you use the product; manufacturers occasionally change recipes, and a trigger food may be added to the new recipe. Several terms indicate that egg products have been used in manufacturing processed foods. Terms that imply egg protein is present include:

Albumin

Globulin

Lecithin

Livetin

Lysozyme

Simplesse™

Vitellin

Words starting with "ova" or "ovo," such as ovalbumin or ovoglobulin

Foods and Ingredients to Avoid

Angel food cake

Cholesterol-free egg substitutes (usually contain egg whites)

Cream pies

Custard

Eggs, egg whites and egg yolks

French toast

Hollandaise sauce

Mayonnaise

Meringue

Pancakes

Phosvitin

Puddings

Silicalbuminate

Soufflés

Surimi

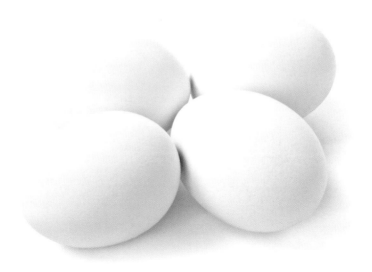

Foods Commonly Containing Eggs

- Baked goods, muffins, rolls and cakes
- Bearnaise sauce and hollandaise sauce
- Beer
- Breaded or battered foods
- Breads, such as challah or others with egg in the dough or an egg glaze
- Broth (clear), consomme or stock clarified with eggs
- Casseroles made with eggs
- Cream-filled chocolates
- Cookies
- Custard
- Divinity and fondant
- Foam in milk toppings on specialty coffee drinks
- Fried food (with eggs used in the batter)
- Fudge
- Ice cream
- Jelly beans (some)
- Marshmallows
- Marzipan
- Mayonnaise and mayonnaise-containing products, such as deli salads
- Meat loaf, meatballs
- Newburgh sauce
- Nougat
- Pastas including those in prepared foods such as soup (non egg pastas may be made on equipment also used for making egg-containing pasta)
- Pretzels
- Root beer
- Salad dressings
- Sausages (some)
- Sherbet
- Sweet rolls and pie crusts (with egg glaze)
- Tartar sauce
- Wine (some are clarified with egg)

Replacing Eggs in Recipes

If the eggs are used for leavening:

- 1½ tablespoons liquid + 1½ teaspoons oil + 1 teaspoon baking powder
- 1 teaspoon baking powder + 1 tablespoon liquid + 1 tablespoon vinegar
- 1 teaspoon yeast + ¼ cup warm water
- ½ teaspoon baking powder +2 tablespoons liquid
- 2 tablespoons flour + 1 ½ tablespoons shortening + ½ teaspoon baking powder + 2 tablespoons liquid

If the eggs are used as a binder:

- 1 packet of plain gelatin + 2 tablespoons warm water
- 1 tablespoon of fruit puree
- 1/3 cup of water blended with 1 tablespoon of flax seeds (for 1 egg)
- Soft tofu

Tips for Chefs

- Substitute mashed avocado, mustard, hummus, red pepper spread or tapenade for mayonnaise on sandwiches.
- Use tofu instead of eggs for a breakfast scramble.
- Use a very clean pan that was not used to cook eggs for a previous guest.

Peanut Allergy

Peanuts are not actually nuts; they are legumes. Also known as groundnuts or monkey nuts, peanuts pose a unique problem because many children love peanut butter and peanut snacks. Some schools ban peanuts when a few children are allergic to them. Exposure can occur in three ways:

- **Direct contact**: The most common exposure is eating peanuts or peanut-containing foods. Sometimes direct skin contact with peanuts can trigger an allergic reaction.

- **Cross contact**: The unintended introduction of peanuts into a product is generally the result of exposure during processing or handling of a food product. Cross contact could come from serving a fruit sherbet with an ice cream scoop that had been previously used for ice cream with nuts.

- **Inhalation**: An allergic reaction may occur if dust or aerosols containing peanuts is inhaled – for example, peanut flour or peanut oil cooking spray.

Ingredients to Avoid

- Peanuts
- Peanut oil

Foods Commonly Containing Peanuts

- African, Chinese, Indonesian, Thai, Vietnamese and Mexican dishes (Thai dipping sauces, salads, pad Thai, etc.)
- Sauces, such as pesto, gravy, mole sauce and peanut sauce
- Artificial nuts (peanuts reflavored as pecans or walnuts)
- Nuts roasted in peanut oil
- Baked goods
- Chocolate candy, peanut brittle and candy bars
- Egg rolls
- Foods that contain extruded, cold-pressed or expelled peanut oil, which may contain some peanut protein
- Ice cream
- Salad dressing
- Seeds, such as sunflower seeds and soy nuts made or processed on equipment shared with peanuts
- Some vegetarian and vegan food products, especially those sold as meat substitutes
- Sweets, such as puddings, cookies and hot chocolate

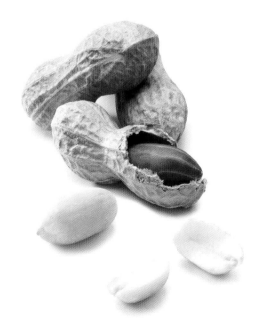

Tree Nut Allergy

Most people allergic to tree nuts are also allergic to peanuts. Water chestnuts are actually part of a plant root and are not nuts. They, like nutmeg, are safe for someone allergic to tree nuts.

Tree nuts

Almonds

Coconuts

Macadamia nuts

Beech nuts

Gingko nuts

Pecans

Brazil nuts

Hazelnuts/filberts

Pinenuts

Cashews

Hickory nuts

Pistachios

Chestnuts

Lychee nuts

Walnuts

Foods Commonly Containing Tree Nuts

- Barbecue sauce
- Breading for chicken or fish
- Cereals
- Chocolate candies, nougat, macaroons, marzipan
- Cookies and desserts
- Crackers
- Foie gras (sometimes pistachios)
- Honey and chestnut honey
- Mandelonas (peanuts soaked in almond flavoring)
- Meat-free burgers
- Mexican coffee (uses piñon)
- Mortadella (may contain pistachios)
- Natural flavorings and extracts (pure almond extract)
- Nut butters, nut oils
- Nut-flavored coffee/liqueurs (Amaretto®, Frangelico®)
- Pancakes
- Piecrust, some pies and tarts
- Salads and salad dressings
- Spreads, such as almond paste, chocolate nut, nougat, Nutella® and nut paste

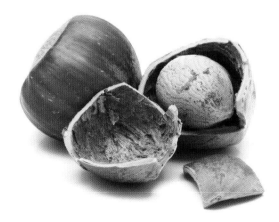

Fish Allergy

Fish and shellfish allergies tend to be severe. People who are allergic to fish should avoid seafood restaurants because of the risk of contamination of non-fish meals. Fish protein can become airborne during cooking.

Foods to Avoid

All fish with fins and scales

All products made with fresh, canned, processed or frozen fish

Foods Commonly Containing Fish

- Asian fish-based sauces
- Imitation fish or shellfish (surimi)
- Barbecue sauce (some are made with Worcestershire)
- Meatloaf and meatballs (may contain Worcestershire sauce)
- Bouillabaisse, chowder, gumbo, jambalaya and cioppino
- Salad dressings
- Steak sauce
- Caesar salad (may contain anchovies in the salad dressing)
- Surimi
- Sushi
- Caponata and sweet/sour relishes that may contain anchovies
- Worcestershire sauce

Shellfish Allergy

Shellfish allergy is one of the most common and severe food allergies. Those with shellfish allergy may have an allergic reaction to only certain kinds of shellfish or may be allergic to all varieties. People with shellfish allergies are often sensitive to iodine as well. Nori rolls and other seaweeds contain high levels of iodine.

Foods to Avoid

All fish with fins and scales

All products made with fresh, canned, processed or frozen fish

Sushi (rolls not including fish may be made with the same equipment as containing sushi)

Common Allergy-Causing Shellfish

Crustaceans	Gastropods
Crabs	Limpets
Crayfish	Periwinkles
Lobster	Snails (escargot)
Langoustines	Abalone
Prawns	**Cephalopods**
Shrimp	Squid
Mollusks	Cuttlefish
Bivalves	Octopus
Clams	
Mussels	
Oysters	
Scallops	

Wheat Allergy

People who are allergic to wheat have a specific intolerance to wheat protein. This allergy is not the same as gluten intolerance (celiac disease). Many wheat-allergic children outgrow this allergy. For those with wheat allergy, alternative grains such as quinoa and rice should be offered. See the following section on gluten-free for grains to use.

Foods and Ingredients to Avoid

All-purpose flour	Graham flour
Bran	Kamut®
Bread (unless wheat-free)	Miller's bran
Breadcrumbs	Modified food starch
Bulgur	Pastry flour
Cake flour	Semolina
Cracked wheat	Spelt
Durum flour	Starch
Enriched flour	Vegetable gum
Gelatinized starch	Wheat germ
Gluten	Whole-wheat flour

Tips for Chefs

When baking with wheat-free flours, a combination of flours usually works best. Experiment with different blends to find one that will give you the texture you are trying to achieve. Blends composed of high proportions of white rice flour, potato starch, arrowroot and tapioca flour and lower proportions of sorghum, millet, garfava and/or brown rice flour yield the best baked items. Gluten-free blends and mixes are available.

Adapting a recipe to be wheat- and dairy-free comes down to four considerations: solutions and proportions of ingredients, acid, protein and a gum. Generally, more leavening is needed in wheat-free products.

Baker's Asthma

Baker's asthma is an allergic reaction to wheat flour and other types of flour. As the name of the disorder suggests, it's a particular problem for bakers or anyone who works with uncooked wheat flours. Inhaling flour rather than eating it causes the allergic reaction. Baker's asthma primarily results in problems breathing. The allergy-causing substance that triggers baker's asthma may be wheat protein or another substance such as a fungus.

Foods Commonly Containing Wheat

- Beer
- Bouillon base and cubes
- Breads (many corn or rye breads also contain some wheat flour) and rolls
- Breakfast bars
- Breakfast cereals
- Candy
- Cakes and muffins
- Coffee substitutes
- Condiments, such as catsup
- Couscous
- Cookies, doughnuts
- Dairy products, such as ice cream
- Deli meat products, cold cuts and sausages
- Farina
- French fries
- Gelatinized starch
- Hot dogs
- Hydrolyzed vegetable protein
- Ice cream
- Imitation crabmeat
- Malt
- Meat, crab or shrimp substitutes
- Modified food starch
- Natural flavorings
- Noodles
- Pancakes, pancake and waffle mixes
- Pasta
- Processed meats
- Sausage
- Soup mixes
- Soy sauce
- Tempura batter
- Vegetable gum
- Waffles
- Wheat germ
- Wheat starch

Saffron Buckwheat Pilaf & Three-Bean Relish with a Spicy Tomato Vinaigrette

Provided by Margaret Condrasky, EdD, RD, CCE
Associate Professor of Food Science and Human Nutrition, Clemson University, Clemson, South Carolina
Recipe by Joel Schaefer, President & Chef, Allergy Chefs, Inc., Dawsonville, Georgia

Yield: 8 cups
Serves: 10 (some dressing remains for another use)

This dish is excellent as an entrée or appetizer. Its many healthy components can be used separately with other items on your menu. The spicy tomato vinaigrette is a good reduced-calorie salad dressing and makes a zesty dip for crudités. It is great for vegans or anyone who wants a healthful option.

Saffron Buckwheat Pilaf — **Yield: 8 cups**

Herb oil or olive oil	2	tablespoons
Diced onions	½	cup
Garlic, minced	2	cloves
Vegetable stock	4	cups
Whole buckwheat groats	2	cups
Bay leaves	2	each
Saffron	$1/8$	teaspoon
Salt	½	teaspoon
Black pepper, freshly ground	¼	teaspoon

Three-Bean Relish — **Yield: 4 ¾ cups**

Black beans	1	15 ounce can
Great northern beans	1	15.5 ounce can
Red beans	1	15.5 ounce can
Sweet onions, caramelized	½	cup
Red bell peppers, diced	½	cup
Green bell peppers, diced	½	cup
Champagne vinaigrette	½	cup

Champagne Vinaigrette — **Yield: ¾ cups**

Champagne vinegar	¼	cup
Extra virgin olive oil	$3/8$	cup
Garlic cloves	2	each
Italian flat parsley	1	tablespoon
Salt	½	teaspoon
Black pepper, freshly ground	¼	teaspoon

Spicy Tomato Vinaigrette — **Yield: 2 cups**

Diced tomatoes, no salt added, undrained	1	14.5 ounce can
Sambal oelek	1	teaspoon
Olive oil	¼	cup
Oregano, fresh, chopped	2	tablespoons
Salt	1	teaspoon
Balsamic vinegar	1	tablespoon

Garnish

Italian flat leaf parsley, fresh, springs	¼	cup

Saffron Buckwheat Pilaf:

1. In a large saucepan, sauté onions and garlic in oil until onions are translucent.
2. Add the vegetable stock and bring to a boil over high heat; quickly stir in the buckwheat, reduce heat to low, add bay leaves and saffron and cover pan tightly.
3. Simmer 15 minutes or until groats are tender and liquid is absorbed. Add salt and pepper to taste. Let sit for 5 minutes and fluff with a fork. Remove bay leaves.

Champagne Vinaigrette:

1. Blend the champagne vinegar, olive oil, garlic cloves and Italian parsley in a blender. Set aside.

Three-Bean Relish:

1. Drain and rinse the beans. Combine the beans, caramelized onions, bell peppers and ½ cup of the champagne vinaigrette. Toss to combine.

Spicy Tomato Vinaigrette:

1. Place all ingredients in a blender and puree.

Assembly:

1. Mold the buckwheat pilaf in 10 3-inch rings or greased ramekins. Unmold on plate. Pour the spicy tomato vinaigrette around the buckwheat. Drizzle remaining dressing lightly around plates. Portion the three-bean relish over the buckwheat. Garnish with fresh Italian parsley.

Per Serving

Calories	360	Cholesterol	0	mg
Fat	15 g	Sodium	575	mg
Saturated Fat	2 g	Carbohydrates	48	mg
Trans Fat	0 g	Dietary Fiber	9	mg
Sugar	6 g	Protein	10	g

Soy Allergy

Read labels carefully. Soybeans have become a major part of processed food products such as baked goods, canned items, cereals, crackers, sauces and soups. Avoiding products made with soybeans can be difficult. Check for soy as an ingredient in anything labeled as vegetarian or vegan; soy products are often added to boost nutrient value. MSG (monosodium glutamate) may be made from corn or soy.

Ingredients to Avoid

Artificial flavorings

Asian flavoring

Bouillon cubes (beef, chicken, vegetable, etc.)

Canned chicken broth

Canned vegetable broth

Edamame

Emulsifier

Glycine max

Hydrolyzed plant protein

Hydrolyzed protein

Hydrolyzed soy protein

Hydrolyzed vegetable protein (HVP)

Lecithin

Miso

Mono- and diglycerides

Monosodium glutamate (MSG)

Natto (fermented soybeans)

Natural flavoring

Plant protein

Protein extender

Protein filler

Shoyu

Sobee® and other soy formulas

Soy albumin

Soy fiber

Soy flour

Soy grits

Soy meal

Soy milk

Soy nut butter

Soy nuts

Soy protein isolate

Soy sauce

Soy sprouts

Soya

Soybeans

Soybean butter

Soybean granules or curds

Tamari

Tempeh

Texturized vegetable protein (TVP)

Tofu

Vegetable gum

Vegetable starch

Worcestershire sauce

Foods Commonly Containing Soy

- Baked goods
- Bread
- Butter substitutes
- Candies
- Canned broths
- Canned soups
- Canned tuna
- Cereal
- Condiments
- Crackers
- Desserts
- Energy bars
- Gravies
- High-protein energy bars and snacks
- Ice cream
- Infant formulas
- Liquid meal replacements
- Low-fat peanut butter
- Margarine
- Meat substitutes
- Salad dressings
- Soups
- Veggie burgers
- Vegetarian sausages and meat substitutes

Tips for Chefs

- Try using paneer (pressed Indian cheese) instead of tofu.
- Substitute rice or cow's milk for soymilk.

For More Information

- *Chef Card Template*. Fairfax, VA: The Food Allergy Research & Education. **https://www.foodallergy. org/chef-card-english**
- Food Allergy Research & Education. **www.foodallergy.org**
- Food and Drug Administration. *Food Allergies: What you Need to Know*. **https://www.fda.gov/ food/ingredientspackaginglabeling/foodaller-gens/ucm079311.htm**
- *Welcoming Guests with Food Allergies*. Fairfax, VA: The Food Allergy & Anaphylaxis Network; 2010. **https://www.foodallergy.org/sites/default/ files/2017-08/welcoming-guests-faan.pdf**

Foods to Avoid for Corn Allergy

Corn is not on the list of the eight top allergens. It affects less than 1% of the American population. Although a rare allergy, it is difficult because a corn derivative, high-fructose corn syrup, is ubiquitous.

Corn-containing foods to avoid include:

Corn chips and tortillas

Corn flakes and other breakfast cereals containing corn

Corn grits, corn flour, cornmeal and polenta

Corn oil, alone or in salad dressings or fried foods

Corn syrup and high fructose corn syrup

Fresh or frozen corn, alone or as an ingredient

Frostings and icings

Instant coffee and drinks

Catsup, jams, gums and candy with corn syrup

Popcorn and corn snacks

Sorbitol and maltodextrin

Yogurt and other foods sweetened with corn syrup

Pizza crust dusted with cornmeal

Soft drinks and sweetened beverages

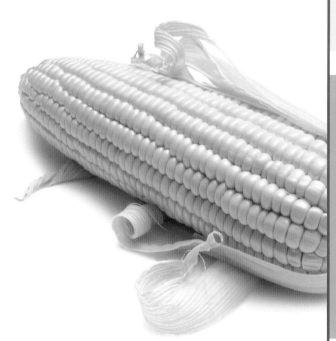

Non-Food Products Made from Corn

Aspirin

Cosmetics

Crayons and chalks

Envelope and stamp glue

Lotions and ointments

Penicillin

Shaving creams

Soaps and cleansers

Toothpastes

Gluten Intolerance

Essentials Expert

Renee Zonka, CEC, RD, CHE, MBA, was managing director and dean of Kendall College in Chicago. She became interested in gluten-free cooking while attending a seminar given by a celiac disease organization at the Culinary Institute of America and when she was an evaluator for a gluten-free cooking class. Her background in science, medicine and healthcare helped her realize how important it is for culinarians to meet this need for their guests. Renee writes extensively and teaches many classes to culinary students, chefs, dietitians and the public on celiac disease and gluten-free recipe development.

Gluten is the protein part of all forms of wheat (including durum, semolina and spelt), rye, barley and grain hybrids such as triticale and kamut. Gluten intolerance is an inherited autoimmune condition also known as *celiac disease*. People with this condition cannot tolerate gluten when it comes in contact with the small intestine. In fact, gluten can eventually destroy their small intestine.

According to a study by the University of Maryland Center for Celiac Research, nearly one of every 141 Americans suffers from celiac disease. [10] Some of them can tolerate small amounts of gluten without reaction. Others have severe symptoms from any contact with gluten. Gluten intolerance is not a wheat allergy, but wheat is the key food to avoid in order to control gluten intolerance. Symptoms of gluten intolerance are abdominal bloating, pain, diarrhea, weight loss and fatigue. Wheat allergy has respiratory and other severe symptoms.

More and more diners are requesting gluten-free food, and the demand for gluten-free retail products is growing. Some food laws, however, make it difficult to know whether or not a food is truly gluten-free. For example, if a snack food contains wheat, it must be labeled, but if it contains vinegar that was derived from wheat, no label is required. So although gluten-free foods have improved dramatically in quantity and quality, people on a gluten-free diet should rely more on whole foods and less on packaged and prepared foods. Gluten-free foods are abundant in nature.

Websites such as **www.allergyeats.com** and others provide lists of restaurants that offer gluten-free menu options or are entirely gluten free.

Key Nutrition Points

- People with gluten intolerance must avoid all foods containing gluten, a protein in many grains.

- A person can develop intolerance to gluten at any time. It can be triggered by physical trauma, pregnancy, infection, severe emotional stress or surgery.

- In people with gluten intolerance, as gluten is ingested, it destroys the finger-like projections (*villi*) of the small intestine. The villi are essential for the absorption of vitamins and minerals and other nutrients.

- Absorption of calcium and lactose are most affected by the change in the lining of the small intestines. Everyone with gluten intolerance should also be tested for osteoporosis and lactose intolerance. Over time, other allergies may occur including soy, corn and dairy.

- When someone with gluten intolerance strictly follows a gluten-free diet, the villi return to normal function. The gluten intolerance remains but can be managed by diet. If the person consumes gluten, the villi will be destroyed once again. Thus, the gluten-free diet is a lifetime commitment.

- Some people with gluten intolerance have no symptoms; others have bloating, cramping, stomachache, diarrhea, weight loss, lactose-intolerance, anemia and fatigue. When gluten is consumed in even minuscule amounts, it can trigger these symptoms.

Best Choices

Food staples of the gluten-free diet include:

- Fruits and vegetables, fresh, frozen and dried
- Meat, fish, poultry (without wheat breading) and eggs
- Potatoes, corn and beans
- Rice, quinoa, buckwheat, millet, flax, sorghum and teff
- Dairy products
- Cereals made without wheat or barley malt
- Lentils and other legumes
- Seeds, such as amaranth, flax, sesame and sunflower
- Specialty foods, such as pasta, bread, crackers, pancakes, pastries and chips made with permitted grains (rice, tapioca, arrowroot, potato, soy or corn flours and starches)

When diners indicate they are gluten intolerant, you must be direct and honest if you do not have gluten-free items on the menu. Here are a few things you can offer:

- Salads made with fresh vegetables and fruits can be served with homemade vinaigrette. Use distilled vinegar. The distilling process destroys and filters out any gluten. Skip the croutons.
- Broth-based soups without noodles are a good alternative to cream or roux-based soups.
- Meat or fish can be broiled, roasted, sautéed, braised, stewed or pan-fried. The most important thing to remember is preparation. No wheat flour can be used for dusting meats when braising or stewing. Sauce cannot be made with a wheat-flour roux. If meat or fish is sautéed, use a clean pan and tongs.
- Sauces that are reduced from liquids are ideal. If the sauce must be thickened, use arrowroot, potato flour, cornstarch or tapioca flour instead of wheat flour.
- Vegetables can be steamed with butter. Tortilla chips or French fries can be prepared in a clean pot with fresh oil. Rice is a gluten-free food, even glutinous (sticky) rice. Many unusual grains are exciting to experiment with for a creative plate, such as amaranth, quinoa, teff, Jobs tears, millet and buckwheat.

- Many desserts have a wheat component. Even the famous flourless chocolate cake should be offered with caution. It is usually baked in a floured pan, and some recipes do contain a tablespoon of flour. A cheese course with dried fruits and nuts is a welcomed treat. Avoid offering bleu cheese from Europe because it may have gluten particles due to the fermentation and aging process.
- Breakfast items include eggs prepared in a variety of ways, homemade hash browns, fresh fruit and 100% juice.

Grains and Starches Allowed in the Gluten-Free Diet

Amaranth
Arrowroot
Beans and bean flours
Buckwheat
Corn, corn flour, popcorn, corn tortillas, cornmeal
Grits, polenta
Taco shells, unseasoned corn tortilla chips
Couscous
Garfava
Millet
Nut flours
Potato flour
Puffed rice, corn or millet
Pure gluten-free oats and oat flour
Quinoa and quinoa flour
Rice (plain), including brown rice, rice flour, rice noodles, rice crackers
Sorghum, sorghum flour
Soy, soy flour
Tapioca, tapioca flour
Teff, teff flour
Wild rice

Foods to Avoid

The gluten-free diet eliminates all foods, beverages and medications made from the ingredients that contain gluten, including items made with any type of wheat flour (all purpose, white or whole wheat). Many ingredients contain hidden gluten. Gluten or wheat is used as a flavoring agent, fermenting agent and stabilizer. As more ready-made foods become available for foodservice, it will be imperative to know all the components. Here is a list of foods that always or usually contain gluten. Some will be obvious, some not.

- Alcohol: beer, ale and lager (usually made from malted barley, though some gluten-free beer is now available); some wines, gin, whiskey and vodka
- Artificial vanilla (pure vanilla is fine)
- Baked beans thickened with flour
- Cooking sprays for baking (may contain wheat flour or starch)
- Breading
- Breads, muffins, biscuits and flour tortillas
- Broths
- Brown rice syrup (frequently made from barley)
- Buckwheat and buckwheat pasta (soba noodles) made with wheat flour
- Cake icings and frostings (made with small amounts of wheat flour or starch)
- Cakes, pies, cobblers and cookies
- Caramel color made from barley
- Cereals and products made from cereal
- Cheese spreads and sauces thickened with wheat starch or protein
- Chocolates and licorice containing wheat flour
- Coating mixes
- Communion wafers
- Crackers
- Croutons
- Dextrin made from wheat
- Flavored coffee mixes that contain a chip-like ingredient made from cookie crumbs
- Flour (products that are primarily an allowed flour but have small amounts of prohibited flours)
- Gravies and sauces

- Hydrolyzed vegetable protein (HVP), texturized vegetable protein (TVP) or hydrolyzed plant protein (HPP), unless made from soy or corn
- Imitation bacon
- Imitation seafood
- Malt products such as malt flavoring, malt vinegar and malt beverages made from barley
- Marinades
- Meat loaf and frozen burgers with breadcrumbs or fillers
- Modified starch or modified food starch (unless arrowroot, corn, potato, tapioca, waxy maize or maize as the grain source)
- Mono- and diglycerides
- Pastas
- Processed meats with fillers or seasoning containing hydrolyzed wheat protein
- Rice cakes and crackers containing some flour
- Rice mixes containing hydrolyzed wheat protein or soy sauce
- Roux and sauces made with roux
- Sauces
- Self-basting poultry
- Snack foods such as seasoned chips, taco chips and soy nuts containing wheat products in seasonings
- Soup bases
- Soy sauce fermented with wheat, and sauces that are made from soy sauce, such as dumpling and teriyaki sauce
- Specialty mustards with wheat flour
- Stuffing
- Tempeh seasoned with soy sauce
- Thickeners
- Vegan sausages
- Vegetarian burgers or meat substitutes (may have wheat gluten, wheat proteins or barley malt)
- Vegetable gum (unless carob bean gum, locust bean gum, cellulose gum, guar gum, gum arabic, gum aracia, gum tragacanth, xanthan gum or vegetable starch)

Grains Containing Gluten

- Wheat in all forms: wheat starch, wheat bran, wheat germ, cracked wheat, hydrolyzed wheat protein
- Barley (all forms including malt)
- Kamut®
- Oats, unless grown and processed without contact with other grains. Pure oats are fine.
- Rye
- Spelt
- Triticale, a cross between wheat and ryes
- Wheat flours (durum, semolina, etc.)

Gluten free doesn't mean bland. In a fine-dining restaurant, chefs take doing gluten-free meals as a creative challenge. Fortunately, gluten-free products are becoming more mainstream. As a dietitian who has gluten intolerance, I pick my restaurants carefully. One place lets me bring in my own brown rice pasta and charges me half price for pasta dishes. I bring my own gluten-free soy sauce when I go out for sushi. Another chef I know keeps a collection of gluten-free ingredients on hand for his regulars. Still another has an area in his kitchen devoted only to gluten-free cooking. This is the kind of commitment it takes – and you will be building a loyal clientele.

Diane Barrera, MPH, RD
Chicago, Illinois

Oats or No Oats

Oats do not contain gluten, but most have been grown, harvested, transported or processed on equipment used for other grains. Assume there has been cross contact and that most oats carry traces of gluten. Some companies, however, have dedicated fields and processing equipment and produce pure oats that are gluten free. See www.glutenfreediet.ca/oats.php.

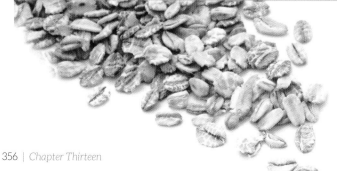

Everyone in the kitchen and front of the house should be educated on gluten intolerance. Eating out is a profound social event that makes us feel good in spirit and mind. People who are gluten intolerant have a difficult time dining out because they are afraid of eating something that will make them ill. A restaurant must remain sustainable. Servicing a group with special needs will develop trust and long-lasting relationships.

Renee Zonka, CEC, RD, CHE, MBA
Kendall College

Gluten-Free Realities

In recent years the gluten-free diet has been advocated for weight loss and general well-being. Many people have heard the hype and choose to be on this diet, some or all of the time, without true or diagnosed gluten intolerance. In this case it is more of a preference than a medical necessity and there will not be medical consequences if a food containing a bit of gluten is eaten. Nevertheless, every foodservice should treat a stated gluten intolerance, or any known allergen, as a serious issue.

In response to consumer demand, there are many gluten-free products available and labeled as such for both consumer and foodservice markets. Items like gluten-free sandwich buns make it fairly to provide a gluten-free meal. However, for those who have celiac disease and are truly gluten intolerant, the issue of cross contamination remains. Spoons, tongs, gloves, knives, etc. can not be used that have been in contact with gluten containing products without careful washing between uses; frying oils for gluten- free foods can't have cooked breaded items, etc. While a list of menu items that do not contain gluten should be available, it is wise to be clear that yours is not a gluten-free kitchen.

In some cases, families with a child who must be on a gluten-free diet, or any other food allergy or intolerance, may choose to bring a meal or snack for the child while the rest of the group enjoys foods from your menu. Others may bring their own crackers, dressings or condiments that they know are safe choices. Be open to this so that guests feel comfortable. If guests call ahead it is sometimes possible to prepare a gluten-free or allergen- free meal but it does take a dedicated effort, not easy at busy serving times.

Tips for Chefs

Gluten-free foods that routinely appear on menus include plain, unsauced steaks, fish fillets, grilled meats, and vegetables that are cooked whole. Fish and meats can be "breaded" with nut meal instead of bread crumbs. Guests who want to eat gluten free usually will ask a lot of questions of the server about method of preparation, cooking liquids and sauces. Servers should be educated on menu items and method of preparation.

Be very careful of cross contamination. Items that are naturally gluten free may share transportation, a production line, a knife, a fryer, a toaster, a strainer or a grill with a gluten-containing grain. This contact will contaminate an item that would otherwise be gluten free. Utensils that have touched bread or bread baskets, spoons that have stirred roux-based soups, and spatulas that have flipped toasted cheese sandwiches will carry some residual gluten. Ovens can be used for gluten-free cooking if the temperature has been raised to 500° F and held for 15 minutes before cooking the gluten-free item.

If you decide to prepare gluten-free food on a regular basis, the kitchen and all equipment should be thoroughly cleaned and allowed to rest for 24 hours. Baking and mixing equipment should be specific for gluten-free items and cordoned off from the rest of the equipment to avoid cross contact. When not in use, equipment should be covered in plastic wrap. Ideally, a specific area should be identified for gluten-free food preparation. [11]

In the front of the house, create a special menu to help guide diners to appropriate choices, or develop a list that service staff can use to make appropriate suggestions. Encourage diners to call ahead to alert the chef to their special needs. Some restaurants ask these diners to make reservations for a time when the kitchen is less busy.

For More Information

- Be Free for Me, **www.befreeforme.com/blog**
- Case S., Drury W. *Gluten Free: The Definitive Resource Guide*. Saskatchewan, Canada: Case Nutrition Consulting; 2016.
- Celiac Disease Center at Columbia University, **www.celiacdiseasecenter.columbia.edu**
- Celiac Disease Foundation, **www.celiac.org**
- Celiac Sprue Association/USA, Inc., **www.csaceliacs.org**
- Coppedge R and The Culinary Institute of America. *Baking for Special Diets*. New York: Wiley, 2016.
- Duane J. *Bake Deliciously! Gluten and Dairy Free Cookbook*. Centennial, CO: Alternative Cook, LLC; 2009. **www.alternativecook.com**.
- Gluten Intolerance Group, ***www.gluten.net***
- Langevin L. *The Anti-Inflammatory Kitchen Cookbook: More Than 100 Healing, Low-Histamine, Gluten-Free Recipes*. New York: Sterling Epicure, 2019.

casebycase | Up on the Farm

Boston Medical Center (BMC)) is a 567-bed teaching hospital and major trauma center located in Boston's historic South End. It is Boston's primary "safety net" hospital; most families in the area are food insecure. Serving vulnerable populations and supporting patients and families holistically while striving to reduce healthcare costs are fundamental to BMC's mission. The hospital not only makes sure patients receive the best medical care, it also offers innovative, hands-on food and nutrition education to help them lead healthier lives.

In 2001, in partnership with the Greater Boston Food Bank, BMC opened the first hospital-based food pantry in the country, providing healthy foods that are often lacking in a family's diet due to cost and accessibility. Since its inception, the pantry has served more than 1 million people and has been a national model for other hospitals.

BMC providers refer individuals with special nutritional needs to the pantry with a prescription for supplemental foods (fresh fruits, vegetables, and meat) that are medically and culturally appropriate for all family members. Originally designed to feed 500 patients per month, the Food Pantry, which is 100 percent funded by philanthropy, has grown to 1,500 square feet, serves 7,000 patients and their families, and distributes close to 12,000 pounds of food every month. Families can drop in at the Food Pantry every two weeks and receive three to four days' worth of food for their household per visit.

Just giving people food, however, does not ensure that they will know how to prepare it. And that's where the on-site Teaching Kitchen comes in. With Culinary Institute of America graduate Tracey Burg, RDN, as culinary nutrition manager, the kitchen offers about 25 classes per month focusing on simple, cost-effective recipes. "Culinary nutrition is a fairly new topic," Tracey explains. "Our classes are free and open to anyone. We talk about disease-specific foods and share healthy cooking techniques." In the summer, the Teaching Kitchen hosts a free culinary camp for children. The Teaching Kitchen also occasionally hosts a BMC Top Chef competition for staff. The prize: a golden spatula.

True to BMC's food-as-medicine philosophy, each cooking class incorporates fresh food from the hospital's roof-top farm, which occupies 2,400 square feet atop the hospital's power plant and yields more than 5,000 pounds of produce a year – fresh local products not only for the Teaching Kitchen, but also for the hospital's foodservice operations, farmers market, and pantry. The farm has other benefits as well. It reduces the hospital's carbon footprint, increases green space, and reduces energy use, including the energy required to transport food.

With its Preventive Food Pantry, Teaching Kitchen and roof-top farm, Boston Medical Center is making a difference in food insecurity and nutrition for special diets in Boston's South End and is providing a model for other hospitals nationwide.

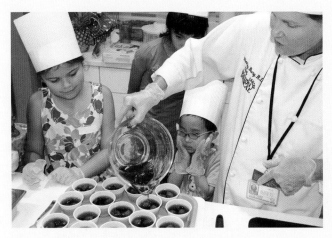 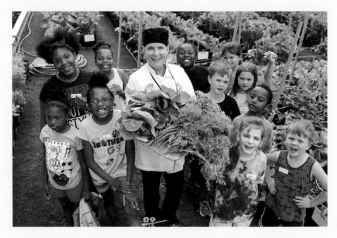

Tracey Burg, RDN, culinary nutrition manager, Boston Medical Center, in the kitchen and at the center's farm with students from the Kids Summer Culinary Camp.

Gluten-Free Fried Chicken

Yield: 10 pieces

Chef Ina Pinkney
This was a popular recipe at the now closed Ina's, Chicago, Illinois

Chicken pieces (thighs, legs or breasts)	10	each
Egg whites	3	each
Transfat free canola oil		

Dry mix coating:

White rice flour	1	pound
Brown rice flour	4	ounces
Tapioca flour or tapioca starch	2	ounces
Potato starch (not potato flour)	1 ½	ounces
Kosher salt	1	teaspoon
Black pepper	½	teaspoon
Garlic powder	1	teaspoon

Marinade:

Buttermilk	2	cups
Kosher salt	1	teaspoon
Black pepper	½	teaspoon
Garlic, minced	2	cloves

Note: For recipes using deep fat frying, nutritional analysis is more accurate than calculated values.

1. Combine white rice flour, brown rice flour, tapioca flour, potato starch, salt, pepper, and garlic powder.

2. Combine buttermilk, salt, black pepper and minced garlic. Soak chicken pieces overnight. Drain the chicken thoroughly before coating.

3. Dredge the chicken pieces in the flour mixture, then dip into lightly beaten egg whites and then back into the flour mixture. It is good to "pack" the mixture on the second dip and shake off any excess.

4. Heat a trans fat-free commercial canola oil to 275° F in a heavy deep pot. Gently place the chicken into the pot (chicken must be completely covered in the oil). Do not overload the pot and do not move the chicken around for at least ten minutes for the crust to set up. At this temperature, a breast will take 20-25 minutes, legs and thighs will take 20 minutes. Remove the chicken and set it on a rack to drain for about 5 minutes.

Per Serving (pieces vary by size, this is an average)

Calories	250	Cholesterol	85	mg
Fat	13 g	Sodium	170	mg
Saturated Fat	2 g	Carbohydrates	5	mg
Trans Fat	0 g	Dietary Fiber	0	mg
Sugar	0 g	Protein	27	g

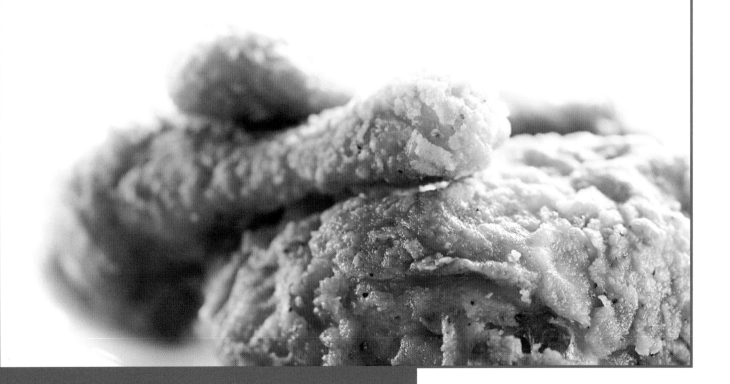

Christmas Beer Cake
Yield: 10 inch bundt cake   Serves: 16

Renee Zonka, CEC, RD, CHE, MBA
former Managing Director and Dean, Kendall College, Chicago, Illinois

Sorghum flour	1 ½	cups
Tapioca flour	½	cup
Potato starch	½	cup
Baking powder	2	teaspoons
Baking soda	1	teaspoon
Salt	½	teaspoon
Xanthan gum	2	teaspoons
Butter, softened	¾	cup
Sugar	1 ½	cup
Eggs, large	3	each
Sour cream	1 ½	cup
Beer, gluten-free*	½	cup
Vanilla	1 ½	teaspoons

Filling and Topping:

Sugar	½	cup
Cinnamon	2	teaspoons
Walnuts, chopped	2/3	cup

1. Preheat oven to 350° F. Prepare a 10-inch tube pan or large bundt pan with nonstick spray.

2. Sift the flours, baking powder, baking soda, salt and xanthan gum in large bowl. Mix well.

3. In a mixing bowl, cream together butter and sugar. Add eggs, sour cream, beer and vanilla. Mix for about 2 minutes. Add dry ingredients and mix until all ingredients are well blended.

4. In a separate bowl, mix sugar, cinnamon and walnuts.

5. Spoon one-third of cake batter into greased pan. Sprinkle on one-third of cinnamon-nut mixture. Spoon on another third of cake batter and again sprinkle on a third of cinnamon-nut mixture.

6. Spoon on remaining third of batter. The cake will expand during baking so do not fill bundt pan to the top.

7. Bake 55-65 minutes until brown and cake tester comes out clean.

8. Cool and turn out of pan. Sprinkle remaining cinnamon-nut mixture on top of cake.

***Note**: If beer is not desired, substitute sparkling water.

Per Serving

Calories	340	Cholesterol	70	mg
Fat	17	g	Sodium	310	mg
Saturated Fat	9	g	Carbohydrates	45	mg
Trans Fat	0	g	Dietary Fiber	2	mg
Sugar	26	g	Protein	4	g

Gluten-Free Brownies
Yield: 24 Brownies

Jean Duane
Alternative Cook, LLC, Centennial, Colorado

Jean Duane, Alternative Cook, is known for her gluten-free cooking. She wrote Bake Deliciously! Gluten and Dairy Free Cookbook. *Jean maintains an active website, www.alternativecook. com,and blog,www.askjeanduane.com, with much information on gluten-free cooking. She shared this delicious recipe for gluten-free brownies.*

Sunflower oil	1	cup
Sugar	1 ½	cups
Eggs, large	4	each
Vanilla	2	teaspoons
Cider vinegar	1	teaspoon
Guar gum	2	teaspoons
Cocoa powder	2/3	cup
Sorghum flour	½	cup
Potato starch	¼	cup
Protein flour (soybean)	¼	cup
Baking powder	¾	teaspoon
Instant coffee crystals	2	teaspoons

1. Beat together the oil, sugar, eggs, vanilla and vinegar.

2. Whisk together the dry ingredients. Mix in the wet ingredients.

3. Put batter into an oiled 9-inch by 12-inch pan and bake at 350° F for 25 minutes.

4. Cool. Cut into 24, 2-inch squares.

Per Serving

Calories	170	Cholesterol	30	mg
Fat	10	g	Sodium	30	mg
Saturated Fat	1.5	g	Carbohydrates	18	mg
Trans Fat	0	g	Dietary Fiber	2	mg
Sugar	13	g	Protein	2	g

Used with permission from: Duane, Jean (2010) Bake Deliciously! Gluten and Dairy Free Cookbook. Centennial, CO: Alternative Cook, LLC. www.alternativecook.com.

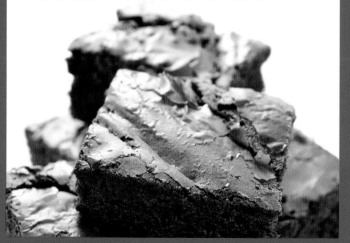

Opportunities for Chefs

Chefs and foodservice professionals prepare foods in a variety of operations, from healthcare facilities to schools to fine-dining establishments. People with special dietary needs are dining every day in all of these settings. This chapter looked at key nutrition points, best food choices, foods to limit and tips for chefs to serve guests who are living with cardiovascular disease, hypertension, cancer, diabetes, digestive disorders, food allergies and celiac disease (gluten intolerance). Being prepared to serve these guests requires that you plan your meals and menus around healthful principles, offer a variety of choices, keep portions reasonable, and be open and willing to train staff to serve guests with special health needs.

Learning Activities

1. Select a menu from a foodservice operation that you work in or visit frequently. Select a particular food allergy. Identify items on the menu that would be appropriate for someone with that food allergy.

2. Develop a weeklong school lunch menu for children on a gluten-free diet.

3. You are catering a function for the local chapter of a diabetes support group (or cardiovascular disease or hypertension). Develop a menu and recipes for this event.

4. Collect two labels of foods from each basic food group. Using the ingredient lists, identify all sources of each of the eight common allergens.

Appendices

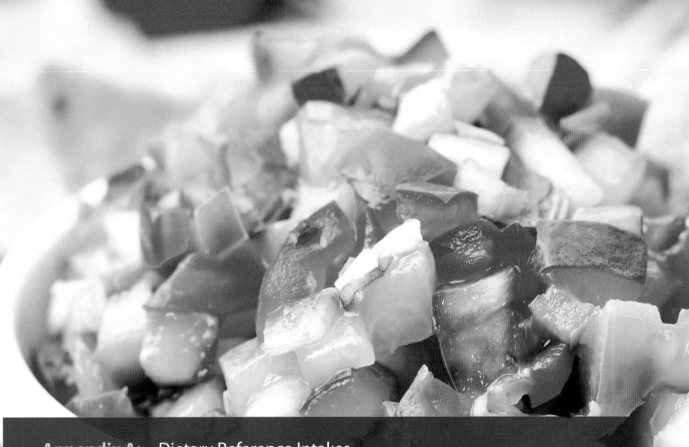

Appendix A

Dietary Reference Intakes (DRIs): Recommended Intakes for Individuals, Macronutrients, Vitamins and Mineral Elements
Food and Nutrition Board, Institute of Medicine, National Academies

	Children 9-18	Males 19-70 years	Females 19-70 years	Males over 70 years	Females over 70 years
Total water (L/day)	2.1 -3.3	3.7	2.7	3.7	2.7
Carbohydrate (g/day)	130	130	130	130	130
Total fiber (g/day)	26-38	30-38	21-25	30	21
Protein (g/day)	34-52	56	46	56	46
Fat	25-35	20-35	20-35	20-35	20-35
Vitamin A (µg/day)	600-900	900	700	900	700
Vitamin C (mg/day)	45-75	90	75	90	75
Vitamin D (µg/day)	15	15	15	20	20
Vitamin E (mg/day)	11-15	15	15	15	15
Vitamin K (µg/day)	60-75	120	90	120	90
Thiamin (mg/day)	.9-1.2	1.2	1.1	1.2	1.1
Riboflavin (mg/day)	.9-1.3	1.3	1.1	1.2	1.1
Niacin (mg/day)	12-16	16	12	16	12
Vitamin B_6 (mg/day)	1.0-1.3	1.3-1.7	1.3-1.5	1.7	1.5
Folate (µg/day)	300-400	400	400	400	400
Vitamin B_{12} (µg/day)	1.8-2.4	2.4	2.4	2.4	2.4
Pantothenic acid (mg/day)	4-5	5	5	5	5
Biotin (µg/day)	20-25	30	30	30	30
Choline (mg/day)	375-550	550	425	550	425
Calcium (mg/day)	1300	1000	1000-1200	1200	1200
Chromium (µg/day)	21-35	30-35	20-25	30	20
Copper (µg/day)	700-890	900	900	900	900
Fluoride (mg/day)	2-3	4	3	4	3
Iodine (µg/day)	120-150	150	150	150	150
Iron (mg/day)	8-15	8	8-18	8	8
Magnesium (mg/day)	240-410	400-420	310-320	420	320
Manganese (mg/day)	1.6-2.2	2.3	1.8	2.3	1.8
Molybdenum (µg/day)	34-43	45	45	45	45
Phosphorus (mg/day)	1250	700	700	700	700
Selenium (µg/day)	40-55	55	55	55	55
Zinc (mg/day)	8-11	11	8	11	8
Potassium (g/day)	4.5-4.7	4.7	4.7	4.7	4.7
Sodium (g/day)	1.5	1.3-1.5	1.3-1.5	1.2	1.2
Chloride (g/day)	2.3	2.0-2.3	2.0-2.3	1.8	1.8

Adapted from **Dietary Reference Intakes (DRIs): Recommended Intakes for Individuals, Vitamins, Dietary Reference Intakes (DRIs): Recommended Intakes for Individuals, Elements** and **Dietary Reference Intakes (DRIs): Recommended Intakes for Individuals, Macronutrients,** Food and Nutrition Board, Institute of Medicine, National Academies

Appendix B

Daily Values
Adults and children over 4 years of age

Food Component	Daily Value
Total fat	78 grams (g)
Saturated fat	20 g
Cholesterol	300 milligrams (mg)
Sodium	2,300 mg
Total carbohydrate	300 g
Dietary fiber	28 g
Protein	50 g
Added Sugars	50 g
Vitamin A	900 micrograms (mcg) RAE
Vitamin C	90 mg
Calcium	1,300 mg
Iron	18 mg
Vitamin D	20 mcg
Vitamin E	15 mg
Vitamin K	120 mcg
Thiamin	1.2 mg
Riboflavin	1.3 mg
Niacin	16 mg NE
Vitamin B_6	1.7 mg
Folate	400 mcg DFE
Vitamin B_{12}	2.4 mcg
Biotin	30 mcg
Pantothenic acid	5 mg
Phosphorus	1,250 mg
Iodine	150 mcg
Magnesium	420 mg
Zinc	11 mg
Selenium	55 mcg
Copper	.9 mg
Manganese	2.3 mg
Chromium	35 mcg
Molybdenum	45 mcg
Chloride	2,300 mg
Potassium	4,700 mg
Choline	550 mg

Source: Food Labeling Guide, U. S. Food and Drug Administration, **https://www.fda.gov/ downloads/Food/GuidanceRegulation/GuidanceDocumentsRegulatoryInformation/ LabelingNutrition/UCM513814.pdf**

https://www.fda.gov/downloads/Food/GuidanceRegulation/GuidanceDocumentsRegulato- ryInformation/LabelingNutrition/UCM513817.pdf

Appendix C

MyPlate and Physical Activity

MyPlate illustrates the five food groups that are the building blocks for a healthy diet using a familiar image – a place setting for a meal. The five food groups are:

Fruits: Focus on fruits.

Vegetables: Vary your veggies.

Grains: Make at least half your grains whole.

Protein: Go lean with protein.

Dairy: Get your calcium-rich foods.

In addition to guiding food choices, *MyPlate* also emphasizes physical activity. Physical activity simply means movement of the body that uses energy. Walking, gardening, briskly pushing a baby stroller, climbing the stairs, playing soccer, or dancing the night away are all good examples of being active. For health benefits, physical activity should be moderate or vigorous intensity.

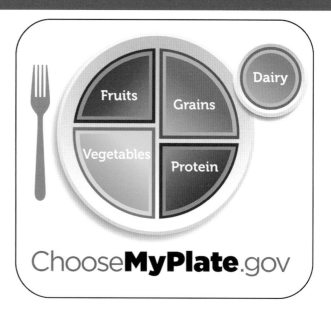

Moderate physical activities include:

- Walking briskly (about 3 ½ miles per hour)
- Bicycling (less than 10 miles per hour)
- General gardening (raking, trimming shrubs)
- Dancing
- Golf (walking and carrying clubs)
- Water aerobics
- Canoeing
- Tennis (doubles)

Vigorous physical activities include:

- Running/jogging (5 miles per hour)
- Walking very fast (4 ½ miles per hour)
- Bicycling (more than 10 miles per hour)
- Heavy yard work, such as chopping wood
- Swimming (freestyle laps)
- Aerobics
- Basketball (competitive)
- Tennis (singles)

You can choose moderate or vigorous intensity activities, or a mix of both each week. Activities can be considered vigorous, moderate, or light in intensity. This depends on the extent to which they make you breathe harder and your heart beat faster.

Only moderate and vigorous intensity activities count toward meeting your physical activity needs. With vigorous activities, you get similar health benefits in half the time it takes you with moderate ones. You can replace some or all of your moderate activity with vigorous activity. Although you are moving, light intensity activities do not increase your heart rate, so you should not count these toward meeting the physical activity recommendations. These activities include walking at a casual pace, such as while grocery shopping, and doing light household chores

Being physically active can help you:

- Increase your chances of living longer
- Decrease your chances of becoming depressed
- Sleep well at night
- Move around more easily
- Have stronger muscles and bones
- Stay at or get to a healthy weight
- Enjoy yourself and have fun

When you are not physically active, you are more likely to:

- Get heart disease
- Get type 2 diabetes
- Have high blood pressure
- Have high blood cholesterol
- Have a stroke

Physical activity and nutrition work together for better health. Being active increases the amount of calories burned. As people age their metabolism slows, so maintaining energy balance requires moving more and eating less.

Some types of physical activity are especially beneficial:

Aerobic activities make you breathe harder and make your heart beat faster. Aerobic activities can be moderate or vigorous in their intensity. Vigorous activities take more effort than moderate ones. For moderate activities, you can talk while you do them, but you can't sing. For vigorous activities, you can only say a few words without stopping to catch your breath.

Muscle-strengthening activities make your muscles stronger. These include activities like push-ups and lifting weights. It is important to work all the different parts of the body - your legs, hips, back, chest, stomach, shoulders and arms.

Bone-strengthening activities make your bones stronger. Bone strengthening activities, like jumping, are especially important for children and adolescents. These activities produce a force on the bones that promotes bone growth and strength.

Balance and stretching activities enhance physical stability and flexibility, which reduces risk of injuries. Examples are gentle stretching, dancing, yoga, martial arts, and t'ai chi.

Source: **www.ChooseMyPlate.gov**

Appendix D

Menu Labeling Rules: Key Facts for Industry

FDA published the final rule for menu labeling on December 1, 2014, and the compliance date was May 7, 2018. The rule requires that certain restaurants and similar retail food establishments provide consumers with calorie and other nutrition information for standard menu items. The goal is to provide consumers with nutrition information in a clear and consistent manner to enable them to make informed and healthy dietary choices for themselves and their families when eating foods away from home.

Overview of the Requirements

The menu labeling rules require covered establishments to:

- Disclose calories for standard menu items listed on menus and menu boards;
- Disclose calories for foods on display and self-service foods that are standard menu items;
- Include on menus and menu boards a succinct statement concerning suggested caloric intake and a statement that additional nutrition information is available upon request; and

- Have the required additional written nutrition information available upon consumer request.

Covered Establishments

Establishments that must meet the requirements of the rule (referred to as covered establishments) are restaurants and similar retail food establishments selling restaurant-type food that are:

- Part of a chain with 20 or more fixed locations;
- Doing business under the same name; and
- Offering for sale substantially the same menu items.

Covered establishments may include:

- Restaurants (quick service and sit-down).
- Grocery and convenience stores.
- Food takeout facilities and delivery services.
- Entertainment venues.
- Cafeterias.
- Coffee shops.
- Superstores.
- Some managed food service operations.

Voluntary Registration

Restaurants or similar retail food establishments that do not meet the requirements of a covered establishment may voluntarily register to be subject to the Federal requirements. State and localities cannot impose additional or different nutrition labeling requirements for food sold at establishments that voluntarily register. Establishments may voluntarily register and renew their registration every other year by submitting FDA Form 3757, available online at the FDA.GOV website at: **https://www.fda.gov/media/116000/download**

Restaurant-Type Foods

The rule defines restaurant-type foods as those that are usually eaten on the premises, while walking away, or soon after arriving at another location, including:

- Meals served at sit-down restaurants.
- Foods purchased at a drive-through.
- Takeout and delivered foods.
- Hot buffet foods.
- Foods ordered from a menu or menu board at a grocery store and intended for immediate consumption.
- Foods that are self-service and intended for immediate consumption.

Foods That Are Generally Covered

- Standard menu items (including alcoholic beverages).
- Combination meals.
- Variable menu items.
- Food on display (including "grab and go" items).
- Self-service food and beverages.

Menus and Menu Boards

The rule defines menus and menu boards as the primary writing from which a customer selects food. An establishment may have more than one primary writing. Primary writings may include:

- Breakfast, lunch and dinner menus.
- Specialty menus (e.g., drink, dessert and catering menus).
- Children's menus.
- Menu boards at a drive-through.
- Electronic menus and menu boards.
- Online menus if the customer can order online or by phone.

Marketing Material

Marketing material (e.g., coupons, posters in store windows, signs on gas pumps, or paper inserts) generally would not be considered a menu or menu board and would not require calorie declarations. Written material of an establishment that does not satisfy the criteria of a primary writing from which a customer makes an order selection (such as a poster on a storefront, a coupon, or other promotional material, banners, billboards and stanchions) would be considered a "secondary writing" of an establishment. If the primary purpose of these materials is to "entice" customers into the covered establishment, they are not considered to be a primary writing, and they would not require calorie declarations.

The Succinct Statement and Statement of Availability

The succinct statement "2,000 calories a day is used for general nutrition advice, but calorie needs vary" must appear on the bottom of menu boards and at the bottom of each page of multi-page menus, and must meet certain size and color requirements.

The statement of availability "Additional nutrition information available upon request." must appear on the bottom of the first page of a menu that lists standard menu items and at the bottom of the menu board, and must meet certain size and color requirements. For information about certain size and color requirements, see the menu labeling final rule and final guidance for industry.

The succinct statement and the statement of availability must be provided for food that is self-service or on display. They may be on an individual sign adjacent to the food itself, or on a separate, larger sign in close proximity to the food. The customer must be able to easily read the sign when making a selection.

Additional Written Nutrition Information

The additional written nutrition information must include:

- Total calories (cal).
- Total fat (g).
- Saturated fat (g).
- Trans fat (g).
- Cholesterol (mg).
- Sodium (mg).
- Total carbohydrate(g).
- Dietary fiber (g).
- Sugars (g).
- Protein (g).

A simplified format may be used for standard menu items (e.g., alcohol and soft drinks) that contain insignificant amounts of six or more of the required nutrients. This format must:

- Include information on total calories, total fat, total carbohydrates, protein, and sodium and any other of the required nutrients that are present in more than insignificant amounts; and
- Include, at the bottom of the list of nutrients, the statement "Not a significant source of _____" (with the blank filled in with the required nutrients that are present in insignificant amounts).

Determination of Nutrient Content of Foods

Covered establishments must have a reasonable basis for the nutrient information for standard menu items. Upon request from FDA, and within a reasonable period of time (4-6 weeks), covered establishments must supply to FDA information used to substantiate the nutrient values.

A reasonable basis may include, but is not limited to:

- Nutrient databases.
- Laboratory analysis.
- Nutrition Facts labels.
- Cookbooks.
- Other reasonable means (e.g., calculations).

Certifications

Upon request from FDA, covered establishments must provide:

- A statement that is signed and dated by a responsible individual who is employed at the covered establishment, its corporate headquarters, or parent entity who can verify that the nutrient information is complete and accurate.
- A statement that is signed and dated by a responsible individual employed at the covered establishment certifying that the covered establishment has taken reasonable steps to ensure that the method of preparation and the amount of the standard menu item offered for sale are the same as that on which the nutrient values were determined.

Source: U.S. Food & Drug Administration, Menu Labeling Requirements. **https://www.fda.gov/Food/GuidanceRegulation/GuidanceDocumentsRegulatoryInformation/LabelingNutrition/ucm515020.htm.** Accessed November 24, 2018

Appendix E

Body Mass Index Table

BMI	Normal weight							Overweight						Obese						
	19	20	21	22	23	24	25	26	27	28	29	30	31	32	33	34	35
Height (inches)								Body Weight (pounds)									
58	91	96	100	105	110	115	119	124	129	134	138	143	148	153	158	162	167
59	94	99	104	109	114	119	124	128	133	138	143	148	153	158	163	168	173
60	97	102	107	112	118	123	128	133	138	143	148	153	158	163	168	174	179
61	100	106	111	116	122	127	132	137	143	148	153	158	164	169	174	180	185
62	104	109	115	120	126	131	136	142	147	153	158	164	169	175	180	186	191
63	107	113	118	124	130	135	141	146	152	158	163	169	175	180	186	191	197
64	110	116	122	128	134	140	145	151	157	163	169	174	180	186	192	197	204
65	114	120	126	132	138	144	150	156	162	168	174	180	186	192	198	204	210
66	118	124	130	136	142	148	155	161	167	173	179	186	192	198	204	210	216
67	121	127	134	140	146	153	159	166	172	178	185	191	198	204	211	217	223
68	125	131	138	144	151	158	164	171	177	184	190	197	203	210	216	223	230
69	128	135	142	149	155	162	169	176	182	189	196	203	209	216	223	230	236
70	132	139	146	153	160	167	174	181	188	195	202	209	216	222	229	236	243
71	136	143	150	157	165	172	179	186	193	200	208	215	222	229	236	243	250
72	140	147	154	162	169	177	184	191	199	206	213	221	228	235	242	250	258
73	144	151	159	166	174	182	189	197	204	212	219	227	235	242	250	257	265
74	148	155	163	171	179	186	194	202	210	218	225	233	241	249	256	264	272
75	152	160	168	176	184	192	200	208	216	224	232	240	248	256	264	272	279
76	156	164	172	180	189	197	205	213	221	230	238	246	254	263	271	279	287

Appendix F

Exchange Lists for Diabetic Menu Planning

The following chart shows the amounts of nutrients in 1 serving from each food list.

Food List	Carbohydrate (grams)	Protein (grams)	Fat (grams)	Calories
Carbohydrates				
Starch: breads, cereals and grains, starchy vegetables, crackers, snacks, beans, peas and lentils	15	0-3	0-1	80
Fruits	15	0	0	60
Milk				
Fat-free, low-fat, 1%	12	8	0-3	100
Reduced-fat, 2%	12	8	5	120
Whole	12	8	8	160
Sweets, desserts and other carbohydrates	15	Varies	Varies	Varies
Nonstarchy vegetables	5	2	0	25
Meat and Meat Substitutes				
Lean	0	7	0-3	45
Medium-fat	0	7	4-7	75
High-fat	0	7	8+	100
Plant-based proteins	Varies	7	Varies	Varies
Fats	0	0	5	45
Alcohol	Varies	0	0	100

Adapted from: *Choose Your Foods: Exchange Lists for Diabetes*, American Diabetes Association and The American Dietetic Association, 2008

Appendix G

Carb Counting

Carb counting (also called "*carbohydrate counting*") is estimating the number of carbohydrate grams in a given meal or snack. Total carbs are tallied on a running basis to ensure that the total doesn't exceed a predetermined dietary goal for the meal and/or day.

An alternative form of carb counting is called "carbohydrate choice" or "simple carb counting." With this method, every 15 grams of carbs are counted as one carbohydrate choice, with a predetermined number of choices allotted daily. While not as precise as carb gram counting, simple carb counting may be preferred by those who like the simplicity.

Both types of carb counting are useful for people with type 1 diabetes who use fast-acting insulin to cover the carb content in their meals. Carb counting allows them to calculate the right amount of insulin to counteract the corresponding blood sugar rise from their meal.

Check food labels for carbohydrate values and to convert to carb choices.

Quick Carb Counting Guide

1 carb choice	=	15 grams carbohydrate
2 carb choices	=	30 grams carbohydrate
3 carb choices	=	45 grams carbohydrate
4 carb choices	=	60 grams carbohydrate
5 carb choices	=	75 grams carbohydrate

1 carb choice = 15 grams carbohydrate	2 carb choices = 30 grams carbohydrates	3 carb choices = 45 grams carbohydrates
1/3 cup cooked rice	2/3 cup cooked rice	1 cup cooked rice
1 slice of bread (1 ounce)	1 small sandwich bun (2 ounces)	1 medium-sized bagel (3 ounces)
1 small piece of fruit	1 large banana	½ cup dried apricots
½ cup fruit juice	1 cup fruit juice	1½ cups fruit juice
1 cup milk or 2/3 cup low-fat yogurt, plain	1 cup chocolate milk	1 cup fruit yogurt

Adapted from *Count Your Carbs: Getting Started*, American Diabetes Association and The American Dietetic Association, 2010

Carbohydrate Counting List

The following foods contain about 15 grams of carbohydrates.

Group	Measure
Breads	1 slice of bread 2 slices of light bread ½ hamburger or hot-dog bun ½ of an English muffin 1 pancake or waffle (4-inch size) 1 corn or flour tortilla (6-inch size)
Cereal and Grains	1/3 cup rice 1/3 cup pasta 1/3 cup bread stuffing ½ cup cooked cereal ½ cup bran cereal ½ cup sugar-frosted cereal 1½ cup puffed cereal ¾ cup unsweetened cereal
Fruit	1 small orange, apple, pear, kiwi, peach, nectarine or banana 1/3 cup baked apple slices 2 small plums or tangerines ½ cup unsweetened applesauce 1/3 of a cantaloupe 1 slice of watermelon or honeydew melon ½ cup fruit cocktail 17 grapes 2 tablespoons of raisins 1¼ cup whole strawberries 1 cup raspberries ½ cup apple, pineapple, grapefruit or orange juice 1/3 cup grape juice, prune juice or cranberry cocktail
Non-starchy vegetables	3 cup raw vegetables 1½ cup cooked of any vegetable not listed on the starchy vegetable list
Starchy vegetables	½ cup corn 1 cup mixed vegetables containing corn or peas ½ cup peas ½ cup mashed potatoes 1 small baked or sweet potato ½ cup winter squash ½ cup cooked dry beans 2/3 cup lima or butter beans
Dairy foods	1 cup milk 1 cup buttermilk 1 cup plain yogurt

Source: American Diabetes Association, **www.diabetes.org**

Appendix H

FODMAP

The term **FODMAPS** is an acronym that stands for fermentable oligosaccharides, disaccharides, mono-saccharides and polyols. They are a collection of poorly absorbed simple and complex sugars that are found in a variety of fruits and vegetables and also in milk and wheat. The fermentation of FODMAPs by bacteria produce the symptoms experienced by people with irritable bowel syndrome. About seventy-five percent of people will experience improvement in symptoms following a reduction of high FODMAP foods. These sugars are found in a wide variety of foods in the diet, and not everyone with irritable bowel syndrome will have symptoms with all of them.

Fermentable

Oligosaccharides (fructans and galacto-oligosaccharides)

Disaccharides (lactose or milk sugars)

Monosaccharides (excess fructose)

And

Polyols (sugar alcohols such as sorbitol, mannitol and xylitol)

High FODMAP Foods

Oligosaccharides		Disaccharides	Monosaccharides	Polyols
Fructans (inulin)	**Galactans**	**Lactose**	**Fructose**	
Wheat	Beans	Dairy products	Fruits	Sweetener Additives:
Onion	Lentils		• Apples	• Sorbitol
Garlic	Legumes		• Mango	• Mannitol
Dried fruits	Pistachios		• Pear	• Xylitol
• Raisins	Cashews		• Watermelon	• Maltitol
• Dates			• Persimmon	Stone fruits
• Figs			Agave	• Apricots
Watermelon			Honey	• Avocado
Persimmon			High-fructose corn syrup	• Cherries
Other vegetables			Vegetables	• Nectarines
• Asparagus			• Artichokes	• Peaches
• Beet			• Asparagus	• Plums
• Brussels sprouts			• Sugar snap peas	Vegetables
• Cabbage				• Cauliflower
• Leek				• Mushrooms
• Legumes				• Snow peas
• Peas				

Appendix I

Recipe Index: Carb Choices and Exchanges

Recipe Name	Carb Choices	Exchanges
Arctic Char with Blistered Cherry Tomatoes in Garlic Olive Oil, pg. 4	1	5 lean meat + 1 nonstarch vegetable
Arugula, Mint, Apple and Seagreens Salad, pg.4	1	1 nonstarch vegetable + 2 fat
Banana Bread, pg. 286	2	1 starch + 1 fruit
Black Bean Quinoa Burgers, pg. 298	1	1 lean meat + 1 starch
Blueberry Cobbler made with Splenda®, pg. 334	1 ½	½ starch + 1 fruit + 1 fat
Blueberry Cobbler made with Splenda® Blend, pg. 334	2	1 starch + 1 fruit + 1 fat
Butternut Squash Soup with Fried Sage Leaves, pg. 265	1	1 starch
Café Rakka Lamb Korma, pg. 237	3	4 medium fat meat + 3 fat + 1 starch + 1 non starchy vegetable
Carmelized Brie, Grilled Figs, Ham, and Kentucky Bibb Lettuce with Fig Vinaigrette, pg. 219	2 ½	2 high fat meat + 2 fat + 1 nonstarchy vegetable + 1 fruit
Chicken Fesenjan with Walnuts and Pomegranate Syrup, pg. 304	1	5 lean meat + 1 fruit
Christmas Beer Cake, pg. 360	3	3 starch + 3 fat
Cold Watermelon Ginger Soup, pg. 292	1	1 fruit
Cucumber Lemon Refresher, pg. 113	0	free
Curried Sweet Potato Salad, pg. 280	3 ½	3 starchy vegetables + 3 fat
Gluten-Free Brownies, pg. 360	1	1 starch + 2 fat
Gluten-Free Fried Chicken, pg. 359	0	4 medium fat meat
Green Goddess Dressing, pg. 85	0	1 fat
"Hint of Mint" Almond Pesto, pg. 328	0	1 ½ fat
Lentil Curry, pg. 308	2	1 medium fat meat + 2 starch
Oven Roasted Cod with Three Colored Peppers and Baby Potatoes, pg. 182	1 ½	4 lean meat + 1 starch + 1 nonstarch vegetable
Panna Cotta, base recipe, pg. 329	1 ½	½ whole milk + 1 starch + 1 fat
Panna Cotta, high-calorie, pg. 329	1	1 starch + 7 fat
Panna Cotta, moderate-calorie, pg. 329	1 ½	½ whole milk + 1 starch + 2 fat
Panna Cotta, reduced-calorie, pg. 329	1	½ 2% milk + ½ starch
Panna Cotta, reduced-calorie, fat-free, pg. 329	1	½ fat-free milk + ½ starch
Peanutty Energy Bars, pg. 286	2	1 medium fat meat + 2 starch
Poached Chicken Breast with Root Vegetables, pg. 246	2	4 lean meat + 2 starch
Quinoa and Butternut Stuffed Poblano Peppers, pg. 199	2 ½	1 starch + 2 starchy vegetable
Roasted Basil Pesto Salmon, Cauliflower Rice, pg. 199	½	5 medium meat + 2 fat + 11 nonstarchy vegetable
Roasted Butternut Squash Quinoa Salad, pg. 264	3	1 starch + 1 starchy vegetable
Roasted Pineapple Cake with Pina Colada Sorbet and Mango Passion Coulis, pg. 65	5	2 fruit + 2 starch
Saffron Buckwheat Pilaf and Three-Bean Relish with Spicy Tomato Vinaigrette, pg. 350	3	1 medium fat meat + 3 starch + 1 fat
Seared Beef Tenderloin with Tomato Confit, Kale and Sage Polenta, pg. 293	1	5 lean meat + ½ starch + 1 nonstarch vegetable
Slow Roasted Glazed Salmon, pg. 95	0	4 lean meat
Spanish Shoemaker, pg. 127	0	0
Spicy Vegetarian Loaf, pg 46	5	2 starch + 2 starchy vegetables + 2 nonstarchy vegetables
Spinach Salad with Green Goddess Dressing, pg. 85	1	2 nonstarch vegetable + 2 fat

Recipe Index: Carb Choices and Exchanges *continued*

Recipe Name	Carb Choices	Exchanges
Sweet Potato and Pineapple Salad, pg. 135	2	1 starch + 1 fruit + 1 fat
Trout Almondine with Mashed Potatoes and Green Beans, pg. 87	3	5 medium fat meat + 2 starch + 1 nonstarchy vegetable + 2 fat
Turkey Meatloaf, pg. 264	½	3 lean meat + ½ starch
Wild Mushroom Farroto, pg. 207	2	2 starch + 1 nonstarch vegetable + 3 fat
Wild Rice Salad, pg. 339	2	1 starch + 1 fruit + 2 fat

References

Chapter 1

1. Fryar CD, Carroll M, Ogden CL. Prevalence of Overweight, Obesity, and Extreme Obesity Among Adults Aged 20 and Over: United States, 1960–1962 Through 2013–2014. National Center for Health Statistics, Centers for Disease Control and Prevention. Retrieved from **https://www.cdc.gov/nchs/data/hestat/obesity_adult_13_14/obesity_adult_13_14.pdf**. Accessed February 21, 2018.

2. Fryar CD, Carroll M, Ogden CL. Prevalence of Overweight and Obesity Among Children and Adolescents Aged 2–19 Years: United States, 1963–1965 Through 2013–2014. National Center for Health Statistics, Centers for Disease Control and Prevention. Retrieved from **https://www.cdc.gov/nchs/data/hestat/obesity_child_13_14/obesity_child_13_14.htm**. Accessed February 21, 2018.

3. Jones J, Saad L. Gallup Poll. Health and Healthcare Poll. November 4-8, 2015. Retrieved from **http://news.gallup.com/poll/186920/fewer-americans-say-lose-weight.aspx**. Accessed February 21, 2018.

4. Atwater WO. *Principles of Nutrition and Nutritive Value of Food*. U.S. Department of Agriculture, Farmers' Bulletin 1902; No.142.

5. National Center for Health Statistics, Centers for Disease Control and Prevention, U.S. Department of Health and Human Services. National Vital Statistics Report. Deaths: Final Data for 2015. November 27, 2017. Retrieved at **https://www.cdc.gov/nchs/data/nvsr/nvsr66/nvsr66_06.pdf**. Accessed February 21, 2018.

6. U.S. Department of Health and Human Services and U.S. Department of Agriculture. 2015 – 2020 *Dietary Guidelines for Americans*. 8th Edition. December 2015. Retrieved from **http://health.gov/dietaryguidelines/2015/guidelines/**. Accessed February 21, 2018.

7. Holman DM, Grossman M, Henley SJ, Peipins LA, Tison L, White MC. Opportunities for cancer prevention during midlife: highlights from a meeting of experts. *Am J Prev Med*. 2014;46(3, Supplement 1):S73–S80. Retrieved from **https://www.ncbi.nlm.nih.gov/pmc/articles/PMC4535330/**. Accessed February 21, 2018.

8. Cordain L, Eaton SB, Sebastian A, Mann N, Lindeberg S, Watkins BA, O'Keefe JA, Brand-Miller J. Origins and evolution of the Western diet: health implications for the 21st century. *Am J Clin Nutri*. 2005;81:341-45.

9. International Food Information Council Foundation. 2017 Food and Health Survey: A Healthy Perspective: Understanding American Food Values. Retrieved from **https://www.foodinsight.org/2017-food-and-health-survey**. Accessed February 21, 2018.

10. Hartman Group. *Culture of Food 2015: New Appetites, New Routines of Food 2015*. Bellevue, WA: Hartman Group, Inc.; 2015.

11. Fulkerson JA, Larso, N, Horning M, and Neumark-Sztainer D. A review of associations between family or shared meal frequency and dietary and weight status outcomes across the lifespan. *J Nutr Educ Behav*. 2014; 46: 2-19.

12. Martin-Biggers, J., Spaccarotella, K., Berhaupt-Glickstein, A., Hongu, N., Worobey, J., and Byrd-Bredbenner, C. Come and get it! A discussion of family mealtime literature and factors affecting obesity risk. Adv Nutr. 2014; 5: 235–247.

13. International Food Information Council Foundation. 2015 Food & Health Survey: Consumer Attitudes Toward Food Safety, Nutrition, & Health. Retrieved from **https://www.foodinsight.org/2015-food-health-survey-consumer-research**. Accessed February 22, 2018.

14. Condrasky M, Hegler. M. Bridging the nutrition gap for chefs. *The National Culinary Review*. 2009;Feb:54-56.

15. Schwartz J, Byrd-Bradbenner C. Portion distortion: typical portion sizes selected by young adults. J Am Diet Assoc. 2006;106:1412-1418.

16. Mintel Group. Healthy Dining Trends – US – March 2017.

Chapter 2

1. Institute of Medicine. 2012. Front-of-Package Nutrition Rating Systems and Symbols: Promoting Healthier Choices. Washington, DC: The National Academies Press. **https://doi.org/10.17226/13221**. Accessed March 1, 2018.

2. Food and Drug Administration, Background Information on Point of Purchase Labeling, October 2009. Available at **www.fda.gov/Food/LabelingNutrition/LabelClaims/ucm187320.htm**. Accessed March 1, 2018.

Chapter 3

1. Sugar and Sweeteners Yearbook Tables, Economic Research Service, U.S. Department of Agriculture. August 4, 2017. Available at **https://www.ers.usda.gov/data-products/sugar-and-sweeteners-yearbook-tables.aspx**. March 1, 2018

2. US Departments of Agriculture and Health and Human Services. 2015-2020 Dietary Guidelines for Americans. 8th ed. Washington, DC: US Government Printing. Available at **http://www. DietaryGuidelines.gov**. Accessed March 1, 2018.

3. Gupta P, Gupta N, Pawar AP, Birajdat SS, Natt AS, Role of Sugar and Sugar Substitutes in Dental Caries: A Review. ISRN Dentistry. 2013; 2013: 519421. Published online 2013 Dec 29. doi: 10.1155/2013/519421. Accessed March 1, 2018.

4. Bellisle F. Effects of diet on behaviour and cognition in children. *Br J Nutr*. 2004; 92(suppl 2):S227-S232.

5. Corwin RL, Grigson PS. Symposium overview—Food addiction: Fact or fiction? JNutr. 2009;139(3):617-619.

6. McGinnis JM, Gootman JA, Kraak VI, Ed. Food Marketing to Children and Youth: Threat or Opportunity? Committee on Food Marketing and the Diets of Children and Youth. Available at **http://www.nap.edu/catalog.php?recordid=11514**. Accessed July 9, 2012

Chapter 4

1. National Academy of Sciences and Institute of Medicine. Dietary Reference Intakes for Energy, Carbohydrate, Fiber, Fat, Fatty Acids, Cholesterol, Protein and Amino Acids. Washington, DC: National Academy Press; 2002.

Chapter 5

1. Dhillon J, Craig BA, Leidy HJ, Amankwaah AF, Anguah KO, Jacobs A, Jones BL, Jones JB, Keeler CL, Keller CEM, McCrory MA, Rivera RL, Slebodnik M, Mattes RD, Tucker RM. The Effects of Increased Protein Intake on Fullness: A Meta-Analysis and Its Limitations. JADA. 2016; 116 (6): 968-983 Available at http://dx.doi.org/10.1016/j.jand.2016.01.003. Accessed March 8, 2018.

2. Ortinau LC, Hoertel HA, Douglas SM, Leidy HJ. Effects of high-protein vs. high- fat snacks on appetite control, satiety, and eating initiation in healthy women. *Nutrition Journal. 2014*;13:97. doi:10.1186/1475-2891-13-97. Accessed March 8, 2018.

3. Hill C. This chart proves Americans love their meat. MarketWatch. December 1, 2016. https://www.marketwatch.com/story/this-chart-proves-americans-love-their-meat-2016-08-15. Accessed February 18, 2019.

4. Liddel M, Yencho M. National Oceanic and Atmospheric Administration. Fisheries of the United States, 2017 Report. September 2018. https://www.fisheries.noaa.gov/resource/document/fisheries-united-states-2017-report. Accessed February 18, 2019.

5. The World Agricultural Supply and Demand Estimates Report (WASDE), WADSE 584. December 2018. www.usda.gov/oce/commodity/wasde/wasde1218.pdf. Accessed February 18, 2019.

Chapter 6

1. National Research Council. Dietary Reference Intakes: The Essential Guide to Nutrient Requirements. Washington, DC: The National Academies Press, 2006. Available at https://www.nap.edu/catalog/11537/dietary-reference-intakes-the-essential-guide-to-nutrient-requirements. Accessed March 9, 2018.

2. National Research Council. Dietary Reference Intakes for Water, Potassium, Sodium, Chloride, and Sulfate. Washington, DC: The National Academies Press, 2005. Available at https://www.nap.edu/catalog/10925/dietary-reference-intakes-for-water-potassium-sodium-chloride-and-sulfate. Accessed March 9, 2018

3. Ding M, Satija A, Bhupathiraju SN, Hu Y, Sun Q, Han J, Lopez-Garcia E, Willett W, van Dam RM, Hu FB, *Association of Coffee Consumption with Total and Cause-Specific Mortality in Three Large Prospective Cohorts*, Circulation. 2015; CIRCULATIONAHA.115.017341. Available at https://doi.org/10.1161/CIRCULATIONAHA.115.017341. Accessed March 9, 2018.

4. Salleh A. Athletes caffeine use reignites scientific debate. ABC Science Online. August 2, 2008. Available at http://www.abc.net.au/news/2008-08-02/athletes-caffeine-use-reignites-scientific-debate/462428. Accessed March 9, 2018.

5. NCAA Banned Drugs List. Available at http://www.ncaa.org/sites/default/files/2017_18_NCAA_Banned_Drugs_20170605.pdf. Accessed March 9, 2018.

6. Chen L, Appel LJ, Loria C, Lin P, Champagne CM, Elmer PJ, Ard JD, Mitchell D, Batch BC, Svetkey LP, Caballero B. Reduction in consumption of sugar-sweetened beverages is associated with weight loss: The PREMIER trial. *Am J Clin Nutr.* 2009; 89:1299-06.

7. Marcus K. Research and findings: A User's Guide to Wine Science. Wine Spectator. Available at www.winespectator.com/wssaccess/show/id/40815. Accessed March 9, 2018

8. Brewers Association. https://www.brewersassociation.org/statistics/number-of-breweries/. Accessed March 9, 2018.

Chapter 7

1. U.S. Department of Health and Human Services and U.S. Department of Agriculture. 2015 – 2020 *Dietary Guidelines for Americans.* 8th Edition. December 2015. Retrieved from http://health.gov/dietaryguidelines/2015/guidelines/. Accessed March 12, 2018.

2. Kushi LH, Doyle C, McCullough M, Rock CL, Demark-Wahnefried W, Bandera EV, Gapstur S, Patel AV, Andrews K, Gansler T, and The American Cancer Society 2010 Nutrition and Physical Activity Guidelines Advisory Committee (2012). American Cancer Society guidelines on nutrition and physical activity for cancer prevention. CA: A Cancer Journal for Clinicians, 62: 30–67. doi: 10.3322/caac.20140. Available at http://onlinelibrary.wiley.com/doi/10.3322/caac.20140/ full. Accessed July 18, 2012.

3. U.S. Department of Agriculture, Agricultural Research Service. 2015. USDA National Database for Standard Reference, Release 28. Nutrient Data Laboratory, Available at http://www.ars.usda.gov/services/docs.htm?docid=8964. Accessed March 26, 2018.

4. Rickman JC, Barrett DM, Bruhn CM. Nutritional comparison of fresh, frozen and canned fruits and vegetables. *J Sci Food Agric.* 2007; 87(7):1185-96.

Chapter 8

1. Mintel. Better-For-You Eating Trends: Spotlight on Real. September 2016. Available at https://store.mintel.com/us-better-for-you-eating-trends-spotlight-on-real-market-report. Accessed March 27, 2018.

2. National Restaurant Association. Chef Survey: What's Hot in 2018. Available at http://www.restaurant.org/News-Research/Research/What-s-Hot. Accessed March 27, 2018.

3. Chefs Collaborative Statement of Principles. http://www.chefscollaborative.org/about/. Accessed March 27, 2018.

4. IBIS World. Food Trucks-US Market Research Report. December 2017. https://www.ibisworld.com/industry-trends/specialized-market-research-reports/consumer-goods-services/food-service-drinking-places/food-trucks.html.

5. Food Truck Operator. Infographic: Why Food Truck Businesses are Revving Up. April 19. 2017. https://www.foodtruckoperator.com/blogs/infographic-food-truck-industry-to-hit-27b/. Accessed March 27, 2018.

6. Rolls BJ, Hermann M. The Ultimate Volumetrics Diet: Smart, Simple, Science-Based Strategies for Losing Weight and Keeping It Off. New York: William Morrow Cookbooks; 2012.

7. U.S. Department of Health and Human Services and U.S. Department of Agriculture. 2015 – 2020 *Dietary Guidelines for Americans.* 8th Edition. December 2015. Retrieved from http://health.gov/dietaryguidelines/2015/guidelines/. Accessed March 28, 2018.

8. Adolphus K, Lawton CL, Dye L. The effects of breakfast on behavior and academic performance in children and adolescents. Frontiers in Human Neuroscience. 2013;7:425. doi:10.3389/fnhum.2013.00425.

9. Wesnes KA, Pincock C, Scholey A. Breakfast is associated with enhanced cognitive function in schoolchildren. An internet based study. Appetite 59, 646–649. 2012.

10. Hollands GJ, Shemilt I, Marteau TM, Jebb SA, Lewis HB, Wei Y, Higgins J, Ogilvie D. Portion, package or tableware size for changing selection and consumption of food, alcohol and tobacco. Cochrane Database of Systematic Reviews 2015, Issue 9. Art. No.: CD011045. DOI: 10.1002/14651858.CD011045.pub2.

12. Ogden CL, Carroll MD, Lawman HG, Fryar CD, Kruszon-Moran D, Kit BK, et al. Trends in Obesity Prevalence Among Children and Adolescents in the United States, 1988-1994 Through 2013-2014. JAMA 2016;315(21):2292-9.

13. Moran AJ, et al. Trends in Nutrient Content of Children's Menu Items in U.S. Chain Restaurants. *American Journal of Preventive Medicine*, Volume 52 , Issue 3 , 284 – 291. 2017. https://doi.org/10.1016/j.amepre.2016.11.007

14. National County of Farmers Market Directory Listing. USDA-AMS-Marketing Services Division. 2017. Available at https://www.ams.usda.gov/sites/default/files/media/CSANewModelsforChangingMarketsb.pdf. Accessed March 28, 2018.

15. Woods T, Ernst M, Tropp D. Community Supported Agriculture – New Models for Changing Markets. U.S. Department of Agriculture, Agricultural Marketing Service, April 2017. Web. Available at https://www.ams.usda.gov/sites/default/files/media/CSANewModelsforChangingMarketsb.pdf. Accessed March 28, 2019.

16. Food, Agriculture, Conservation and Trade Act of 1990. Available at https://www.ers.usda.gov/webdocs/publications/42024/50900_aib624.pdf?v=42079. Accessed March 28, 2018.

17. University of California Sustainable Agriculture Research and Education Program. Available at http://asi.ucdavis.edu/programs/sarep. Accessed March 28, 2018.

18. 2016 Restaurant Industry Forecast, National Restaurant Association. Available at http://www.restaurant.org/Home/old_files/2016-Restaurant-Industry-Forecast. Accessed March 28, 2018.

19. USDA Economic Research Service. Organic Market Overview. https://www.ers.usda.gov/topics/natural-resources-environment/organic-agriculture/organic-market-overview/. Accessed March 28, 2018.

20. Hartman Group. Organic & Natural 2016. Bellevue, WA: Hartman Group, Inc.; 2016.

21. Smith-Spangler C, Brandeau ML, Hunter GE, Bavinger JC, Pearson M, Eschbach PJ, et al. Are Organic Foods Safer or Healthier Than Conventional Alternatives?: A Systematic Review. *Ann Intern Med*. 2012;157:348–366. doi: 10.7326/0003-4819-157-5-201209040-00007.

22. Dangour AD, Dodhia SK, Hayter A, Allen E, Lock K, Uauy R. Nutritional quality of organic foods: A systematic review. *Am J Clin Nutri*. 2009;90:680-85.

23. Benbrook C, Zhao X, Yanez J, Davies N, Andrews P. New evidence confirms the nutritional superiority of plant-based organic foods. The Organic Center. Available at http://www.organic-center.org/reportfiles/NutrientContentReport.pdf. Accessed March 28, 2018.

24. Institute of Food Technologists. Functional Foods. Available at http://www.ift.org/Knowledge-Center/Read-IFT-Publications/Science-Reports/Scientific-Status-Summaries/Functional-Foods/. Accessed March 28, 2018.

25. Crowe KM. et al. Position of the Academy of Nutrition and Dietetics: Functional Foods. JADA. 2013; 113: 1096-1103.

Chapter 9

1. International Food Information Council Foundation. 2012 Food & Health Survey: Consumer Attitudes toward Food Safety, Nutrition and Health. Available at: www.foodinsight. org/Resources/Detail.aspx?topic=2012_IFIC_Foundation_ Food_Health_Survey_Media_Resources. Accessed August 5, 2012.

2. 2010 Mintel Healthy Dining Trends Survey press release.

3. Mintel Group. Healthy Dining Trends – US – May 2012. Scope and Themes. Available at http://oxygen.mintel.com/ sinatra/oxygen/display/id=623040/display/id=622993. Accessed May 30, 2012.

4. Hartman Group. Reimagining Health + Wellness Lifestyle and Trends Report 2010. June 2010. Available at http:// hartman-group.com/publications/reports/reimagininghealth-wellness-lifestyle-and-trends-report-2010. Accessed September 1, 2012.

5. Librairie Larousse's Gastronomic Committee. Larousse Gastronomique. Updated. New York: Clarkson Potter Publishers; 2009.

6. Mattes RD. The taste for salt in humans. *Am J Clin Nutr*. 1997;65(suppl):692S-97S.

7. Beauchamp GK. Sensory and receptor responses to umami: An overview of pioneering work. *Am J Clin Nutr*. 2009;90(3):723S-27S.

8. Mattes RD, Hollis J, Hayes, D, Stunkard J., Appetite: measurement and manipulation misgivings, *J Am Diet Assoc*. 2005;105:S87-S97.

9. Nasser J. Taste, food intake and obesity. Obes Rev. 2001;2:213-18.

10. Rolls BJ, Barnett RA. Volumetrics: Feel Full on Fewer Calories. New York: Harper Collins; 1999.

11. Gerstein DE, Woodward-Lopez G, Evans AE, Kelsey K, Drewnowski A. Clarifying concepts about macronutrients' effects on satiation and satiety. *J Am Diet Assoc*. 2004;104(7):1151-53.

12. Page K, Dorenburg A. The Flavor Bible: The Essential Guide to Culinary Creativity, Based on the Wisdom of America's Most Imaginative Chefs. New York: Little Brown & Co.; 2008.

13. Report of the Dietary Guidelines Advisory Committee on the Dietary Guidelines, 2010. Available at www.cnpp.usda.gov/DGAs2010-DGACReport.htm. Accessed September 1, 2012.

14. Dickinson BD, Havas S. For the Council on Science and Public Health, American Medical Association. Reducing the population burden of cardiovascular disease by reducing sodium intake. *Arch Intern Med*. 2007;167(14):1460-68.

15. The Salt Institute. Available at www.saltinstitute.org. Accessed August 9, 2012.

Chapter 10

1. FDA Food Code, Chapter 3: Food. Available at http://www.fda.gov/Food/FoodSafety/RetailFoodProtection/Food01Code/FoodCode2009/default.htm. Accessed July 22, 2102.

2. Gil MI, Aguayo E, Kader AA. Quality changes and nutrient retention in fresh-cut versus whole fruits during storage. *J Agril Food Chem*. 2006;54(12):4284-96.

3. U.S. Department of Agriculture, Agricultural Research Service. 2009. Table of Nutrient Retention Factors, Release 6. Nutrient Data Laboratory. Available at www.nal.usda.gov/fnic/foodcomp/Data/retn6/retn06.pdf. Accessed August 4, 2012.

Chapter 11

1. Patient Protection and Affordable Care Act. Public Law 111-148. Available at **https://www.congress.gov/111/plaws/publ148/PLAW-111publ148.pdf**. Accessed April 10, 2018.

2. AP-GfK Poll: Americans support menu labeling in restaurants, grocery stores. December 31, 2014. Available at **ap-gfkpoll.com/featured/findings-from-our-latest-poll-11**. Accessed April 10, 2018.

3. U.S. Food and Drug Administration. Food Labeling Guide. Available at **https://www.fda.gov/food/guidanceregulation/guidancedocumentsregulatoryinformation/ucm2006828.htm**. Accessed April 10, 2018.

4. NPD Group. A Generational Study: The Evolution of Eating. 2016. Available at **https://www.npd.com/latest-reports/fbc-consumption-evolution-of-eating/**. Accessed April 10, 2018.

Chapter 12

1. State of the Plate: 2015 Study on America's Consumption of Fruits and Vegetables, 2015. Produce for Better Health Foundation. Available at **https://pbhfoundation.org/about/res/pbh_res/**. Accessed May 11, 2018.

2. Centers for Disease Control and Prevention, National Center for Chronic Disease Prevention and Health Promotion. Youth Risk Behavior Surveillance System-United States, 2015. Available at **https://www.cdc.gov/healthyyouth/data/yrbs/pdf/2015/ss6506_updated.pdf**. Accessed May 11, 2018.

3. Condon E, Drilea S, Lichtenstein C, Mabli J, Madden E, and Niland K. (2015). Diet Quality of American School Children by National School Lunch Participation Status: Data from the National Health and Nutrition Examination Survey, 2005-2010. Prepared by Walter R. McDonald & Associates, Inc. for the Food and Nutrition Service. Available at **https://fns-prod.azureedge.net/sites/default/files/ops/NHANES-NSLP05-10-Summary.pdf**. Accessed May 11, 2018.

4. US Departments of Agriculture and Health and Human Services. 2015-2020 *Dietary Guidelines for Americans*. 8th ed. Washington, DC: US Government Printing. Available at **http://www. DietaryGuidelines.gov**. Accessed May 11, 2018.

5. Ohlund I, Lind T, Hernell O, Silfverdal S-A, Karlsland Akeson P. Increased vitamin D intake differentiated according to skin color is needed to meet requirements in young Swedish children during winter: a double-blind randomized clinical trial. *Am J Clin Nutr*. 2017. Available at: **doi: 10.3945/ajcn.116.147108**. Accessed May 11, 2018.

6. Cetron M, Davies O. 52 Trends Shaping Tomorrow's World. World Future Society Website. Available at **https://www.wfs.org/specialreports**. Published 2010. Accessed August 28, 2015.

7. U.S. Department of Commerce, Economics and Statistics Administration, U.S. Census Bureau. Ortman JM, Velkoff VA, Hogan H. An aging nation: The older population in the United States. Population Estimates and Projections. Current Population Reports. Issued May 2014. (Page 3). Available at **https://www.census.gov/prod/2014pubs/p25-1140.pdf** . Accessed December 14, 2014.

8. Stevenson DG, Cohen MA, Tell EJ, Burwell B. The complementarity of public and private long-term care coverage. Health Affairs. 2010 Jan-Feb; 29(1):96–101. (Page 98).

9. CDC. National Diabetes Statistics Report: Estimates of Diabetes and Its Burden in the United States, 2017. Available at **https://www.cdc.gov/diabetes/pdfs/data/statistics/national-diabetes-statistics-report.pdf**. Accessed May 11, 2018.

10. Position of the American Dietetic Association: Individualized Nutrition Approaches for Older Adults in Health Care Communities, *J Acad Nutr Diet*. 2018;118(4):724-735.

11. Practice Paper of the American Dietetic Association: Individualized Nutrition Approaches for Older Adults in Health Care Communities, *J Am Diet Assoc*. 2010;110:1554-1563.

12. Pioneer Network Food and Dining Clinical Standards Task Force. New Dining Practice Standards. 2011. Available at **http://www.pioneernetwork.net/Data/Documents/NewDiningPracticeStandards.pdf**

13. White JV, Guenter P, Jensen G, Malone A, Schofield M. Academy of Nutrition and Dietetics Malnutrition Work Group, et al. Consensus statement of the Academy of Nutrition and Dietetics/American Society for Parenteral and Enteral Nutrition: Characteristics recommended for the identification and documentation of adult malnutrition (undernutrition). *J Acad Nutr Diet*. 2012;112(5):730–738.

14. Position of the American Dietetic Association, Dietitians of Canada and the American College of Sports Medicine: Nutrition and Athletic Performance. *J Acad Nutr Diet*. 2016;116(3):501-528.

15. Rodriguez NR, Vislocky LM, Gaine PC. Dietary protein, endurance exercise, and human skeletal-muscle protein turnover. Curr Opin Clin Nutr Metab Care. 2007;10:40-45.

16. National Center for Health Statistics. Health, United States, 2016. Available at **http://www.cdc.gov/nchs/hus.htm**. Accessed May 11, 2018.

17. International Food Information Council Foundation. 2017 Food & Health Survey: Consumer Attitudes Toward Food Safety, Nutrition, & Health. Available at **www.foodinsight.org/Resources/Detail.aspx?topic=2011_Food_Health_Survey_Consumer_Attitudes_Toward_Food_Safety_Nutrition_Health**. Accessed May 30, 2012.

18. Hill JO. Can a small-changes approach help address the obesity epidemic? A report of the Joint Task Force of the American Society for Nutrition, Institute of Food Technologists, and International Food Information Council. *Am J Clin Nutr*. 2009; 89:477-84.

19. Nishida C, Uauy R, Kumanyika S, Shetty P. The Joint WHO/FAO Expert Consultation on diet, nutrition and the prevention of chronic diseases: process, product and policy implications. Public Health Nutrition. 2004;7:245-50.

20. Yasmin MR, Kamensky V, Manson JE, Silver B, Rapp SR, Haring B, Beresford SAA, Snetselaar L, Wassertheil-Smoller S. Artificially Sweetened Beverages and Stroke, Coronary Heart Disease, and All-Cause Mortality in the Women's Health Initiative. Stroke. 2019; 50: 01-08. DOI: 10.1161/STROKEAHA.118.023100

21. Vegetarian Resource Group. How Many Adults in the U.S. are Vegetarians and Vegan? Available at **https://www.vrg.org/nutshell/Polls/2016_adults_veg.htm**. Accessed May 11, 2018.

22. Vegetarian Resource Group. How Many Adults Eat Vegetarian and Vegan Meals When Eating Out? Available at **https://www.vrg.org/nutshell/Polls/2016_adults_veg.htm**. Accessed May 11, 2018.

23. Pew Research Center. A portrait of Jewish Americans: Findings from a Pew Research Center Survey of US Jews. October 2013. **http://www.pewforum.org/2013/10/01/jewish-american-beliefs-attitudes-culture-survey/**. Accessed February 21, 2019.

Chapter 13

1   Benjamin EJ, Virani SS, Callaway CW, Chang AR, Cheng S, Chiuve SE, Cushman M, Delling FN, Deo R, de Ferranti SD, Ferguson JF, Fornage M, Gillespie C, Isasi CR, Jimenez MC, Jordan LC, Judd SE, Lackland D, Lichtman JH, Lisabeth L, Liu S, Longenecker CT, Lutsey PL, Matchar DB, Matsushita K, Mussolino ME, Nasir K, O'Flaherty M, Palaniappan LP, Pandey DK, Reeves MJ, Ritchey MD, Rodriguez CJ, Roth GA, Rosamond WD, Sampson UKA, Satou GM, Shah SH, Spartano NL, Tirschwell DL, Tsao CW, Voeks JH, Willey JZ, Wilkins JT, Wu JHY, Alger HM, Wong SS, Muntner P; on behalf of the American Heart Association Council on Epidemiology and Prevention Statistics Committee and Stroke Statistics Subcommittee. Heart disease and stroke statistics 2018 update: a report from the American Heart Association [published online ahead of print January 31, 2018]. Circulation. DOI: 10.1161/CIR.0000000000000558. Accessed May 14, 2018.

2. Cancer Trends Progress Report. National Cancer Institute, NIH, DHHS, Bethesda, MD, February 2018, **https://progressreport. cancer.gov**. Accessed May 14, 2018.

3. National Diabetes Statistics Report, 2017: Estimates of Diabetes and Its Burden in the United States. National Center for Chronic Disease Prevention and Health Promotion. Available at **https://www.cdc.gov/diabetes/pdfs/data/statistics/national-diabetes-statistics-report.pdf**. Accessed May 14, 2018.

4. The Culinary Institute of America. Worlds of Healthy Flavors, 2010. Available at **www.ciaprochef.com/wohf/index.html**. Accessed August 4, 2012.

5. Dickinson BD, Havas S. for the Council on Science and Public Health. Reducing the population burden of cardiovascular disease by reducing sodium intake. Arch Intern Med.2007;167(14):1460-68.

6. Mattes RD, Donnelly D. Relative contributions of dietary sodium sources. *J Am Coll Nutr.* 1991;10(4):383-93.

7. Institute of Medicine of the National Academies. A Population-Based Policy and Systems Change Approach to Prevent and Control Hypertension. Washington, DC: The National Academies Press. Board on Population Health and Public Health Practice Committee on Public Health Priorities to Reduce and Control Hypertension in the US Population; 2010.

8. Rock CL, Doyle C, Demark-Wahnefried W, Meyerhardt J, Courneya KS, et al. CA: A Cancer Journal for Clinicians. 2012; 62(4):243-74. Available at **http://onlinelibrary.wiley.com/doi/10.3322/caac.21142/epdf**. Accessed March 17, 2016.

9. Center for Disease Control and Prevention. NCHS Summary Health Statistics: National Health Interview Survey, 2016. Available at **https://ftp.cdc.gov/pub/Health_Statistics/NCHS/NHIS/SHS/2016_SHS_Table_C-2.pdf**. Accessed May 15, 2018.

10. Rubio-Tapia A, Ludvigsson JF, Brantner TL, Murray JA, Everhart JE. The prevalence of celiac disease in the United States. *American Journal of Gastroenterology*. 2012;107(10):1538–1544.

11. Beyond Celiac. GREAT Gluten-Free Kitchens. Available at **https://www.beyondceliac.org/kitchens/**. Accessed May 15, 2018.

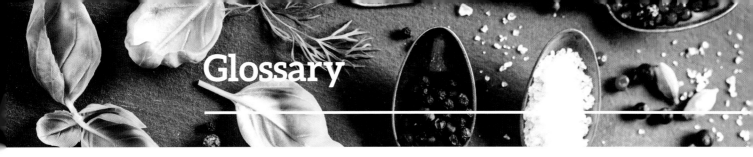

Glossary

Absorption The process by which nutrients pass from the digestive tract, through the intestinal walls, and into the bloodstream.

Acceptable Macronutrient Distribution Range (AMDR) A range of intake for carbohydrates, fats and proteins that reduces risk of chronic disease while providing intakes of essential nutrients. If an individual's intake is outside the AMDR, the risk for chronic diseases and/or insufficient intakes of essential nutrients is increased.

Added sugars Sugars, syrups and other caloric sweeteners that are added to foods during processing or preparation or consumed separately. Added sugars do not include naturally occurring sugars such as those in milk or fruits. Names for added sugars include: brown sugar, corn sweetener, corn syrup, dextrose, fructose, fruit juice concentrates, glucose, high-fructose corn syrup, honey, invert sugar, lactose, maltose, malt syrup, molasses, raw sugar, turbinado sugar and sucrose.

Adequate Intake (AI) A recommended average daily nutrient intake level based on estimates of average nutrient intake by healthy people. AI is used when the Recommended Dietary Allowance cannot be determined.

Adipose tissue Fat tissue in the body.

Adobo seasoning A seasoning mix used in Latin American and Southwest American cooking.

Allergy An immune reaction to an ordinarily harmless substance.

Amino acids The building blocks of protein. Chains of amino acids link together to form proteins.

Anaphylaxis An allergic reaction that, in severe cases, can be fatal within minutes either from swelling that shuts off airways or from a dramatic drop in blood pressure.

Animal protein Protein from animal products such as meat, poultry, seafood, eggs, milk and milk products. Animal proteins tend to be higher quality because they contain all the essential amino acids humans need. They are more digestible than most vegetable sources of protein.

Antibodies Proteins generally found in the blood that detect and destroy invaders such as bacteria and viruses.

Aromatics Plant ingredients such as garlic, citrus zest, herbs and spices used to enhance the taste and fragrance of food.

Artificial sweetener A man-made chemical substance that provides sweetness without providing calories or carbohydrates.

Atherosclerosis A disease in which plaque builds up in the arteries, limiting the flow of oxygen-rich blood through the body; can lead to a heart attack or stroke.

Baker's asthma Common occupational respiratory diseases caused by exposure to antigens from flour and/or grain dust in bakeries.

Baking Surrounding food with hot, dry air in a closed environment, usually an oven; a dry-heat cooking method.

Barbecue Grilling food over a wood or charcoal fire. A marinade or sauce is often brushed on the item during cooking.

Batch cooking Preparing small containers of food several times throughout a service period so a fresh supply of cooked items is always available.

Bile A digestive fluid made in the liver and stored in the gall bladder that aids in fat digestion in the intestines; made of cholesterol, bile salts and bilirubin.

Bioavailability The ability of a nutrient to be absorbed; influenced by the condition of the small intestine and presence of other substances needed to transport nutrients through the intestine into the bloodstream.

Biotin A water-soluble vitamin essential for the metabolism of proteins and carbohydrates and in the production of hormones and cholesterol.

Blanching Briefly boiling foods in water; a technique generally used as the first part of a combination cooking method, such as to remove peels from fruits or vegetables.

Body mass index (BMI) A measure of body weight relative to height. BMI is a tool that is often used to determine if a person is at a healthy weight, overweight or obese, and whether a person's health is at risk due to his/her weight. The formula used to calculate BMI is:

$$BMI = \frac{\text{Weight in Pounds} \times 703}{\text{Height in Inches} \times \text{Height in inches}}$$

A BMI of 18.5 to 24.9 is considered healthy. A person with a BMI of 25 to 29.9 is considered overweight; a person with a BMI of 30 or more is considered obese. See Appendix E for a table on Body Mass Index.

Boiling Cooking food by transferring heat from very hot water (around 212° F) to food. The water has large, rolling bubbles rising to the surface.

Bouquet garni A small bunch of herbs, flavorful foods and/or spices tied with string; used to flavor stocks, braises and other preparations. The standard ingredients are parsley stems, thyme, celery and bay leaves. The bouquet is discarded after flavor is imparted to the foods.

Braising Browning food in hot fat and then covering it with liquid and cooking slowly over low heat.

Broiling A dry-heat cooking method using heat radiating from an overhead source.

Broth A flavorful liquid made by simmering water with meat, vegetables and/or spices and herbs.

Calcium A mineral needed by the body to maintain bone health and to regulate functions of the heart, muscles and nerves. Dairy products such fat-free or low-fat milk, yogurt and cheeses are the best sources of calcium.

Calorie A unit of heat in food that produces energy to sustain the body's various functions, including metabolic processes and physical activity. Food calories come from carbohydrates, proteins, fats and alcohol. Carbohydrates and proteins have 4 calories per gram; fat has 9 calories per gram; and alcohol has 7 calories per gram.

Cancer Abnormal cells that create a malignant and invasive growth or tumor that may recur after removal and can spread to other sites.

Capsaicin The chemical compound that puts the heat or pungency in chiles.

Carbohydrate A macronutrient that includes sugars, starches and fibers. Carbohydrates are a major source of energy in the diet. Simple carbohydrates are sugars and complex carbohydrates include both starches and fiber. Carbohydrates provide 4 calories per gram.

Cardiovascular disease Diseases of the heart and blood vessel system (arteries, capillaries, veins) within a person's entire body. The most common cardiovascular disease is atherosclerosis.

Caramelization The process of browning sugar using heat. Sugar caramelizes at approximately 320° F to 360° F.

Celiac disease An immune reaction to gluten, a protein found in wheat, rye and barley. The disease causes damage to the lining of the small intestine and prevents absorption of nutrients; also called celiac sprue or nontropical sprue.

Cholesterol A fat-like substance that is both made by the body and found naturally in animal foods such as meat, fish, poultry, eggs and dairy products. Some cholesterol is needed for hormone and vitamin production and to make bile. Cholesterol is carried through the blood in small units called lipoproteins. There are two types of cholesterol carriers: low-density lipoproteins (LDL) and high-density lipoproteins (HDL). When cholesterol levels are too high, some of the cholesterol is deposited in the walls of the blood vessels. Over time, the deposits can build up and cause the blood vessels to narrow and blood flow to decrease. Both cholesterol in food and saturated fat tend to raise blood cholesterol, which increases the risk for heart disease.

Coenzyme A small molecule that works with an enzyme to promote the enzyme's activity. Many coenzymes have B vitamins as part of their structure.

Complementary protein A combination of foods, each of which supplies amino acids. The amino acids lacking (or an insufficient supply) in one food are supplied by amino acids found in the second food. Together they supply all the amino acids necessary to build body proteins.

Complete protein A food source that provides all of the essential amino acids in amounts that can be used in the body to create other proteins.

Complex carbohydrates Starches and fiber with many linked sugar units. Complex carbohydrates are usually not sweet. Some fibers are not digested and aid in elimination.

Coulis A thick puree of fruit or vegetables.

Cross-contamination The spread of bacteria, viruses or other harmful agents (like gluten for some individuals) from one surface to another surface.

Deep-frying A dry-heat cooking method submerging food, usually coated first in breading or batter, into very hot fat. Deep-frying creates a crispy-coated surface on the food product.

Deglaze Swirling or stirring a liquid, such as stock or wine, in a pan to dissolve cooked food particles on the bottom of the pan. The resulting mixture usually is used as a base for a sauce.

Dehydration A process of reducing the moisture in foods to levels that inhibit the microbial growth that causes them to rot. Dehydration is done either by heat of the sun or at approximately 120° F to 140° F.

Diabetes mellitus A disease that occurs when the body is not able to form or use blood glucose (sugar) properly. Blood sugar levels are controlled by insulin, a hormone in the body that helps move glucose from the blood to muscles and other tissues. Diabetes occurs when the pancreas does not make enough insulin or the body does not respond to the insulin that is made. There are several types of diabetes mellitus.

Diet What a person eats and drinks. The term diet is also used to mean any type of restricted eating plan.

Dietary Approaches to Stop Hypertension (DASH) A dietary pattern that emphasizes potassium-rich vegetables and fruits and low-fat dairy products; includes whole grains, poultry, fish and nuts and is reduced in red meat, sweets and sugar-containing beverages. As a result, the DASH diet is rich in potassium, magnesium, calcium and fiber and reduced in total fat, saturated fat and cholesterol. It also is slightly increased in protein. This nutrient-rich diet has been shown to lower blood pressure and LDL cholesterol.

Dietary cholesterol A substance found in foods of animal origin, including meat, fish, poultry, eggs and dairy products. Used by the body to produce hormones, vitamin D and bile. Excesses of dietary cholesterol may lead to atherosclerosis over time.

Dietary fiber Complex carbohydrates with chemical bonds that cannot be broken down during digestion by humans. This nondigestible carbohydrate is found in foods such as whole-grain products, fruits, vegetables and legumes (such as dry beans and peas).

Dietary Guidelines for Americans The federal government's science-based advice to promote health and reduce risk of chronic diseases through nutrition and physical activity. The guidelines are developed jointly by the U.S. Department of Agriculture and Health and Human Services and are updated every five years.

Dietary pattern A description of the types of foods and beverages generally consumed on average, over time. For example:
Plant-based – A pattern in which the majority of protein comes from plant products, though some animal products can be included.
Vegetarian – A pattern that is exclusively or almost exclusively composed of plant foods. Some vegetarians may consume specified animal products, such as eggs, milk and milk products (lacto-ovo vegetarians) and processed foods containing small amounts of animal products.
Vegan – A pattern that is exclusively composed of plant foods.

Dietary Reference Intakes (DRIs) Amounts of nutrients based on scientific data. DRIs expand upon and replace the former Recommended Dietary Allowances (RDAs). Sets of DRI data include:
- Acceptable Macronutrient Distribution Ranges (AMDR)
- Adequate Intakes (AI)
- Estimated Average Requirements (EAR)
- Recommended Dietary Allowance (RDA)
- Tolerable Upper Intake Level (UL)

Digestion The process the body uses to break food down in the digestive tract into simple substances for energy, growth and cell repair.

DVs (Daily Values) Healthful levels for daily consumption of nutrients determined by public health experts and based on a 2,000-calorie diet. These values are found in the footnote of the Nutrition Facts label and do not change from product to product.

Electrolyte balance The equilibrium among elements that regulate cell activity by providing positive and negative ions.

Electrolytes Positive and negative ions including sodium, chloride, potassium and sulfate.

Emulsifiers Ingredients that bind together foods or liquids that normally do not mix, such as oil and water. Emulsifiers are used to stabilize solutions so fat and water ingredients do not separate.

Endorphins Peptide compounds in the brain that raise the threshold for pain and produce a feeling of well being.

Energy balance The balance between calories consumed through eating and drinking and those expended through physical activity and metabolic processes. Energy consumed must equal energy expended for a person to remain at the same body weight. Weight gain will result from excess calorie intake and/or inadequate physical activity. Weight loss will occur when a calorie deficit exists, which can be achieved by eating less, being more physically active or a combination of the two.

Energy density The amount of energy per unit of weight of a food, usually expressed as calories per 100 grams.

Energy expenditure The amount of energy, measured in calories, that a person uses. Calories are used to breathe, circulate blood, digest food, maintain posture and be physically active.

Energy nutrients Substances found in foods that can be broken down in the body and used for energy as well as for the growth, repair and replacement of tissues. These substances include carbohydrates, protein and fat. Alcohol provides energy but is not a nutrient.

Enrichment The addition of specific nutrients (iron, thiamin, riboflavin and niacin) to refined grain products to replace nutrient losses that occur during processing/refining.

Enzymes Specialized protein substances that act as catalysts to regulate the speed of the many chemical reactions within cells.

Essential fatty acids (EFA) Fatty acids that cannot be manufactured by the body and must come from food.

Estimated Average Requirement (EAR) The average daily nutrient intake estimated to meet the requirement of half the healthy individuals in a particular life stage and gender group.

Estimated Energy Requirement (EER) The average calorie intake to maintain weight of a healthy adult of a particular age, gender, weight, height and level of physical activity.

Extraction The process of removing juice from fruits and vegetables.

Fat A nutrient that supplies the body with essential fatty acids and calories. Fat is the most concentrated source of calories. Fats in foods are generally triglycerides – linked fatty acids that may be monounsaturated, polyunsaturated, saturated or a combination of these. Fat is stored in the body as adipose tissue. Oil is fat in liquid form.

Fiber Nondigestible carbohydrates and lignin that are part of the structure of plants. Dietary fiber is the fiber naturally occurring in foods, and functional fiber is specific types of nondigestible carbohydrate that have beneficial physiological effects in humans.

Flavor The sensation produced when food comes into the mouth; a result of the complex interplay of experiences from all the senses – smell, taste, touch, sight and sound.

Flavor enhancers Spices, herbs, seasonings and food preparation techniques that improve the taste and aroma of foods.

Fluids All the liquids and water in beverages and foods.

Folate A water-soluble vitamin that works with vitamin B_{12} to help form red blood cells. Folate is necessary for the production of DNA, which controls tissue growth and cell function. Low levels of folate are linked to birth defects such as spina bifida. Folic acid, folacin and folate are slightly different forms of the same vitamin.

Food allergy An abnormal response to a food triggered by the body's immune system.

Food environment The overall food supply and the settings from which a person can obtain food, such as the home, food retail establishments, restaurants, schools and worksites.

Food insecurity The limited availability of nutritionally adequate and safe foods or uncertain ability to acquire acceptable foods in socially acceptable ways. Lack of funds to buy enough food is the most common cause of food insecurity.

Food security Access by all people at all times to enough food for an active, healthy life. Food security includes the ready availability of nutritionally adequate and safe foods, and an ability to acquire acceptable foods in socially acceptable ways (e.g., without resorting to emergency food supplies, scavenging, stealing or other coping strategies).

Foodborne disease Disease caused by consuming foods or beverages contaminated with disease-causing bacteria or viruses. Many different disease-causing microbes, or pathogens, can contaminate foods. Poisonous chemicals or other harmful substances can cause foodborne diseases if they are present in food. The most common foodborne infections are those caused by the bacteria *Campylobacter*, *Salmonella* and *E. coli* O157:H7, and by a group of viruses called calicivirus, also known as Norwalk and Norwalk-like viruses.

Fortification The addition of nutrients to food that did not have these nutrients in their natural state. Milk is fortified with vitamins A and D; some juices are fortified with calcium.

Glucose A simple sugar that is the building block of most carbohydrates. Digestion causes some carbohydrates to break down into glucose. After digestion, all carbohydrates are converted to glucose, which is carried in the blood and goes to cells where it is used for energy or stored as glycogen or body fat.

Gluten A protein found in wheat, rye and barley. In people with celiac disease, gluten damages the lining of the small intestine or causes sores on the skin.

Glycerol A chemical compound that links combinations of fatty acids to form fats.

Glycogen A chain of glucose molecules used for glucose storage in the body, primarily in the liver. The body has limited stores of glycogen, which is released to maintain blood levels of glucose necessary for brain and nervous system cells.

Grill A dry-heat cooking method of heating food from a source (electricity, burning gas or charcoal) below the cooking surface.

Healthy diet A diet that emphasizes a variety of fruits, vegetables, whole grains and fat-free and low-fat milk products; includes lean meats, poultry, fish, beans, eggs and nuts. A healthy diet is low in saturated and trans fats, cholesterol, salt (sodium) and added sugars; and stays within daily calorie needs for a person's recommended weight.

Healthy weight A range of body weight based on gender, age and frame size that is least likely to be linked with weight-related health problems. People above and below healthy weight have increased health risks.

Heirloom plant An open-pollinated (by birds, insects, wind or other mechanisms) plant that was grown in an earlier era.

Herbs The edible leaves of aromatic plants; available fresh, dried and, in some cases, frozen.

Heritage animals Animals that have unique genetic traits, were raised many years ago and are typically grown in a sustainable manner.

Heterocyclic amines Substances in the muscle protein of red meat, poultry or seafood that react under high heat to form carcinogenic compounds.

High blood pressure Another term for hypertension. Blood pressure rises and falls throughout the day. An optimal blood pressure is less than 120/80 mm Hg. When blood pressure stays high – greater than or equal to 140/90 mm Hg – hypertension is diagnosed. With high blood pressure, the heart works harder, arteries are stressed and chances of a stroke, heart attack and kidney problems are greater. Prehypertension is blood pressure between 120 and 139 for the top number or between 80 and 89 for the bottom number. If blood pressure is in the prehypertension range, it is likely that a person will develop high blood pressure unless action is taken to prevent it.

High-density lipoprotein (HDL) A specific fat-protein substance in the bloodstream that transports cholesterol to the liver. HDL is commonly called "good" cholesterol. High levels of HDL cholesterol lower the risk of cardiovascular disease. An HDL level of 60 mg/dl or greater is considered high and is protective against heart disease. An HDL level less than 40 mg/dl is considered low and increases the risk for developing heart disease.

High-fructose corn syrup A sugar syrup made from corn that contains high amounts of the monosaccharide fructose, a sugar sweeter than glucose.

Hormones Chemical messenger proteins that help regulate body functions. Examples of hormones are thyroxin, insulin, estrogen and growth hormone.

Hunger The uneasy or painful sensation caused by a lack of food; the recurrent and involuntary lack of access to food.

Hydrogenation A chemical process in which hydrogen is added to fat to alter and stabilize the fat, which generally turns an oil to a semisolid or solid fat. In hydrogenation, some fat is turned into trans fats.

Hypertension See "high blood pressure."

Inactive lifestyle Lifestyle including only light physical activity during standard day-to-day life, such as getting dressed, preparing food, talking with others and attending class, with much of the time spent sitting.

Infuse To steep an aromatic or flavorful item such as an herb in liquid to extract its flavor.

Inherently healthy foods Foods that are high in nutrients and phytochemicals and low or moderate in calories in their unprocessed or minimally processed forms.

Insoluble fiber Carbohydrates with chemical bonds that are not soluble in water. They usually remain in the digestive tract and are not broken down by digestion for energy. Insoluble fibers provide bulk and aid elimination. Wheat bran and whole grains provide insoluble fiber.

Iron A mineral nutrient that helps build and renew the part of red blood cells (hemoglobin) that carries oxygen to cells.

Jus líe Meat juice thickened lightly with cornstarch or arrowroot.

Kilocalorie (Kcal) 1,000 calories. A food calorie is actually a Kcal.

Lactose intolerance The body's inability to make lactase, the enzyme necessary to digest lactose, which is the natural sugar found in milk. Symptoms are distention, pain and diarrhea.

Lecithin A fatty substance occurring in animal and plant tissues. In cooking, it can be used as an emulsifier and to prevent sticking. Brain and nervous system cells contain lecithin.

Lipids Organic compounds, including fats, oils, sterols and triglycerides, that are insoluble in water. Together with carbohydrates and proteins, lipids constitute the principal macronutrients and energy sources.

Lipoprotein Compounds made up of fat bound to protein that carry fats and fat-like substances, such as cholesterol, in the blood.

Locavore Someone who exclusively or primarily eats foods from his/her local or regional area from a determined radius from home (usually 100 or 250 miles, depending on location).

Low-calorie A specific nutrient content claim about a food indicating 40 calories or less per standard serving.

Low-density lipoprotein (LDL) A unit made up of proteins and fats that carry cholesterol in the body. High levels of LDL cholesterol cause a buildup of cholesterol-containing plaque in the arteries. LDL is commonly called "bad" cholesterol. High levels of LDL increase the risk of heart disease. An LDL level less than 100 mg/dl is considered optimal; 100 to 129 mg/dl is considered near or above optimal; 130 to 159 mg/dl is considered borderline high; 160 to 189 mg/dl is considered high; and 190 mg/dl or greater is considered very high.

Macrominerals Minerals required by humans in amounts of 100 mg/day or more.

Macronutrients Nutrients present in foods in substantial quantities that provide energy; includes carbohydrate, fat and protein.

Maillard reaction A reaction that occurs when heat is applied to a food that contains carbohydrate and protein; causes browning and development of flavor as in toasting or roasting.

Marinate Soaking or coating a food in a seasoned liquid to infuse flavors and tenderize the food prior to cooking.

Metabolism All of the chemical processes that occur in cells of the body that turn food into energy the body can use.

Microminerals Minerals required by humans in amounts of less than 100 mg/day.

Micronutrients A term that includes both vitamins and minerals needed in small quantities necessary for life and health.

Minerals Inorganic substances that include calcium, iron, zinc, chromium, copper, fluoride, iodine, magnesium, manganese, molybdenum, phosphorus, potassium, selenium and sodium. Some minerals regulate body processes while others become part of body tissues.

Minimally processed food Food processed for food safety or storage that retains most of its inherent physical, chemical, sensory and nutritional properties. Many minimally processed foods are as nutritious as the food in its unprocessed form. Plain frozen vegetables or frozen fish are examples of minimally processed foods.

Mirepoix A combination of chopped vegetables used to give flavor to stocks, sauces and gravies as well as to simmered, braised and stewed dishes. The standard ratio is 2 parts onion, 1 part carrot and 1 part celery.

Moderate alcohol consumption Daily consumption of up to 1 drink per day for women and up to 2 drinks per day for men, with no more than 3 drinks in any single day for women and no more than 4 drinks in any single day for men. One drink is defined as 12 fluid ounces of regular beer, 5 fluid ounces of wine or 1.5 fluid ounces of distilled spirits.

Monounsaturated fat A fat that has one double bond in its carbon chain. Monounsaturated fat is found in canola oil, olives and olive oil, nuts, seeds, and avocados. Monounsaturated fats may help lower cholesterol and reduce heart disease risk. Monounsaturated fat has the same number of calories as other types of fat and can still contribute to weight gain if eaten in excess.

MyPlate *MyPlate* is the visual image developed by the U.S. Department of Agriculture as a guide to healthful eating.

MyPyramid *MyPyramid: Steps to a Healthier You* was the infographic developed by the U.S. Department of Agriculture to guide healthful eating and active living. It has been replaced by *MyPlate*.

Niacin A water-soluble B vitamin that helps maintain healthy skin and nerves. As a supplement in high doses, niacin has cholesterol-lowering effects but some side effects.

Nitrates Compounds containing nitrogen and oxygen. Some nitrates are used as food preservatives. At high concentrations, nitrates can have harmful effects on humans and animals.

Nonessential amino acids Amino acids that the body is able to produce from other amino acids to meet its requirements.

Non-heme iron The form of iron found in plants that is less well absorbed than iron from animal sources.

Nutrient-dense foods Foods that are naturally rich in vitamins, minerals and phytochemicals; lean or low in solid fats; without added solid fats, sugars, starches or sodium; and retain naturally occurring components such as fiber. All vegetables, fruits, whole grains, fish, eggs and nuts prepared without added solid fats or sugars are considered nutrient-dense, as are lean or low-fat forms of fluid milk, meat and poultry prepared without added solid fats or sugars. Nutrient-dense foods provide substantial amounts of vitamins and minerals (micronutrients) and relatively few calories per standard serving; also called "healthful foods."

Nutrients Compounds supplied by food that are required by the body to maintain life. Carbohydrates, fat, protein, vitamins, minerals and water are nutrients.

Nutrition The study of food and diet.

Nutrition Facts label The part of the food label that lists the serving size, servings per container, calories per serving and information on some nutrients in a standard format.

Obesity Excess body fat. Because total body fat is difficult to measure, a ratio of body weight to height (body mass index or BMI) is often used instead. An adult who has a BMI of 30 or higher is considered obese. See "body mass index."

Oils Fats that are liquid at room temperature. Oils come from many different plants and from fish. Common oils include canola, corn, olive, peanut, safflower, soybean and sunflower. Foods that are naturally high in oils include nuts, olives, fish and avocados.

Omega-3 fatty acids Polyunsaturated essential fatty acids found in fish, flax, canola oil, pumpkin seeds and walnuts. A diet rich in omega-3 fatty acids raises HDL cholesterol levels and may help to prevent cardiovascular disease.

Omega-6 fatty acids Polyunsaturated essential fatty acids found largely in plant and vegetable oils including soy, corn and safflower oils.

Omega-9 fatty acids Nonessential polyunsaturated fatty acid that can be created chemically or by the human body from unsaturated fat.

Osteoporosis The thinning of bone tissue and loss of bone density over time. A diet inadequate in calcium and other minerals, vitamin D and protein plus hormonal deficits contribute to the development of osteoporosis, which leads to weakened bones that break easily.

Overweight A body mass index (BMI) of 25 to 29.9. Body weight comes from fat, muscle, bone and body water. Although BMI correlates with amount of body fat, BMI does not directly measure body fat. As a result, some people, such as muscular athletes, may have a BMI that categorizes them as overweight even though they do not have excess body fat.

Oxalic acid An organic acid, found in some leafy vegetables, that binds calcium and inhibits its absorption.

Pan-fry A dry-heat cooking method in which food is cooked quickly in a shallow pan with some hot fat.

Pantothenic acid A water-soluble vitamin essential for the metabolism of food. Pantothenic acid plays a role in the production of hormones and cholesterol.

Papillae The bumps on top of the tongue that help grip food and move it around while chewing; contain the taste buds.

Peptide bonds Chemical bonds that link two amino acids.

Percent Daily Values (%DVs) The percentage of the Daily Values found in a specific serving of a food. %DVs are based on Daily Value recommendations for key nutrients in a 2,000-calorie diet. %DVs help determine if a serving of food is high or low in a nutrient. Created for food labels, %DVs make it easier to compare the amount of nutrients in a food and to know which foods contribute a lot or little to meeting the daily need for key nutrients.

Phospholipids Chemical structures combining a fat with a phosphorus compound. Phospholipids circulate in the bloodstream and can be used for energy by most types of cells.

Physical activity Any form of exercise or movement. Physical activity may include planned activities such as walking, running, strength training, basketball or other sports. Physical activity may also include daily activities such as household chores, yard work, walking the dog, etc. It is recommended that adults get at least 30 minutes of moderate-intensity physical activity daily for general health benefits. Children should get at least 60 minutes of moderate-intensity physical activity most days of the week. Moderate-intensity physical activity is any activity that uses as many calories as walking 2 miles in 30 minutes.

Phytic acid A phosphorus-containing compound, found in the outer husks of grains, that binds with iron, calcium and other minerals and inhibits absorption of these nutrients.

Phytochemicals Certain organic components of plants that are thought to promote human health. Fruits, vegetables, grains, legumes, nuts and teas are rich sources of phytochemicals. Also called phytonutrients.

Plant sterols and stanols Naturally occurring substances found in plants that may reduce risk for heart disease by blocking the absorption of cholesterol in the small intestine. They are present in small quantities in many fruits, vegetables, vegetable oils, nuts, seeds, cereals and legumes.

Plaque Deposits composed primarily of cholesterol that collect on the inner walls of blood vessels and narrow the vessels, increasing risk of heart attacks and strokes.

Poach A moist-heat cooking method in which food is submerged into a hot liquid (approximately 160° F to 180° F).

Polycyclic aromatic hydrocarbons Compounds produced when meats are grilled or broiled over a direct flame; thought to be cancer causing.

Polyunsaturated fat A triglyceride in which most of the fatty acids have two or more points of unsaturation. Polyunsaturated fats are found in greatest amounts in corn, soybean and safflower oils and in many types of nuts.

Portion The amount of food eaten in one eating occasion.

Portion size The amount of a food served or to be eaten in one eating occasion. A portion is not a standardized amount. The amount served as a portion is subjective and varies.

Prebiotics Nondigestible food ingredients that are helpful in stimulating the growth or activity of beneficial bacteria in the colon.

Probiotics Live microorganisms added to food to promote intestinal health; also called "friendly bacteria."

Processed food Any food other than a raw agricultural commodity. Any food that has been washed, cleaned, milled, cut, chopped, heated, pasteurized, blanched, cooked, canned, frozen, dried, dehydrated, mixed, packaged or undergone any procedure that alters it from its natural state is a processed food. Processing also may include the addition of other ingredients to the food, such as preservatives, flavors, nutrients and other food additives or food ingredients. Processing may reduce, increase or have no affect on the nutritional characteristics of raw agricultural products.

Protein Large molecules composed of many amino acids. This essential macronutrient helps build all parts of the body, including muscle, bone, skin and blood. Protein provides 4 calories per gram and is abundant in foods such as meat, fish, poultry, eggs, dairy products, beans, nuts and tofu.

Recommended Daily Allowance (RDA) The average daily dietary nutrient intake needed to meet the nutrient requirement of nearly all (97% to 98%) healthy individuals of a particular life stage and gender group.

Reduce or reduction To cook a liquid long enough to reduce its original volume, concentrating the flavor, color and amount of the original liquid.

Refined grains Grains and grain products processed to remove the bran, germ and/or endosperm; any grain product that is not a whole grain. Many refined grains are low in fiber but enriched with thiamin, riboflavin, niacin and iron and fortified with folic acid.

Registered Dietitian (RD) A person who has studied diet and nutrition at a college program approved by the Academy of Nutrition and Dietetics (formerly The American Dietetic Association), completed 900 hours of supervised practical experience accredited by the Accreditation Council for Education in Nutrition and Dietetics and passed an exam to earn the RD credential.

Riboflavin A water-soluble vitamin that is part of the B-complex. Riboflavin is important for the production of red blood cells and many chemical reactions within cells.

Roast A dry-heat cooking method in which food is surrounded with hot air, either in an oven or over a fire; usually applies to meat, poultry, game, vegetables or potatoes.

Satiety The pleasant feeling of fullness after eating.

Saturated fat A fat composed primarily of saturated fatty acids; found in high-fat dairy products (like cheese, whole milk, cream, butter and regular ice cream), meats, lard, palm oil and coconut oil. Eating a diet high in saturated fat raises blood cholesterol and risk of heart disease. The *Dietary Guidelines for Americans* recommend limiting saturated fat to 7% of calories.

Saute A dry-heat cooking method in which heat is transferred from a hot pan to the food with a small amount of fat; usually done at very high temperatures.

Sear Browning food surfaces quickly over very high heat; usually the first step in a combination cooking method.

Serum cholesterol A lipid that travels in the blood as part of particles containing both lipids and proteins (lipoproteins). High serum cholesterol levels can be caused by genetics and internal production of cholesterol and/or from the cholesterol in foods eaten. High serum cholesterol levels increase the risk of atherosclerosis.

Serving size A standardized amount of a food in volume or weight, such as a cup or an ounce, used to provide information about food, such as on the Nutrition Facts label, in diabetic exchanges or in dietary guidance. Standard serving sizes aid comparisons among similar foods. Portion size consumed may differ from the standard serving size.

Servings per container Total number of servings in a food package based on the standard serving size for that type of food as listed in the Federal Register; listed on the Nutrition Facts label directly below the serving size.

Shortfall nutrients Nutrients that are consumed in amounts low enough to be of concern for adults and children. Shortfall nutrients identified in the *Dietary Guidelines for Americans, 2010* for children include vitamins A, C, D and E, and calcium, phosphorus and magnesium. Shortfall nutrients in adults are vitamins A, C, D, E and K, and choline, calcium, magnesium, potassium and dietary fiber.

Simmer Cooking food in a hot liquid that is heated to just below the boiling point. Small bubbles may rise to the surface of the liquid, but the liquid is much calmer than boiling.

Simple carbohydrates Sugars, monosaccharides or disaccharides that are usually sweet. Glucose, fructose and sucrose are examples.

Slurry Starch dispersed in a cold liquid to prevent it from forming lumps when added to hot liquid as a thickener.

Smoke roasting Method for cooking and flavoring food by exposing it to smoke in a closed container.

Sodium A mineral nutrient that helps balance the movement of fluid in and out of body cells, regulate blood pressure and transmit nerve impulses. Table salt is 40% sodium and 60% chloride. Most Americans eat too much sodium.

SoFAS An abbreviation for solid fats and added sugars. This term is used when calculating the number of calories that come from these two food components together. Limits for the amount of calories from SoFAS are included in U.S. Department of Agriculture food patterns and guidance beginning in 2010.

Solid fats Fats that are usually not liquid at room temperature. Solid fats are found in most animal foods but also can be made from vegetable oils through hydrogenation. Some common solid fats are butter, beef fat (tallow, suet), pork fat (lard), stick margarine and shortening. Foods high in solid fats include many cheeses, creams, whole milk, ice creams, well-marbled cuts of meats, regular ground beef, bacon, sausages and many baked goods (such as cookies, crackers, doughnuts, pastries and croissants). Most solid fats contain saturated fat, cholesterol and/or trans fats.

Soluble fiber Food components that readily dissolve in water and often impart gummy or gel-like characteristics to foods, such as pectin. Soluble fibers are indigestible by human enzymes but may be broken down to absorbable products by bacteria in the digestive tract.

Sous vide Method of cooking that is intended to maintain the integrity of ingredients by heating them for a long period at relatively low temperatures sealed in an airtight plastic bag placed in hot water.

Sphincter (esophageal) The muscular ring at the opening between the esophagus and stomach.

Starches Many glucose units linked together. Examples of foods containing starch include breads, pastas, potatoes, dry beans and peas, and grains (e.g., rice, oats, wheat, barley and corn).

Steam or steaming A moist-cooking method in which food is exposed directly to vaporized liquid, usually by placing it in a basket or rack above a boiling liquid in a covered pan or in a commercial steamer.

Sterols A type of fat with a specific ring-like chemical structure, the most abundant being cholesterol.

Stock A liquid made by simmering bones and flavorful ingredients in water to extract flavor and color. Stock is often a base for soups and sauces and can be used for cooking grains.

Sugar A simple carbohydrate composed of 1 unit (a monosaccharide, such as glucose and fructose) or 2 joined units (a disaccharide, such as lactose and sucrose). There are many forms of sugar; their names often end in -ose.

Sugar substitute A calorie-free sweetener that does not contain carbohydrates.

Supplement A product that provides concentrated nutrients such as vitamins, minerals, amino acids and fiber. Herbal products and many other chemicals that have (or are purported to have) health benefits are also sold as supplements. A dietary supplement can be taken by mouth as a pill, capsule, tablet or liquid.

Sustainable agriculture An integrated system of plant and animal production practices having a site-specific application that will, over the long term, satisfy human food and fiber needs, enhance environmental quality and natural resources, make the most efficient use of nonrenewable resources, sustain the economic viability of farm operations and enhance the quality of life for farmers and society as a whole.

Sweat To cook a food such as onions over low heat in a small amount of fat or stock, covered, until the food releases its own juices and becomes limp and tender.

Thiamin A water-soluble B vitamin that helps cells change carbohydrates into energy; essential for heart function and healthy nerve cells.

Tolerable Upper Intake Level (UL) The highest daily intake of a nutrient likely to pose no risk of adverse health effects for nearly all individuals in a particular life stage and gender group. As intake increases above the UL, the potential risk of adverse health effects increases.

Trans fatty acids A fat that is produced when oil is turned into solid fat through a chemical process called hydrogenation that rearranges molecules in the structure of fatty acids. Eating trans fatty acids raises blood cholesterol and risk of heart disease. Most trans fats are created by food processing, and trans fat levels must be listed on food labels. Trans fatty acids are found in some margarines and shortenings and in some commercial baked foods like cookies, crackers, muffins and cereals.

Triglycerides Three fatty acids joined to a glycerol molecule; the most common form of fat in foods.

Type 1 diabetes Previously known as "insulin-dependent diabetes mellitus," or "juvenile diabetes." Type 1 diabetes is a life-long condition in which the pancreas does not make insulin. To treat the disease, a person must get insulin from an external source, follow a specific eating plan, exercise daily and test blood sugar several times a day. Type 1 diabetes usually, but not always, begins before the age of 30.

Type 2 diabetes Previously known as "noninsulin-dependent diabetes mellitus" or "adult-onset diabetes." Type 2 diabetes is the most common form of diabetes mellitus. People with type 2 diabetes produce insulin, but either do not make enough insulin or their bodies do not efficiently use the insulin they make. Although Type 2 diabetes commonly occurs in adults, an increasing number of children and adolescents who are overweight also develop type 2 diabetes.

Umami A savory, meaty taste often associated with glutamate in foods and monosodium glutamate.

Unsaturated fat A fat that is composed primarily of unsaturated fatty acids. Unsaturated fats include polyunsaturated and monounsaturated fats. Most vegetable oils, nuts, olives, avocados and fatty fish such as salmon contain unsaturated fat.

Vegetable protein Protein from plants such as legumes, dry beans, grains, nuts, seeds and vegetables. Vegetable proteins tend to have lower protein quality than animal proteins because they are usually lacking one or more of the essential amino acids. Soybean products provide relatively complete protein from vegetable sources.

Villi Tiny, fingerlike projections on the inside surface of the small intestine that increase surfaces for nutrient absorption.

Vitamin A A fat-soluble vitamin that helps form and maintain healthy teeth, bones, soft tissue, mucous membranes and skin.

Vitamin B$_{12}$ A water-soluble vitamin, like the other B vitamins, that is important for metabolism. Vitamin B$_{12}$ also helps form red blood cells and maintain the central nervous system.

Vitamin B$_6$ A water-soluble vitamin also called pyridoxine, pyridoxal or pyridoxamine. The more protein consumed, the more vitamin B$_6$ needed to help the body use it. Vitamin B$_6$ helps form red blood cells and maintain brain function.

Vitamin C A water-soluble vitamin; also called ascorbic acid. Vitamin C is an antioxidant that promotes healthy teeth and gums, connective tissues between cells and wound healing. Vitamin C helps the body absorb iron from plant sources.

Vitamin D A fat-soluble vitamin known as the "sunshine vitamin," because the body can make it after being in the sun. Many people do not make enough vitamin D and need more from their diet or from supplements. Vitamin D helps the body absorb calcium and is needed for the normal development and maintenance of healthy teeth and bones and other body functions. Vitamin D has several forms – calciferol, cholecalciferol (D$_3$) and ergocalciferol (D$_2$). Most milk is fortified with vitamin D.

Vitamin E A fat-soluble vitamin that is an antioxidant; also known as tocopherol. Vitamin E plays a role in the formation of red blood cells and helps the body use vitamin K.

Vitamin K A fat-soluble vitamin that that helps blood coagulate; also known as phylloquinone.

Vitamins Nutrients that do not provide energy or build body tissue but are needed in small quantities to help regulate body processes. Vitamins include biotin, choline, folate, niacin, pantothenic acid, riboflavin, thiamin, vitamin A, vitamin B$_6$, vitamin B$_{12}$, vitamin C, vitamin D, vitamin E and vitamin K.

Waist circumference A measurement of the waist in inches or centimeters. Women with a waist measurement of more than 35 inches and men with a waist measurement of more than 40 inches have a higher risk of developing obesity-related health problems, such as diabetes, high blood pressure and heart disease.

Weight control Achieving and maintaining a healthy weight by eating healthful foods and being physically active.

Weight-cycling A pattern of losing and gaining weight over and over again; commonly called "yo-yo dieting."

Whole grains Grains and grain products made from the entire grain seed, usually called the kernel, which consists of the bran, germ and endosperm. If the kernel has been cracked, crushed or flaked, it must retain nearly the same relative proportions of bran, germ and endosperm as the original grain in order to be called whole grain. Whole grains are a good source of dietary fiber, vitamins, minerals and complex carbohydrates.

Index (See also Glossary on pages 383-392)

Y

Z